11·99

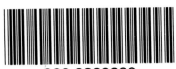

369 0289829

This book is due for return on or before the last date shown below.

2012
YEAR BOOK OF
OTOLARYNGOLOGY–
HEAD AND NECK SURGERY®

The 2012 Year Book Series

Year Book of Anesthesiology and Pain Management™: Drs Chestnut, Abram, Black, Gravlee, Lien, Mathru, and Roizen

Year Book of Cardiology®: Drs Gersh, Cheitlin, Elliott, Gold, Graham, and Thourani

Year Book of Critical Care Medicine®: Drs Dries, Zanotti-Cavazzoni, Latenser, Martinez, Rincon, and Zwank

Year Book of Dermatology and Dermatologic Surgery™: Dr Del Rosso

Year Book of Diagnostic Radiology®: Drs Elster, Abbara, Oestreich, Offiah, Rosado de Christenson, Stephens, and Strickland

Year Book of Emergency Medicine®: Drs Hamilton, Bruno, Handly, Minczak, Mullin, Quintana, and Ramoska

Year Book of Endocrinology®: Drs Schott, Apovian, Clarke, Eugster, Meikle, Oetgen, Ovalle, Schteingart, and Toth

Year Book of Hand and Upper Limb Surgery®: Drs Yao, Adams, Isaacs, Lee, and Rizzo

Year Book of Medicine®: Drs Barker, Garrick, Gersh, Khardori, LeRoith, Panush, Talley, and Thigpen

Year Book of Neonatal and Perinatal Medicine®: Drs Fanaroff, Benitz, Donn, Neu, Papile, Polin, and Van Marter

Year Book of Neurology and Neurosurgery®: Drs Klimo, Minagar, Gandhi, House, Kevill, Liu, Mazia, Panagariya, Ragel, Riesenburger, Robottom, Schwendimann, Shafazand, Uhm, and Yang

Year Book of Obstetrics, Gynecology, and Women's Health®: Drs Dungan and Shulman

Year Book of Oncology®: Drs Arceci, Bauer, Chiorean, Gordon, Lawton, Murphy, Thigpen, and Tsao

Year Book of Ophthalmology®: Drs Rapuano, Cohen, Flanders, Hammersmith, Milman, Myers, Nagra, Nelson, Penne, Pyfer, Sergott, Shields, Talekar, and Vander

Year Book of Orthopedics®: Drs Morrey, Huddleston, Rose, Swiontkowski, and Trigg

Year Book of Otolaryngology-Head and Neck Surgery®: Drs Sindwani, Balough, Franco, Gapany, and Mitchell

Year Book of Pathology and Laboratory Medicine®: Drs Raab and Bissell

Year Book of Pediatrics®: Dr Stockman

Year Book of Plastic and Aesthetic Surgery™: Drs Miller, Gosman, Gurtner, Gutowski, Ruberg, Salisbury, and Smith

2012

The Year Book of OTOLARYNGOLOGY– HEAD AND NECK SURGERY®

Editor-in-Chief
Raj Sindwani, MD, FACS, FRCS(C)

Associate Editors
Ben J. Balough, CAPT, MC, USN
Ramon A. Franco, Jr, MD
Markus Gapany, MD, FACS
Ron B. Mitchell, MD

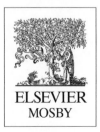

ELSEVIER
MOSBY

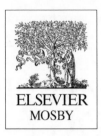

ELSEVIER
MOSBY

Vice President, Continuity: Kimberly Murphy
Editor: Jessica McCool
Production Supervisor, Electronic Year Books: Donna M. Skelton
Electronic Article Manager: Emily Ogle
Illustrations and Permissions Coordinator: Dawn Vohsen

Composition by TNQ Books and Journals Pvt Ltd, India

Printed and bound by CPI Group (UK) Ltd, Croydon, CR0 4YY

Transferred to Digital Print 2012

Editorial Office:
Elsevier
Suite 1800
1600 John F. Kennedy Blvd.
Philadelphia, PA 19103-2899

International Standard Serial Number: 1041-892X
International Standard Book Number: 978-0-323-08888-6

Editorial Board

Editor-in-Chief
Raj Sindwani, MD, FACS, FRCS(C)
Section Head, Rhinology, Sinus and Skull Base Surgery, Head and Neck Institute, Cleveland Clinic Foundation, Cleveland, Ohio

Associate Editors
Ben J. Balough, MD
Otology-Neurotology, The Permanente Medical Group, Sacramento, California
Ramon A. Franco, Jr, MD
Associate Professor, Department of Otology and Laryngology, Harvard Medical School; Director, Division of Laryngology, Medical Director of the Voice and Speech Laboratory, Massachusetts Eye and Ear Infirmary, Boston, Massachusetts
Markus Gapany, MD, FACS
Associate Professor of Otolaryngology, University of Minnesota; Chief of Otolaryngology, Minneapolis VA Medical Center; Paparella Ear, Head, and Neck Institute, Minneapolis, Minnesota
Ron B. Mitchell, MD
William Beckner Distinguished Chair in Otolaryngology, Professor of Otolaryngology and Pediatrics, Chief of Pediatric Otolaryngology, UT Southwestern Medical Center, Children's Medical Center Dallas, Dallas, Texas

Table of Contents

Journals Represented

Journals represented in this YEAR BOOK are listed below.

Acta Oto-Laryngologica
Acta Oto-Laryngologica Supplementum
AJR American Journal of Roentgenology
Alimentary Pharmacology & Therapeutics
Allergy
American Journal of Otolaryngology
American Journal of Respiratory and Critical Care Medicine
American Journal of Rhinology & Allergy
American Journal of Surgery
American Surgeon
Anesthesia & Analgesia
Annals of Otology Rhinology & Laryngology
Annals of Surgical Oncology
Archives of Facial Plastic Surgery
Archives of Otolaryngology Head & Neck Surgery
Canadian Journal of Surgery
Cancer
Chest
Cleft Palate-Craniofacial Journal
Clinical Endocrinology
European Respiratory Journal
Head & Neck
International Journal of Cancer
International Journal of Radiation Oncology Biology Physics
Journal of Allergy and Clinical Immunology
Journal of American Association for Pediatric Ophthalmology and Strabismus
Journal of Applied Physiology
Journal of Clinical Endocrinology & Metabolism
Journal of Clinical Oncology
Journal of Clinical Pathology
Journal of Laryngology and Otology
Journal of Neurosurgery
Journal of Otolaryngology Head & Neck Surgery
Journal of Plastic, Reconstructive & Aesthetic Surgery
Journal of Surgical Research
Journal of the American Academy of Dermatology
Journal of Trauma
Journal of Ultrasound in Medicine
Laryngoscope
Neuroradiology
New England Journal of Medicine
Oral Oncology
Otology & Neurotology
Pediatric Emergency Care
Pediatric Radiology
Pediatrics
Plastic and Reconstructive Surgery

Radiotherapy & Oncology
Thyroid
Transplantation
Ultrasound in Obstetrics & Gynecology

STANDARD ABBREVIATIONS

The following terms are abbreviated in this edition: acquired immunodeficiency syndrome (AIDS), cardiopulmonary resuscitation (CPR), central nervous system (CNS), cerebrospinal fluid (CSF), computed tomography (CT), deoxyribonucleic acid (DNA), electrocardiography (ECG), health maintenance organization (HMO), human immunodeficiency virus (HIV), intensive care unit (ICU), intramuscular (IM), intravenous (IV), magnetic resonance (MR) imaging (MRI), ribonucleic acid (RNA), and ultrasound (US).

NOTE

The YEAR BOOK OF OTOLARYNGOLOGY–HEAD AND NECK SURGERY is a literature survey service providing abstracts of articles published in the professional literature. Every effort is made to assure the accuracy of the information presented in these pages. Neither the editors nor the publisher of the YEAR BOOK OF OTOLARYNGOLOGY–HEAD AND NECK SURGERY can be responsible for errors in the original materials. The editors' comments are their own opinions. Mention of specific products within this publication does not constitute endorsement.

To facilitate the use of the YEAR BOOK OF OTOLARYNGOLOGY–HEAD AND NECK SURGERY as a reference tool, all illustrations and tables included in this publication are now identified as they appear in the original article. This change is meant to help the reader recognize that any illustration or table appearing in the YEAR BOOK OF OTOLARYNGOLOGY–HEAD AND NECK SURGERY may be only one of many in the original article. For this reason, figure and table numbers will often appear to be out of sequence within the YEAR BOOK OF OTOLARYNGOLOGY–HEAD AND NECK SURGERY.

Preface

Like previous editions, the 2012 YEAR BOOK OF OTOLARYNGOLOGY—HEAD AND NECK SURGERY contains abstracts and insightful commentaries that are sure to stimulate, inspire, provoke, and entertain our readers.

The format and content of the YEAR BOOK series are features unique to this publication. This body of articles has been hand selected from over 350 national and international journals by our Associate Editors, who then dissect, evaluate, and frame the articles which they have chosen. In so doing, these renowned thought leaders place their indelible signatures on each edition of the YEAR BOOK. Since so much of this publication hinges on the work and opinions of these individuals, I wanted to take the opportunity to provide a little background information about our team of experts:

Recently retired after a 22-year career in the United States Navy, Dr Ben Balough joined The Permanente Medical Group of Northern California in September 2011. There he serves as the regional otology and neuro-otology consultant for the central and Sacramento Valleys of Northern California, encompassing a large geographic area and diverse patient population. His training includes undergraduate and medical school at the University of Southern California, residency at the Naval Medical Center in San Diego, and fellowship at the Michigan Ear Institute. His military career included tours as a flight surgeon for tactical jet aircraft, staff surgeon and later department chairman for Otolaryngology-Head and Neck Surgery at the Naval Medical Center San Diego, and Deputy Director for Clinical Research with the Navy Bureau of Medicine and Surgery.

Dr Markus Gapany, MD, received his medical degree from the Hebrew University—Hadassah Medical School. He took his surgery training at SUNY—Downstate Medical Center, and otolaryngology—head and neck surgery training at the University of Iowa Hospitals and Clinics, which he completed in 1991. In 1992, he completed his fellowship training in head and neck oncologic and reconstructive surgery at the University of Cincinnati Medical Center, and the same year joined the Department of Otolaryngology at the University of Minnesota. Dr Gapany is board certified in adult and pediatric otolaryngology as well as head and neck tumor and facial plastic and reconstructive surgery. He is a Fellow of the American College of Surgeons and a Fellow of the American Society of Head and Neck Surgeons. He is an Associate Professor of Otolaryngology at the University of Minnesota and Chief of Otolaryngology—Head and Neck Surgery at the Minneapolis VA Medical Center. Dr Gapany's expertise includes head and neck tumor surgery, reconstructive and plastic surgery of head, neck, and face, and thyroid and parathyroid surgery. Special expertise includes minimally invasive, microvascular and laser surgery as well as implantation of vagus nerve stimulator device (VNS) for epilepsy and depression.

Ramon Franco, Jr, MD, is the Director of the Division of Laryngology and Medical Director of the Voice and Speech Laboratory at the Massachusetts Eye and Ear Infirmary. He is an Associate Professor within the Department of Otology and Laryngology, Harvard Medical School. He completed his Otolaryngology residency at the State University of New York at Brooklyn program (2000) before completing a Laryngology-Professional Voice Fellowship at Harvard Medical School/Massachusetts Eye and Ear Infirmary in 2001. He has a laryngology practice treating professional singers/performers with laryngeal cancer, hoarseness from unilateral vocal fold paralysis, and airway reconstruction for airway stenosis. He has helped to pioneer outpatient–awake treatment of various laryngeal disorders with the pulsed dye laser including papillomatosis and recurrent keratosis, as well as treatment of idiopathic subglottic stenosis using steroids. He is an active researcher with interests in the molecular biology of premalignant laryngeal lesions, elucidating the pathogenesis of idiopathic subglottic stenosis, developing a new sutureless method to bond epithelium, photodynamic treatment of recalcitrant keratosis, pulsed dye laser treatment, and developing a 3D system to evaluate vocal fold mucosal wave.

Ron Mitchell, MD, is a Professor of Otolaryngology and Pediatrics at UT Southwestern Medical Center. He is Chief of Pediatric Otolaryngology and Director of the Sleep Disorder Program at UT Southwestern Medical Center/ Children's Medical Center Dallas. He holds the William Beckner, MD, Distinguished Chair in Otolaryngology. Dr Mitchell's area of expertise is in sleep-disordered breathing/obstructive sleep apnea (OSA) in children. He has published over 70 manuscripts and 20 book chapters and is an editor for a book entitled *Pediatric Otolaryngology for the Clinician.* He serves on many national and international committees and has had several grants to study sleep disorders in children.

I would like to acknowledge and sincerely thank Drs Balough, Gapany, Franco, and Mitchell for their contributions to the continued success of the Year Book of Otolaryngology-Head and Neck Surgery.

Raj Sindwani, MD, FACS, FRCS(C)

1 Allergy and Immunology

General

Allergy-related outcomes in relation to serum IgE: Results from the National Health and Nutrition Examination Survey 2005-2006

Salo PM, Calatroni A, Gergen PJ, et al (Natl Insts of Health, Research Triangle Park, NC; Rho, Inc, Chapel Hill, NC; Natl Insts of Health, Bethesda, MD; et al)

J Allergy Clin Immunol 127:1226-1235, 2011

Background.—The National Health and Nutrition Examination Survey (NHANES) 2005-2006 was the first population-based study to investigate levels of serum total and allergen-specific IgE in the general US population.

Objective.—We estimated the prevalence of allergy-related outcomes and examined relationships between serum IgE levels and these outcomes in a representative sample of the US population.

Methods.—Data for this cross-sectional analysis were obtained from NHANES 2005-2006. Study subjects aged 6 years and older (n = 8086) had blood taken for measurement of total IgE and 19 specific IgE levels against common aeroallergens, including *Alternaria alternata*, *Aspergillus fumigatus*, Bermuda grass, birch, oak, ragweed, Russian thistle, rye grass, cat dander, cockroach, dog dander, dust mite (*Dermatophagoides farinae* and *Dermatophagoides pteronyssinus*), mouse and rat urine proteins, and selected foods (egg white, cow's milk, peanut, and shrimp). Serum samples were analyzed for total and allergen-specific IgE by using the Pharmacia CAP System. Information on allergy-related outcomes and demographics was collected by questionnaire.

Results.—In NHANES 2005-2006, 6.6% reported current hay fever, and 23.5% had current allergies. Allergy-related outcomes increased with increasing total IgE levels (adjusted odds ratios for a 10-fold increase in total IgE level of 1.86 [95% CI, 1.44-2.41] for hay fever and 1.64 [95% CI, 1.41-1.91] for allergies). Increased levels of plant-, pet-, and mold-specific IgE contributed independently to allergy-related symptoms. The greatest increase in odds was observed for hay fever and plant-specific IgE (adjusted odds ratio, 4.75; 95% CI, 3.83-5.88).

Conclusion.—In the US population self-reported allergy symptoms are most consistently associated with increased levels of plant-, pet-, and mold-specific IgE.

▶ Despite the increasing morbidity of allergic conditions, allergy-related outcomes (other than asthma) have been less well characterized in population-based studies. The National Health and Nutrition Examination Survey (NHANES), which is a major survey program of the National Center for Health Statistics, included an allergy component in the 2005–2006 survey. This article reports the findings from the new Allergy component in which total immunoglobulin E (IgE) and specific IgE levels to a panel of 19 allergens were measured in the survey participants who also answered demographic and allergy-related questions by questionnaire. NHANES 2005–2006 was the first population-based study to assess levels of serum IgE specific to a wide variety of indoor, outdoor, and food allergens in the general US population. This large-scale cross-sectional study included more than 8000 subjects (aged 6 years and older). The NHANES 2005–2006 demonstrated that a large proportion of the US population has allergies. Almost 50% of the population is sensitized to at least 1 allergen, and more than 50% who are given a diagnosis of allergy reported active symptoms. The reported symptoms were most consistently associated with plant-, pet-, and mold-specific IgE. Sensitization to dust mites, however, which is also highly prevalent in the population, was not strongly associated with these outcomes. NHANES data provided important information on sensitization patterns, but additional studies are needed to put some of these findings into a better clinical context. The authors do a good job of highlighting some of the weaknesses of this study and cross-sectional methodology in general. The group concluded that allergy-related outcomes are most strongly associated with increased levels of plant-, pet-, and mold-specific IgE and noted that although increases in total IgE levels might contribute independently to allergy-related outcomes, the magnitude of the effect is quite small.

R. Sindwani, MD

Evidence for intranasal antinuclear autoantibodies in patients with chronic rhinosinusitis with nasal polyps

Tan BK, Li Q-Z, Suh L, et al (Northwestern Univ Feinberg School of Medicine, Chicago; Univ of Texas Southwestern, Dallas)
J Allergy Clin Immunol 128:1198-1206, 2011

Background.—Chronic rhinosinusitis (CRS) with nasal polyps is an inflammatory condition of the nasal passage and paranasal sinuses characterized by T_H2-biased inflammation with increased levels of B-cell activating factor of the TNF family (BAFF), B lymphocytes, and immunoglobulins. Because high levels of BAFF are associated with autoimmune diseases, we assessed for evidence of autoimmunity in patients with CRS.

Objectives.—The objective of this study was to investigate the presence of autoantibodies in sinonasal tissue from patients with CRS.

Methods.—Standardized nasal tissue specimens were collected from patients with CRS and control subjects and assayed for immunoglobulin production, autoantibody levels, tissue distribution of immunoglobulins, and binding potential of antibodies in nasal tissue with a multiplexed autoantibody microarray, ELISA, and immunofluorescence.

Results.—Increased levels of several specific autoantibodies were found in nasal polyp tissue in comparison with levels seen in control tissue and inflamed tissue from patients with CRS without nasal polyps ($P < .05$). In particular, nuclear-targeted autoantibodies, such as anti-dsDNA IgG and IgA antibodies, were found at increased levels in nasal polyps ($P < .05$) and particularly in nasal polyps from patients requiring revision surgery for recurrence. Direct immunofluorescence staining demonstrated diffuse epithelial and subepithelial deposition of IgG and increased numbers of IgA-secreting plasma cells not seen in control nasal tissue.

Conclusions.—Autoantibodies, particularly those against nuclear antigens, are present at locally increased levels in nasal polyps. The presence of autoantibodies suggests that the microenvironment of a nasal polyp promotes the expansion of self-reactive B-cell clones. Although the pathogenicity of these antibodies remains to be elucidated, the presence of increased anti-dsDNA antibody levels is associated with a clinically more aggressive form of CRS with nasal polyps requiring repeated surgery.

▶ An evolving contemporary concept is that chronic rhinosinusitis (CRS) is a clinical syndrome associated with persistent inflammation of the nasal and paranasal sinus mucosa that has several different subtypes. The 2 most agreed-to variants are CRSwNP and CRSsNP, which have clinically and morphologically different characteristics and even treatment approaches. CRSwP is thought of as a distinct type of CRS characterized by TH2-biased inflammation with increased levels of B-cell—activating factor, B lymphocytes, immunoglobulins, and a relation to atopy. This study is an example of the growing basic science evidence that is helping to establish the distinctions within CRS as a syndrome. Nasal tissue specimens collected from CRS patients and controls were assayed for immunoglobulin production, autoantibody levels, tissue distribution of immunoglobulins, and binding potential of antibodies. The study found significantly increased levels of several specific autoantibodies (in particular anti-dsDNA IgG and IgA antibodies) in nasal polyp tissue in comparison with levels seen in control tissue and CRSwNP. This was particularly noted in nasal polyps from patients requiring revision surgery. The presence of autoantibodies locally in polyp tissues suggests a unique microenvironment in patients with polyps that distinguishes this type of CRS from others and promotes expansion of B-cell clones, which the authors suggest may be associated with a more aggressive form of CRS (requiring revision surgery). More work is required in this exciting area.

R. Sindwani, MD

Subcutaneous immunotherapy and pharmacotherapy in seasonal allergic rhinitis: A comparison based on meta-analyses

Matricardi PM, Kuna P, Panetta V, et al (Charité Med Univ, Berlin, Germany; Barlicki Univ Hosp, Lodz, Poland; et al)
J Allergy Clin Immunol 128:791-799, 2011

Background.—Allergen-specific subcutaneous immunotherapy (SCIT) of seasonal allergic rhinitis (SAR) is usually considered a "second-line," slow-acting, disease-modifying treatment.

Objective.—We sought to test whether SCIT is as effective as antisymptomatic treatment in the control of symptoms in patients with SAR in the first year of treatment.

Methods.—We reviewed meta-analyses with 5 or more randomized, double-blind, placebo-controlled trials of SCIT or antisymptomatic treatment in patients with SAR. We then selected trials measuring the total nasal symptom score (TNSS), the total symptom score (TSS), or both during the first pollen season after treatment initiation. Efficacy was determined as the percentage reduction in TSSs and TNSSs obtained with active treatment compared with placebo (relative clinical impact [RCI]) and the standardized mean difference (SMD) of treatment versus placebo (effect size [ES]).

Results.—The weighted mean RCI of SCIT on TNSSs ($-34.7\% \pm 6.8\%$) was higher than those of mometasone ($-31.7\% \pm 16.7\%$, $P < .00001$) and montelukast ($-6.3\% \pm 3.0\%$, $P < .00001$). The weighted mean RCI of SCIT on TSSs ($-32.9\% \pm 12.7\%$) was higher than that of desloratadine ($-12.0\% \pm 5.1\%$, $P < .00001$). The overall ES of SCIT in terms of TNSSs (SMD, -0.94; 95% CI, -1.45 to -0.43) was similar to that of mometasone (SMD, -0.47; 95% CI, -0.63 to -0.32; $P > .05$) and higher than that of montelukast (SMD, -0.24; 95% CI, -0.33 to -0.16; $P < .05$). The overall ES of SCIT in terms of TSSs (SMD, -0.86; 95% CI, -1.17 to -0.55) was comparable with that of desloratadine (SMD, -1.00; 95% CI, -1.68 to -0.32; $P > .05$).

Conclusions.—Our data provide indirect but consistent evidence that SCIT is at least as potent as pharmacotherapy in controlling the symptoms of SAR as early as the first season of treatment (Fig 3).

▶ This provocative study questions traditional thinking and approaches to the management of seasonal allergic rhinitis (SAR) by asking, "Is allergen-specific subcutaneous immunotherapy (SCIT) really less efficient than pharmacotherapy in the short-term control of seasonal allergic rhinitis (SAR) symptoms?" Based on their data, derived from analyzing meta-analyses, the answer was a surprising "No." Although SCIT is considered by most to be a second-line treatment to be initiated only if pharmacotherapy is unsuccessful, not accepted, or not tolerated by patients experiencing allergic rhinitis, the results of this review of meta-analyses suggest that perhaps this should not be the case. The authors point out that whereas pharmacotherapy reduces the symptoms of allergic rhinitis without modifying its natural history, SCIT can also effectively reduce symptoms

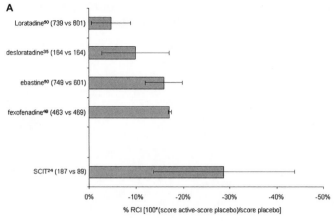

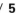

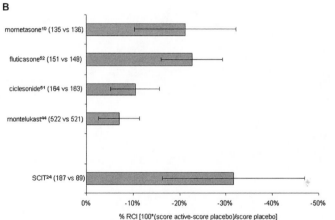

FIGURE 3.—Comparison of the RCI among different treatments. *Meta-analysis of 3 highly homogeneous trials. The numbers of patients receiving active treatment or placebo are reported in *parentheses*. RCI = [100 × (score active−score placebo)/score placebo]; treatment period. Differences between SCIT and other treatments were not significant after Bonferroni correction for multiple comparisons. (Reprinted from The Journal of Allergy and Clinical Immunology, Matricardi PM, Kuna P, Panetta V, et al. Subcutaneous immunotherapy and pharmacotherapy in seasonal allergic rhinitis: a comparison based on meta-analyses. *J Allergy Clin Immunol*. 2011;128:791-799. Copyright 2011 with permission from Elsevier.)

in SAR as well as alter the disease process itself. In fact, as shown in Fig 3, the findings of this article suggest that SCIT is at least as effective as nasal corticosteroids, oral antihistamines, and other drugs (the usual first-line and fast-acting treatments for SAR) in relieving symptoms in patients with SAR as early as the first season after initiation.

The authors point out that many factors, such as safety, costs, feasibility, and compliance, contribute to the characterization of the roles of various therapeutic options in disease management, but they propose that early consideration of SCIT be included in the options. Trials directly comparing the antisymptomatic effects of pharmacotherapy versus SCIT in patients with SAR would be needed to confirm the indirect evidence brought forward by this article. An explicit cost-benefit analysis of the 2 modalities would also be useful.

R. Sindwani, MD

2 Head and Neck Surgery and Tumors

Basic and Clinical Research

Anatomic distribution of cervical lymph node spread in parotid carcinoma
Chisholm EJ, Elmiyeh B, Dwivedi RC, et al (Royal Marsden Hosp, London, UK)
Head Neck 33:513-515, 2011

Background.—The pattern of distribution of cervical nodal involvement from primary parotid carcinomas has not been extensively described.

Methods.—All cases of parotid carcinoma over a 10-year period treated at our institution were reviewed. Data from the patients with cervical metastases were analyzed. These findings were pooled with previously published data on topography of cervical lymph nodes from parotid carcinomas.

Results.—Of 80 cases, 15 had cervical metastases (N+) in our series. When pooled with the data from all other reports, a total of 66 N+ cases were available for analysis. Twenty-eight percent of cases had involvement of level I, 59% had level II, 52% had level III, 38% had level IV, and 41% had level V. There were frequent skip metastases to level V but all were ipsilateral.

Conclusion.—The diffuse distribution of cervical nodal metastases does not support a high echelon neck dissection or radiotherapy fields limited to the upper chain in the management of cervical nodal disease.

▶ Parotid cancers are rare, and information on the distribution of cervical metastases is very sparse. This is, therefore, a welcome study that sheds some light on the topography of cervical nodal disease. The empirical approach that I have taken for years when surgically managing parotid carcinoma with clinical and radiographic N0 disease was intraoperative frozen sections of lymph nodes from zones IA and IIA (essentially a supraomohyoid neck dissection). When intraoperative sampling was negative for metastases, zones III, IV, and V were not dissected. When frozen sections showed metastases, a complete cervical lymphadenectomy was performed. The data of this study, however, do not support such an approach; apparently, the spread of parotid carcinoma may be diffused and not follow a predictable pattern of spread from upper echelon lymph nodes to lower echelon lymph nodes. The authors report skipped metastases to lower level lymph nodes without involvement of the upper level lymph nodes. The data of this study support a complete cervical lymphadenectomy in parotid carcinoma even with N0 necks.

M. Gapany, MD

A meta-analysis of the randomized controlled trials on elective neck dissection versus therapeutic neck dissection in oral cavity cancers with clinically node-negative neck
Fasunla AJ, Greene BH, Timmesfeld N, et al (Philipps-Univ of Marburg, Germany)
Oral Oncol 47:320-324, 2011

There is still no consensus on the optimal treatment of the neck in oral cavity cancer patients with clinical N0 neck. The aim of this study was to assess a possible benefit of elective neck dissection in oral cancers with clinical N0 neck. A comprehensive search and systematic review of electronic databases was carried out for randomized trials comparing elective neck dissection to therapeutic neck dissection (observation) in oral cancer patients with clinical N0 neck. A meta-analysis of the studies which met our defined selection criteria was performed using disease-specific death as the primary outcome, and the relative risk (RR) of disease-specific death was calculated for each of the identified studies. Both fixed-effects (Mantel–Haenszel method) and random-effects models were applied to obtain a combined RR estimate, although between-study heterogeneity was not found to be significant as indicated by an I^2 of 8.5% ($p = 0.350$). Four studies with a total of 283 patients met our inclusion criteria. The results of the meta-analysis showed that elective neck dissection reduced the risk of disease-specific death (fixed-effects model RR = 0.57, 95% CI 0.36–0.89, $p = 0.014$; random-effects model RR = 0.59, 95% CI 0.37–0.96, $p = 0.034$) compared to observation. This reduction in disease-specific death rate supports the need to perform elective neck dissection in oral cancers with clinical N0 neck.

▶ This is a unique meta-analysis of existing randomized trials comparing elective neck dissection versus observation (with neck dissection for salvage) in early oral cavity cancer with clinical N0 necks. Only 4 such studies were identified. This meta-analysis confirmed the commonly held opinion that elective neck dissection offers improved regional control compared with surgery for salvage. It also demonstrated, however, a disease-specific survival advantage in the elective neck dissection group. Does this mean that every early oral cavity cancer with clinically negative neck should undergo elective neck dissection? Probably not—there is a substantial body of literature that supports the value of tumor thickness as a useful predictive parameter for determining the risk of regional metastases in early oral cavity cancer. Tumors reaching thickness of 4 mm may have a 25% to 30% risk for occult cervical metastases and should undergo prophylactic neck dissection, whereas tumors with thickness of less than 3 mm are considered safe for observation. Most head and neck surgeons use the thickness criterion in daily practice.

M. Gapany, MD

Evaluation of human papillomavirus testing for squamous cell carcinoma of the tonsil in clinical practice
Thavaraj S, Stokes A, Guerra E, et al (King's College London Dental Inst, UK; Univ of Brasilia, Brazil; et al)
J Clin Pathol 64:308-312, 2011

Background.—Oncogenic human papillomavirus (HPV)-associated oropharyngeal squamous cell carcinoma (SCC) is a subtype of head-and-neck cancer with a distinct clinical and prognostic profile. While there are calls to undertake HPV testing for oropharyngeal SCCs within the diagnostic setting and for clinical trials, there are currently no internationally accepted standards.

Methods.—142 tonsil SCCs were tested using p16 immunohistochemistry (IHC), high-risk HPV DNA in situ hybridisation (ISH) and HPV DNA polymerase chain reaction (PCR; GP5+/6+ primers).

Results.—There were high levels of agreement between pathologists for p16 IHC and HPV ISH scoring; however, around 10% of HPV ISH cases showed some interobserver discrepancy that was resolved by slide review. The combination of p16 IHC and HPV ISH classified 53% of the samples as HPV-positive, whereas the combination of p16 IHC and HPV PCR classified 61% of the samples as HPV-positive. By employing a three-tiered, staged algorithm (p16 IHC/HPV ISH/HPV PCR), the authors were able to classify 98% of the cases as either HPV-positive (p16 IHC+/HPV DNA+; 62%) or HPV-negative (p16 IHC−/HPV DNA−; 35%).

Conclusions.—The current study suggests that using a combination of p16 IHC/HPV ISH/HPV PCR, in a three-tiered, staged algorithm, in conjunction with consensus reporting of HPV ISH, leads to less equivocal molecular classification. In order to ensure consistent reporting of this emerging disease, it is increasingly important for the head-and-neck oncology community to define the minimum requirements for assigning a diagnosis of 'HPV-related' oropharyngeal SCC in order to inform prognosis and for stratification in clinical trials.

▶ Evidence has been mounting that human papillomavirus (HPV) infection constitutes an independent etiologic factor for causing oropharyngeal cancer and that HPV-associated oropharyngeal cancer has different epidemiologic, biologic, and clinical characteristics from non-HPV cancer. There are more than 200 different HPV genotypes described, which, according to their association with uterine cervical carcinogenesis, are classified as high, intermediate, or low oncogenic risk. It is therefore important for prognostic and clinical trial purposes to determine carcinogenic risk of HPV infection in oropharyngeal cancer. A merely positive result for HPV DNA on polymerase chain reaction (PCR) amplification only demonstrates the presence of HPV viral genome and does not necessarily imply its role in carcinogenesis. In situ hybridization (ISH) techniques permit identification of infections in which HPV DNA is integrated into the host genome, and expression of p16 is considered a good indicator of HPV carcinogenicity. This study suggests that molecular classification of oropharyngeal cancers for HPV involvement can be feasible using routine p16 immunohistochemistry (IHC) along with detection of high-risk HPV using ISH and/or PCR. Furthermore, using a 3-tiered diagnostic algorithm incorporating p16 IHC, HPV ISH, and HPV PCR can further improve molecular HPV classification.

M. Gapany, MD

Clinical utility of PET/CT in the evaluation of head and neck squamous cell carcinoma with an unknown primary: A prospective clinical trial
Rudmik L, Lau HY, Matthews TW, et al (Univ of Calgary, Canada)
Head Neck 33:935-940, 2011

Background.—Metastatic head and neck squamous cell carcinoma with an unknown primary is an uncommon but important problem. PET/CT, as an adjunct to diagnosis, is potentially useful but has never been studied in a prospective, single-blinded clinical trial.

Methods.—In all, 20 subjects with cervical metastases from an unknown head and neck primary were enrolled in a prospective clinical trial. A standard protocol was used in both clinic and operating room (OR). Study surgeons were blinded to the PET/CT result upon completion of the standard work-up.

Results.—PET/CT increased the detection of a primary site from 25% to 55% (5 vs 11 subjects). This difference was statistically and clinically significant ($p = .03$, McNemar's test). There was 1 false negative PET/CT scan.

Conclusions.—An unknown primary should be diagnosed only after a complete head and neck examination, flexible endoscopy, and CT or MRI. PET/CT performed prior to panendoscopy will increase the diagnostic yield in the unknown head and neck primary population, leading to more targeted, and less morbid, treatment.

▶ There is a growing body of literature confirming the important role that positron emission tomography/computed tomography (PET/CT) can play in the workup of patients with cervical lymph node metastasis from an unknown primary tumor. The standard evaluation of such patients usually includes CT or magnetic resonance imaging (MRI) of the head and neck, CT of the chest, office and operative endoscopy with targeted biopsies of the tongue base and nasopharynx, and tonsillectomy. PET/CT is gaining popularity because of reported improvement in sensitivity over CT and MRI only. Recent studies have reported that PET/CT imaging can detect unknown primary tumors in 29% of cases, while changing the therapeutic plans in 25% of patients because of detection of primary tumor or distant metastases. In this prospective clinical trial, PET/CT facilitated the detection of unknown primary tumor by elevating the detection rate from 25% using standard workup to 55% utilizing PET/CT.

In my opinion, the data in the literature are very supportive of routine use of PET/CT as part of workup of patients with unknown primary source. In our practice, PET/CT has become an integral part of such a workup.

M. Gapany, MD

Role of panendoscopy to identify synchronous second primary malignancies in patients with oral cavity and oropharyngeal squamous cell carcinoma
Rodriguez-Bruno K, Ali MJ, Wang SJ (Univ of California—San Francisco)
Head Neck 33:949-953, 2011

Background.—Tobacco use increases the risk for squamous cell carcinoma (SCC) of the upper aerodigestive tract. The reported incidence of synchronous second primary tumors in head and neck cancer is approximately 10%. Therefore, patients with oral cancer have routinely undergone "panendoscopy" consisting of direct laryngoscopy, bronchoscopy, and esophagoscopy. Recent studies indicate increasing numbers of upper aerodigestive tumors occurring in nonsmoking populations who may have a lesser risk for second primary tumors. The purpose of this study was to evaluate the utility of performing "panendoscopy" to identify second primary tumors in these patient populations.

Methods.—A retrospective study of 64 consecutive patients at a university head and neck surgery practice was performed. A cohort of patients with oral cavity or oropharyngeal SCC with no tobacco history who underwent diagnostic panendoscopy were compared with similarly staged patients with a current or past history of tobacco use. Operative reports were examined for synchronous primaries, and epidemiologic data were collected. Subgroup analysis of incidence of synchronous primaries with regard to smoking status, age, sex, T classification, N classification, and location of primary tumor was also carried out. Student's *t* test statistical analysis was used to ascertain significance.

Results.—No synchronous second primary malignancies were discovered in the nonsmoking patients. In all, 12.1% of smoking patients were diagnosed with synchronous primary cancers on panendoscopy, and this difference was significant ($p = .0392$).

Conclusions.—Routine panendoscopy of the upper aerodigestive tract in patients who have never smoked is unlikely to result in identification of synchronous second primary tumors.

▶ The role of surgical panendoscopy as part of the workup for newly diagnosed head and neck cancer is clearly declining. First, routine rigid bronchoscopy for identifying synchronous pulmonary malignancy has been called into question because of very low yield. More recently, the indication for routine rigid esophagoscopy has been challenged, because synchronous esophageal tumors are very rare, and because the complication rate from rigid esophagoscopy was not insignificant; therefore, in the absence of localizing symptomatology, routine esophagoscopy was difficult to justify. We practically were left with operative pharyngo-laryngoscopy and not true panendoscopy—a term that was historically used to describe complete rigid endoscopic evaluation of the upper aerodigestive tract.

This selected article further challenges the need for routine surgical endoscopy in human papillomavirus—associated oropharyngeal and oral cancers in nonsmokers and nondrinkers. I will go even further to state that there are very few indications left for operative endoscopy even in smokers with newly diagnosed head and neck cancers. In general, office fiberoptic endoscopy (including transnasal office esophagoscopy, when indicated) appears to be a safer and more economic diagnostic procedure that is gradually replacing traditional operative endoscopy. In combination with new imaging modalities, such as computed tomography and positron emission tomography, proper staging and screening for occult synchronous or metastatic disease is feasible without a trip to the operating room in the majority of cases. The few exceptions include metastatic cancers with unknown primary source and tumors that are not readily accessible for in-office biopsy, such as some pyriform sinus and tongue base cancers.

M. Gapany, MD

Cognitive functioning after radiotherapy or chemoradiotherapy for head-and-neck cancer

Gan HK, Bernstein LJ, Brown J, et al (Princess Margaret Hosp, Toronto, Ontario, Canada)
Int J Radiat Oncol Biol Phys 81:126-134, 2011

Purpose.—To perform a comprehensive cognitive function (CF) assessment in patients who were relapse free after curative intent radiotherapy (RT) or chemoradiotherapy for squamous cell carcinoma of the head and neck.

Methods and Materials.—Patients underwent neuropsychological tests to assess their objective CF; completed questionnaires to assess subjective CF, quality of life, and affect; and underwent blood tests to assess hematologic, biochemical, endocrine, and cytokine status. Retrospectively, the dosimetry of incidental radiation to the brain was determined for all patients, and the dose intensity of cisplatin was determined in those who had undergone chemoradiotherapy.

Results.—A total of 10 patients were enrolled (5 treated with radiotherapy only and 5 with radiotherapy and cisplatin). The mean time from the end of treatment was 20 months (range, 9–41). All patients were able to complete the assessment protocol. Of the 10 patients, 9 had impaired objective CF, with memory the most severely affected. The severity of memory impairment correlated significantly with the radiation dose to the temporal lobes, and impaired dexterity correlated significantly with the radiation dose to the cerebellum, suggesting that these deficits might be treatment related. Patients receiving cisplatin appeared to have poorer objective CF than patients receiving only RT, although this difference did not achieve statistical significance, likely owing to the small sample size. Consistent with the published data, objective CF did not correlate with subjective CF or quality of life. No association was found between objective CF and patients' affect, hematologic, biochemical, endocrine, and cytokine status.

Conclusion.—Neuropsychological testing is feasible in squamous cell carcinoma of the head-and-neck survivors. The findings were suggestive of treatment-related cognitive dysfunction. These results warrant additional investigation.

▶ Impaired cognitive function is known to be common among head and neck cancer patients. Long years of tobacco and alcohol abuse and poor general health are definitely contributing factors. Some studies have even shown correlation between decreased cognitive function and advanced stage of the disease.[1] This selected pilot study is the first to claim that the treatment itself (ie, radiochemotherapy for organ preservation) can contribute to significant impairment of the cognitive function. Although results of this study should be interpreted cautiously, because of its limited cohort and faulty design (no pretreatment neuropsychologic testing was done on the individuals enrolled in the study), the results are alarming. Increasingly, oropharyngeal cancer is becoming a human papillomavirus—linked disease of nonsmoking, nondrinking individuals of younger age, who are productive and have an excellent chance for cure. If indeed aggressive radiochemotherapy can significantly impair their cognitive function, then the paradigm for therapy should be carefully reconsidered, taking the negative effects on the cognitive function into consideration. This argument, however, has to be put on hold until more substantial data emerge from well-designed, prospective studies.

M. Gapany, MD

Reference

1. Rohlender NH, Wysluch A, Maurer P, et al. Decreased cognitive functioning in patients with advanced oral squamous cell carcinoma. *Oral Oncol.* 2011;47: 993-997.

Carcinoma of unknown primary in the head and neck: comparison between positron emission tomography (PET) and PET/CT
Keller F, Psychogios G, Linke R, et al (Friedrich Alexander Univ of Erlangen—Nuremberg, Germany)
Head Neck 33:1569-1575, 2011

Background.—Comparison of the diagnostic validity of positron emission tomography (PET) alone with integrated PET and CT (PET/CT) in the search for occult primary tumors in patients with cancer of unknown primary (CUP) site in the head and neck.

Methods.—Thirty-nine consecutive patients with clinical CUP were investigated with PET and 38 patients with PET/CT. After initial diagnostic panendoscopy and histological confirmation of the cervical lymph node metastasis, either PET or PET/CT scanning was performed.

Results.—Integrated PET/CT had a significantly higher overall detection rate than dedicated PET alone (55.2% vs 30.8%; $p = .039$) and positive prediction rate (93.3% vs 46.1%; $p = .01$).

Conclusion.—Integrated PET/CT showed to be superior to PET in the detection of the primary site of clinically occult tumors in CUP syndrome. However, a negative result should still be investigated further by means of panendoscopy with tonsillectomy and blind biopsies.

▶ There is a growing body of literature confirming the important role that positron emission tomography (PET) imaging can play in the workup of patients with cervical lymph node metastasis from an unknown primary tumor. The standard evaluation of such patients usually includes computed tomography (CT) or magnetic resonance imaging of the head and neck, CT of the chest, office and operative endoscopy with targeted biopsies of the tongue base, nasopharynx and tonsillectomy. This selected retrospective study has compared the efficacy of PET imaging as compared with CT-PET coregistration in detecting unknown primary tumors. A multitude of previous studies have documented the advantage of CT-PET coregistration as compared with PET alone in improving diagnostic validity of PET imaging. This study confirmed this observation for unknown primary head and neck tumors as well. In my opinion, the data in the literature are very supportive of routine use of CT-PET as part of workup of patients with unknown primary source. In our practice, CT-PET has become an integral part of such a workup.

M. Gapany, MD

Human Papillomavirus Type 16 Oropharyngeal Cancers in Lymph Nodes as a Marker of Metastases

Mirghani H, Moreau F, Lefèvre M, et al (Univ Pierre et Marie Curie Paris VI, France)
Arch Otolaryngol Head Neck Surg 137:910-914, 2011

Background.—Oropharyngeal squamous cell carcinomas (OSCCs) are associated with high-grade human papillomavirus (HPV) infection in 20% to 30% of cases. HPV-16 DNA has been detected in cervical lymph node metastases of HPV-16⁺ OSCC. However, the meaning of HPV-16 DNA detection in lymph nodes remains controversial. Does the presence of HPV-16 DNA in lymph nodes correlate with their metastatic involvement, or is it just a consequence of the filter function of lymph nodes?

Methods.—Viral load quantification using reverse transcriptase–polymerase chain reaction was retrospectively performed in primary tumors and in cervical lymph nodes, originating from levels IIa, IIb, and III, in 11 patients with HPV-16⁺ OSCC and in 3 control patients with HPV-16⁻ OSCC.

Results.—A total of 45 lymph node levels were analyzed. HPV-16 DNA was not detected in HPV-16⁻ OSCC lymph nodes. No statistically significant difference was found between primary tumors and metastatic lymph nodes viral load ($P>.01$). The viral load value was significantly higher in metastatic lymph nodes than in tumor-free lymph nodes ($P<.01$). Among 27 tumor-free lymph node levels, the viral load value was undetectable in 16, low or medium ($<10^5$ copies per million cells) in 8, and high ($>10^5$ copies per million cells) in 3.

Conclusions.—HPV-16 DNA detection in lymph nodes of patients affected with HPV-16⁺ oropharyngeal cancer is indicative of metastatic involvement. Tumor-free lymph nodes with a high viral load value would suggest the presence of occult lymph nodes metastasis and the opportunity to use HPV-16 DNA as a metastatic marker. Further investigations are needed.

▶ Human papillomavirus (HPV)-associated oropharyngeal cancer is on the rise and is bound to reach epidemic proportions. Most recent epidemiologic data from the United States show that 70% of oropharyngeal cancers are HPV positive. Unpublished data (personal communication) from the Stockholm area in Sweden show incidence of infection in 90% of oropharyngeal cancers. We are still in the process of learning the tumor biology of this cancer, and many questions on the behavior of this tumor remain unanswered.

This selected article presents some very interesting information about the HPV-16 viral load in cervical lymph nodes in patients with HPV-positive oropharyngeal cancers. While all metastatic lymph nodes in this study carried a viral load close to those found in primary tumors, some pathologically negative lymph nodes were also found to be highly positive for HPV DNA. It is very likely (although unproven) that those clinically and pathologically negative but HPV-positive lymph nodes might actually represent the so-called occult metastases. This is a very interesting observation, which still has to be confirmed in further studies, but could potentially have important clinical implications.

M. Gapany, MD

Reevaluation of Gastroesophageal Reflux Disease as a Risk Factor for Laryngeal Cancer
Francis DO, Maynard C, Weymuller EA, et al (Veterans Affairs Puget Sound Health Care System, Seattle, WA; Univ of Washington, Seattle; et al)
Laryngoscope 121:102-105, 2011

Objectives/Hypothesis.—The relationship between gastroesophageal reflux disease (GERD) and laryngeal cancer has not been fully elucidated. This case-control study investigates whether GERD increases the odds of developing these malignancies.

Study Design.—Case-control study.

Methods.—Rates of GERD among cases of laryngeal cancer identified in the Veterans Health Administration outpatient care files (year 2000–2006) were compared with controls. Cases (N = 14,449) were frequency matched 1:1 with controls. Multivariate logistic regression was used to determine the association between GERD and cancer.

Results.—After adjusting for tobacco and/or alcohol use, there was no association between GERD and laryngeal cancer (adjusted odds ratio, 1.01; 95% confidence interval, 0.92-1.12, *P* = .780). Although an association was found when time from GERD diagnosis to malignancy was less than 3 months, it disappeared when this period was extended further.

Conclusions.—In this population, there was no increased risk of laryngeal cancer among patients with GERD. However, in subsite analysis, a possible relationship between GERD and glottic cancer was observed. Reverse causality must be considered in future studies assessing the relationship between reflux and laryngeal cancer to limit misclassification bias.

▶ Several recent studies have suggested that laryngopharyngeal reflux (LPR) could be a predisposing condition for laryngeal cancer. Some authors went as far as recommending lifelong prophylactic therapy with proton pump inhibitors (PPI) against LPR in all patients treated for laryngeal cancer. Based on those initial reports, I felt that the potential benefits of treating laryngeal cancer patients preventatively for reflux far outweighed the risks and made it a policy to prescribe PPIs routinely. The association between LPR and laryngeal cancer, however, appeared to be weak, and some later studies actually found none. Furthermore, the newest data in the literature have suggested that long-term use of PPIs actually were not as innocuous as previously thought and were associated with serious side effects. Thus, the case for PPI prophylaxis in laryngeal cancer patients no longer appeared appealing. This selected case-control study again failed to show any association between laryngeal cancer and LPR. Therefore, until solid data prove to the contrary, there is not enough scientific evidence to link LPR to cancer of the larynx.

M. Gapany, MD

Accuracy of whole-body PET and PET-CT in initial M staging of head and neck cancer: A meta-analysis
Xu G-Z, Zhu X-D, Li M-Y (Cancer Hosp of Guangxi Med Univ, Nanning, People's Republic of China)
Head Neck 33:87-94, 2011

Background.—A meta-analysis was conducted to evaluate the accuracy of whole-body positron emission tomography (PET) and PET-CT in initial M staging of head and neck cancer.

Methods.—After a systematic review of English language studies, sensitivity, specificity, and other measures of whole-body PET and PET-CT were pooled. Summary receiver operating characteristic (SROC) curves were also used to summarize overall test performance.

Results.—Eight PET and 7 PET-CT studies were identified. The pooled sensitivity estimates for PET and PET-CT were 0.848 (95% confidence interval [CI], 0.776–0.905) and 0.875 (95% CI, 0.787–0.936). The pooled specificity estimates were 0.952 (95% CI, 0.933–0.967) and 0.950 (95% CI, 0.931–0.964). The Q* index estimates for PET-CT (0.9409) were not significantly higher than for PET (0.9154; $p > .05$).

Conclusion.—Whole-body PET and PET-CT have good diagnostic performance in initial M staging of head and neck cancer; although PET-CT tends to have higher accuracy than PET.

▶ The aim of this meta-analysis was to assess the diagnostic value of computed tomography/positron emission tomography (CT/PET) for M staging of newly diagnosed head and neck cancer. This is an important question, because the additional cost of this imaging modality must be weighed against its potential benefits. Multiple studies of this relatively new imaging modality in head and neck cancer have shown it to be of value in 4 clinical settings: staging, radiation planning, response to therapy, and posttherapy surveillance. It is too costly and therefore impractical to obtain so many CT/PET studies on 1 patient at different stages of therapy for head and neck cancer. Maximal "bang for the buck" is therefore a good way to look at this question. This selected study confirms the value of CT/PET for detecting distant metastases and second primary tumors in newly diagnosed head and neck cancer. Does this mean that a CT/PET should be obtained in every new case of head and neck cancer? The answer is a resounding no.

In my practice, patients who have a low risk for distant metastases, have a clearly defined head and neck cancer on clinical examination and on an anatomic imaging study (CT and/or MRI), and have normal CT scan of the chest do not undergo routine CT/PET imaging. This imaging modality is reserved for tumors at high risk for distant metastases, for patients with particularly advanced disease, or for patients who show suspicious lesions of the chest on CT scan.

M. Gapany, MD

Tumor Depth as a Predictor of Lymph Node Metastasis of Supraglottic and Hypopharyngeal Cancers

Tomifuji M, Imanishi Y, Araki K, et al (Natl Defense Med College, Tokorozawa, Saitama, Japan; Keio Univ School of Medicine, Tokyo, Japan)
Ann Surg Oncol 18:490-496, 2011

Background.—The relationship between the histological parameters of primary lesions and lymph node metastasis in supraglottic and hypopharyngeal cancers has not been elucidated. This analysis is important to evaluate the requirement for additional elective neck dissection when clinically node-negative cancers are treated by transoral surgery.

Methods.—This study included 40 previously untreated patients with supraglottic and hypopharyngeal cancers who underwent transoral en bloc tumor resection in two academic tertiary referral centers. Nodal status was confirmed by neck dissection for cases with findings or suspicion of lymph node metastases or by observation of clinically node-negative cases for more than 1 year. Patients' medical records and pathological features were analyzed retrospectively. The correlation of histological parameters with lymph node metastases, including occult metastases, was evaluated by univariate and multiple logistic regression analyses.

Results.—Univariate analysis showed that lymph node metastasis was correlated with tumor depth ($P = 0.00087$) and venous invasion ($P = 0.027$). Multiple logistic regression analysis showed that it was significantly correlated only with tumor depth ($P = 0.007$).

Conclusions.—Tumor depth is the most useful parameter for predicting lymph node metastases. In clinically node-negative cases, when tumor depth exceeds 1 mm, elective neck dissection must be considered and, when it is less than 0.5 mm, regular clinical follow-up is recommended. Patients with tumor depth between 0.5 and 1 mm should be carefully observed, since they also have a chance of developing nodal metastasis. Venous invasion also indicates high rates of nodal metastasis, therefore elective neck dissection must be considered for these cases.

▶ In oral cancer, the only significant prognostic factor that predicts the risk for cervical nodal metastases appears to be the depth of tissue invasion or, in other words, tumor thickness. Although the correlation between occult cervical metastasis and tumor thickness was fairly well documented in several studies, there is no agreement as to the critical cutoff thickness beyond which the risk of neck metastases is greatly increased. Most authors agree, however, that 4 mm could serve as a safe cutoff thickness. In the past, the criterion of depth of invasion has not been applied to tumors of supraglottic larynx or hypopharynx for 2 main reasons: one is that the incidence of occult disease in cervical lymph nodes for tumors in these anatomic locations is so high that prophylactic neck dissection was recommended in all cases tackled surgically; second is that early cancers of the supraglottis and hypopharynx have been lately treated with radiochemotherapy. With the advent of transoral, minimally invasive operations (laser-assisted microscopic, robot-assisted, or fiberoptic), the question of elective neck dissection following conservative resection became much more relevant. As this study convincingly shows, depth of invasion appears to be a consistent prognostic determinant for prediction of cervical lymph node metastases in supraglottic and hypopharyngeal cancers, similar to oral cavity tumors. Depth of invasion in this study was measured from the level of the basement membrane, suggesting a cutoff of 1 mm for elective neck dissection. Tumors with depth of invasion of less than 0.5 mm appeared to be safe for observation. Validation of these parameters in more extensive studies are needed before routine application in clinical practice can be unequivocally recommended.

M. Gapany, MD

When to Manage Level V in Head and Neck Carcinoma?
Naiboğlu B, Karapinar U, Agrawal A, et al (Haydarpasa Numune Education and Res Hosp, Istanbul, Turkey; Denizli Military Hosp, Turkey; the Ohio State Univ, Columbus)
Laryngoscope 121:545-547, 2011

Objectives/Hypothesis.—As superselective neck dissection strategy is gaining popularity to minimize postoperative morbidity and better life quality, we investigated the metastatic nodal status of level V neck lymph node group for head and neck squamous cell carcinoma in various primary sites. We have also aimed to display the impact of involvement of other nodal groups on level V.

Study Design.—Retrospective review of histopathologic examination of case series at a comprehensive cancer center.

Methods.—The study group was composed of 107 patients who under-went a type of neck dissection including level V among 243 patients. The impact of primary site and metastatic nodal status of other levels on metas-tasis to level V involvement were evaluated.

Results.—The most common primary tumor site was oropharynx (n = 43), followed by oral cavity (n = 32), larynx (n = 16), carcinoma of unknown primary (n = 10), and hypopharynx (n = 6). General pathologic N positivity for all levels was 78.3% (76 of 97) when 10 carcinoma of unknown primary patients were excluded. Level V was involved in 13 of 107 (12.1%) patients. Level V was not involved in any patient when the other levels were not involved (0 of 21). Even when considering only N+ patients, the ratio of N positivity for level V is still <20% (13 of 86, 15.1%).

Conclusions.—Because level V was not involved in any patient when the other levels were not involved, it might be reasonable to preserve level V especially in clinically and intraoperatively N0 patients.

▶ This article serves as a good reminder to head and neck surgeons that metas-tases to level V of the neck are rare. The literature-reported incidence ranges between 4.8% and 7.4%, whereas in this study, which analyzed a selected group of patients, the incidence was slightly higher (12.1%). In N0 necks, the incidence of level V metastases is very rare. It is also very rare in N+ necks from cancer of the oral cavity. The incidence of level V metastases increases in N+ necks from laryngo-pharyngeal cancer.

The classic technique of dissecting level V involves raising the skin flap to the edge of the trapezius muscle, incising the superficial layer of the deep cervical fascia along the posterior edge of the sternocleidomastoid muscle (SCM), then tracing and dissecting cranial nerve (CN) IX as it crosses the posterior trigone of the neck, followed by dissection of the level V lymph nodes. This technique is likely to devascularize a long segment of CN IX, resulting in increased incidence of shoulder dysfunction.

I use a technique that allows selective dissection of accessory lymph nodes, as well as lymph nodes along the transverse cervical artery and supraclavicular fossa, through a standard selective neck dissection approach. It is essentially extension of the submuscular recess dissection inferior to CN IX, which is performed posterior to the rootlets of the cervical plexus, staying under the SCM. It allows a selective dissection of the entire level V when indicated, and adds very little time and morbidity to the operation.

M. Gapany, MD

General

Human papillomavirus infections in laryngeal cancer
Torrente MC, Rodrigo JP, Haigentz M Jr, et al (Universidad de Chile, Santiago de Chile; Instituto Universitario de Oncología del Principado de Asturias, Oviedo, Spain; Montefiore Med Ctr, Bronx, NY; et al)
Head Neck 33:581-586, 2011

Although the association and clinical significance of human papillomavirus (HPV) infections with a subset of head and neck cancers, particularly for oropharyngeal carcinoma, has recently been well documented, the involvement of HPV in laryngeal cancer has been inadequately evaluated. Herein we review the currently known associations of HPV infections in diseases of the larynx and their potential for oncogenicity. Using several methods of detection, HPV DNA has been detected in benign (papillomatosis), indolent (verrucous carcinoma), and malignant (squamous cell carcinoma) lesions of the larynx. Consistent with the known oncogenic risk of HPV infections, common HPV types associated with laryngeal papillomatosis include low-risk HPV types 6 and 11, with high-risk HPV types 16 and 18 more commonly present in neoplastic lesions (verrucous carcinoma and squamous cell carcinoma). Although a broad range of prevalence has been noted in individual studies, approximately 25% of laryngeal squamous cell carcinomas harbor HPV infections on meta-analysis, with common involvement of high-risk HPV types 16 (highest frequency) and 18. Preliminary results suggest that these high-risk HPV infections seem to be biologically relevant in laryngeal carcinogenesis, manifested as having viral DNA integration in the cancer cell genome and increased expression of the p16 protein. Despite this knowledge, the clinical significance of these infections and the implications on disease prevention and treatment are unclear and require further investigation.

▶ Evidence has been mounting that human papillomavirus (HPV) infection constitutes an independent etiologic factor for causing oropharyngeal cancer and that HPV-associated oropharyngeal cancer has different epidemiologic, biologic, and clinical characteristics from non-HPV cancer. Furthermore, there is ample evidence in the literature that links HPV tumor status with relatively favorable clinical course of tonsillar cancer. Although high-risk HPV DNA has been detected in a large proportion of laryngeal cancers, the etiologic association between laryngeal carcinoma and HPV infection has not been clearly established. It is also unclear whether HPV positivity imparts laryngeal cancers with different tumor biology or different response to therapy as compared with HPV-negative tumors. This selected contemporary review article provides a good source of information on the latest findings and developments pertaining to HPV infection and laryngeal cancer. It is definitely worth reviewing for otolaryngologists who treat laryngeal and/or other head and neck cancer and general otolaryngologists who want to stay abreast with latest development in our specialty.

M. Gapany, MD

Central compartment dissection in laryngeal cancer
Medina JE, Ferlito A, Robbins KT, et al (The Univ of Oklahoma Health Sciences Ctr; Univ of Udine, Italy; Southern Illinois Univ School of Medicine, Springfield, IL; et al)
Head Neck 33:746-752, 2011

We report here a review of the literature intended to clarify the nomenclature and boundaries of the nodes in the "central compartment" of the neck, the frequency with which tumors from the different laryngeal sites metastasize to these nodes, and the indications for central compartment node dissection in the treatment of cancers of the larynx. From this review, we conclude that, until consensus is reached about grouping of the lymph nodes in this area, it is best to refer to these nodes by their anatomic location, ie, prelaryngeal, pretracheal, or paratracheal lymph nodes. It is also advisable to describe dissection of these nodes as selective neck dissection (SND) with an annotation about the specific lymph node groups removed. Metastases in prelaryngeal and paratracheal lymph nodes in patients with squamous cell carcinoma of the larynx are associated with increased tumor recurrence, more frequent metastases in lymph nodes of the lateral compartment of the neck, and decreased survival. If untreated, they may lead to the development of peristomal recurrence. Therefore, elective treatment of level VI nodes is recommended in patients with squamous cell carcinomas of the subglottic region, advanced glottis carcinomas with subglottic extension, and in certain advanced carcinomas of the supraglottic region.

▶ This is an excellent review article by an international team of highly respected experts in the field of head and neck oncology on the seldom discussed topic of central compartment metastases in laryngeal cancer. The article reviews the contemporary nomenclature used to describe the lymph node groups in the central neck compartment, their anatomy, and prevalence of cervical lymph node metastases in the central neck compartment from the laryngeal cancer and their prognostic implications. Presence of central compartment metastases is associated with higher rates of recurrence, peristomal recurrence, and higher incidence of metastases to the lateral compartments of the neck. The authors therefore recommend elective surgical treatment of the central compartment lymph nodes in patients with subglottic cancers, patients with advanced glottis cancers with subglottic extension, and advanced cancers of the supraglottis. They also describe the recommended technique for selective central compartment neck dissection. This article is highly recommended for review to surgeons who treat cancer of the larynx.

M. Gapany, MD

Current Practice Patterns in the Management of Glottic Cancer in Canada: Results of a National Survey

Makki FM, Williams B, Rajaraman M, et al (Dalhousie Univ, Halifax, NS)
J Otolaryngol Head Neck Surg 40:205-210, 2011

Objective.—In this study, we sought to determine current trends in the management of glottic cancer in Canada. We further sought to determine the approach to margin status following treatment of glottic cancer.

Methods.—An online survey was distributed to all head and neck (H&N) surgeons and all radiation oncologists (ROs) in Canada. Respondents were asked to choose management recommendations for a series of tumour descriptions and to offer their opinion of margin evaluation. The results were compiled and analyzed using descriptive statistics for frequencies and chi-square analysis for comparison between H&N surgeons and ROs.

Results.—The survey attained a response rate of 60% among H&N surgeons and 20% among ROs. There was a significant difference in choice of management for T1a, T1b, T2a, and T2b tumours, with ROs heavily favouring radiation therapy and H&N surgeons' opinions divided between radiation therapy and transoral laser microsurgery (TLM). There was no significant difference of opinion in the treatment of T3 and T4a tumours. The size of an adequate margin was significantly different between ROs and H&N surgeons, as was the management of a positive margin.

Conclusion.—Compared to previous surveys, this study reflects a move toward TLM as the preferred treatment for T1a glottic cancer among H&N surgeons, whereas ROs continue to favour radiation therapy. The results also show a split in opinions among H&N surgeons with respect to TLM versus radiation therapy for early-stage glottic tumours. The study underscores a difference of opinion between specialties regarding the management of glottic cancer and the need for a definitive comparison study to guide recommendations.

▶ In the past 2 decades the treatment of glottis cancer has undergone dramatic changes. For advanced cancer, the organ preservation approach has gained popularity over total laryngectomy, whereas therapy for early glottic cancers has shifted significantly in favor of transoral laser microsurgery. Despite these advances, no consensus has been reached regarding the best therapeutic options for a given stage of cancer, and the choice of the therapeutic modality largely depends on the specialty of the practitioner (head and neck surgeon vs radiation oncologist) as well as personal preference.

This selected article is an interesting epidemiologic survey of physicians in Canada (both surgeons and radiation oncologists) regarding their choice of recommended therapy for each stage of glottis cancer. The results are telling: as expected, in general, most surgeons prefer surgery, whereas most radiation oncologists prefer radiotherapy. It is interesting, however, that although surgeons prefer to treat T1a tumors with transoral laser microsurgery and are evenly split between laser microsurgery and radiotherapy for T1b tumors, radiation oncologists prefer to treat all tumors with radiation. It would be very interesting to see a similar study conducted in the United States. I suspect, however, that the results would be very similar.

M. Gapany, MD

Differential Diagnosis of Cystic Neck Lesions
Sira J, Makura ZGG (Leeds General Infirmary, England)
Ann Otol Rhinol Laryngol 120:409-413, 2011

Objectives.—In patients less than 40 years of age who present with an upper anterior triangle cystic mass, branchial cyst is the presumed clinical diagnosis. Squamous cell malignancy is the important differential diagnosis in a patient more than 40 years of age. We sought to identify the range of lesions that can be clinically mistaken for, and removed as, branchial cysts.

Methods.—We performed retrospective reviews of 29 neck masses removed as branchial cysts and 47 solitary neck masses diagnosed as cancer between January 2003 and January 2008 across two teaching hospitals in Leeds, England.

Results.—Of the 29 lesions removed, 23 (79.3%) were confirmed to be branchial cysts. The remainder comprised 2 thyroid papillary carcinomas (6.9%) and 4 benign lesions (13.6%; laryngocele, neurilemmoma, parotid gland cyst, and cystadenoma). Of the 47 cases of metastatic cancer, 3 lesions (6.4%) were clinically mistaken as branchial cysts but were subsequently diagnosed as squamous cell carcinomas.

Conclusions.—When presented with a solitary lateral cystic mass, clinicians should consider the possibility of squamous cell carcinoma in patients more than 40 years of age, and thyroid papillary cancer should be considered particularly in the younger age groups. In our series, 30.8% of the neck lesions believed to be branchial cysts in patients over 40 were malignant, in contrast to 5.3% of those lesions in patients under 40.

▶ This article was selected because it serves as a great reminder to otolaryngologists that a cystic mass in the neck, even with benign radiographic and histopathologic features, may still represent a metastatic squamous cell carcinoma, most often from the oropharynx, masquerading as a branchial cyst. In patients older than 40 years, the incidence of metastatic squamous cell cancer in cystic lesion of the neck is even higher. According to this study, 1 in every 3 cystic masses in the older-than-40 age group is malignant metastasis. Others have reported the incidence to be as high as 80%. It is particularly important to be aware of this problem, because the human papillomavirus (HPV)-associated oropharyngeal cancer is on the rise. One of the unique features of HPV-associated squamous cell carcinoma is a tendency to present with an otherwise asymptomatic neck mass and inconspicuous primary cancer in the oropharynx. Benign-appearing squamous epithelial cells in the fine-needle aspiration, therefore, cannot be taken as an absolute proof of a benign process in the neck mass. In patients older than 40 years, direct laryngoscopy and targeted to the oropharynx biopsies should be performed first, and if negative, an excision of the neck mass and potential neck dissection should be planned next.

M. Gapany, MD

Review of Thromboprophylaxis in Otolaryngology—Head and Neck Surgery

Jaggi R, Taylor SM, Trites J, et al (Dalhousie Univ, Halifax, NS)
J Otolaryngol Head Neck Surg 40:261-265, 2011

Research Type.—Translational.

Objective.—To review and tabulate the incidence of thromboembolic complications following head and neck surgery.

Study Design.—Review.

Methods.—Articles were identified using the *MEDLINE* database search engine. The relevant articles were reviewed and any thromboembolic complications were tabulated.

Results.—Six articles, published between 1976 and 2007, were identified that reported on thromboembolic complications following head and neck surgery. Of these articles, four were retrospective reviews and two were prospective. Four of the studies looked at various methods of routine prophylaxis, which included several combinations of low-dose heparin, low-molecular-weight heparin, graduated compression stockings, and intermittent pneumatic compression devices. Two studies were simply investigating complications in general following head and neck surgery.

Conclusions.—Head and neck cancer patients are likely at higher risk than commonly thought, and venous thromboembolism is likely much more common than what is clinically evident. It is important to develop an institutional system of risk stratification to correspond to standardizations of thromboprophylaxis that are generally accepted. Although many institutions are already attempting to do so, such as we have outlined above by extrapolating from other surgical departments, it is important to show these relationships with head and neck patients specifically to justify the high cost of these various therapies.

▶ Thromboembolic complications in head and neck surgery are relatively rare and therefore receive little attention in our literature. This selected article is a review of recently published articles on this subject. The authors were able to find 6 studies on thromboembolic complications in head and neck surgery, of which only 1 was from the United States. No clear recommendations for thromboprophylaxis can be deducted from this published material, but one thing is clear: proper thromboprophylaxis does significantly reduce the rate of thromboembolic complications in head and neck surgery.

Many head and neck surgeons follow their institutional guidelines for thromboprophylaxis. In our medical center, the guidelines for thromboprophylaxis are flexible, allowing each service to choose its preferred methods, as long as such prophylaxis is implemented. We use thromboprophylaxis only in head and neck oncologic surgery; it consists of pneumatic compression stockings (PCS) and early mobilization. Only patients undergoing microvascular reconstruction, in addition to PCS, are given either low molecular weight heparin or low-dose heparin prophylaxis.

M. Gapany, MD

Cutaneous squamous cell carcinoma of the head and neck metastasizing to the parotid gland—A review of current recommendations
O'Hara J, Ferlito A, Takes RP, et al (Newcastle upon Tyne Hosps, Newcastle, UK; Univ of Udine, Italy; Radboud Univ Nijmegen Med Ctr, The Netherlands; et al)
Head Neck 33:1789-1795, 2011

Cutaneous squamous cell carcinoma (SCC) of the head and neck may metastasize in up to 5% of patients, with the parotid lymph nodes the most frequent site for spread. Metastases frequently show delayed presentation after the primary cancer had been treated. The optimum treatment should be surgery followed by adjuvant radiotherapy, with an appropriate parotidectomy, and preservation of the facial nerve if not involved by tumor and treatment to the neck. In a clinically N0 neck, levels I to III should be cleared for facial primaries, levels II to III for anterior scalp and external ear primaries, and levels II to V for posterior scalp primaries. Approximate 5-year disease-specific survival (DSS) after treatment was 70% to 75%. Patients with immunosuppression, in particular transplant recipients, are at high risk of developing aggressive metastatic cutaneous SCC. Modifications of the staging systems have demonstrated the prognostic benefits of accurately staging parotid and/or neck nodal disease.

▶ Cutaneous squamous cell carcinomas are considered relatively well-behaved tumors, with slow progression rate and relatively low incidence of regional lymph node metastases (2%–5%). Cutaneous squamous cell carcinoma of the head and neck, on the other hand, can be a formidable cancer, a fact that is often overlooked by dermatologists and dermatologic surgeons. It is therefore very important to identify high-risk head and neck skin cancers and manage them within the framework of a multidisciplinary team, much like other head and neck cancers. High-risk head and neck skin cancers are defined as tumors originating in the H-zone of the face, which includes upper and lower eyelids, temple, preauricular region, angle of the mandible, pinna, postauricular sulcus, nasolabial sulcus, nares, alar rims, glabella, and medial canthus. Tumors originating in the H-zone are often deeply invasive, are difficult to eradicate, and have higher recurrence rates. It is thought that predisposing factors to spread of these tumors include high density of nerve fibers, proximity to periosteum and perichondrium, and direct facial muscle insertion into the dermis. Furthermore, tumors larger than 2 cm in diameter and tumors with poor differentiation, aggressive growth pattern, depth of invasion exceeding 4 mm, and those with perineural, vascular, and lymphatic invasion should be classified as high risk and handled more aggressively, with wide local excision and consideration for regional lymph node sampling.

This article is an excellent review of current recommendations for management of cutaneous head and neck cancer with high risk for metastases to the parotid gland and cervical lymph nodes.

M. Gapany, MD

Human Papillomavirus and Rising Oropharyngeal Cancer Incidence in the United States

Chaturvedi AK, Engels EA, Pfeiffer RM, et al (Natl Cancer Inst, Rockville, MD; et al)
J Clin Oncol 29:4294-4301, 2011

Purpose.—Recent increases in incidence and survival of oropharyngeal cancers in the United States have been attributed to human papillomavirus (HPV) infection, but empirical evidence is lacking.

Patients and Methods.—HPV status was determined for all 271 oropharyngeal cancers (1984-2004) collected by the three population-based cancer registries in the Surveillance, Epidemiology, and End Results (SEER) Residual Tissue Repositories Program by using polymerase chain reaction and genotyping (Inno-LiPA), HPV16 viral load, and HPV16 mRNA expression. Trends in HPV prevalence across four calendar periods were estimated by using logistic regression. Observed HPV prevalence was reweighted to all oropharyngeal cancers within the cancer registries to account for nonrandom selection and to calculate incidence trends. Survival of HPV-positive and HPV-negative patients was compared by using Kaplan-Meier and multivariable Cox regression analyses.

Results.—HPV prevalence in oropharyngeal cancers significantly increased over calendar time regardless of HPV detection assay (P trend <.05). For example, HPV prevalence by Inno-LiPA increased from 16.3% during 1984 to 1989 to 71.7% during 2000 to 2004. Median survival was significantly longer for HPV-positive than for HPV-negative patients (131 v 20 months; log-rank $P < .001$; adjusted hazard ratio, 0.31; 95% CI, 0.21 to 0.46). Survival significantly increased across calendar periods for HPV-positive ($P = .003$) but not for HPV-negative patients ($P = .18$). Population-level incidence of HPV-positive oropharyngeal cancers increased by 225% (95% CI, 208% to 242%) from 1988 to 2004 (from 0.8 per 100,000 to 2.6 per 100,000), and incidence for HPV-negative cancers declined by 50% (95% CI, 47% to 53%; from 2.0 per 100,000 to 1.0 per 100,000). If recent incidence trends continue, the annual number of HPV-positive oropharyngeal cancers is expected to surpass the annual number of cervical cancers by the year 2020.

Conclusion.—Increases in the population-level incidence and survival of oropharyngeal cancers in the United States since 1984 are caused by HPV infection.

▶ This very important article highlights the epidemic proportions human papilloma virus (HPV)-positive oropharyngeal cancer is reaching in the United States. If this trend continues (and every epidemiologic indicator suggests that it will), then in 20 years HPV-positive oropharyngeal cancer will become the most commonly diagnosed head and neck cancer, surpassing the current incidence of HPV-associated cancer of the uterine cervix. The only effective way to get control of this epidemic would be instituting prophylactic screening for premalignancy and early HPV vaccination, similar to prophylaxis of cervical cancer. Unfortunately, there are no prophylactic screening programs in place for oropharyngeal cancer and no clear-cut policy by the Centers for Disease Control and Prevention (CDC) regarding oropharyngeal HPV infection. The US Food and Drug Administration—approved vaccine for HPV-related cervical cancer prevention has not yet been seriously considered for oropharyngeal cancer prophylaxis, while we are learning more about the incidence, epidemiology, and biological behavior of this malignancy. Meanwhile, a very significant (although currently unknown) proportion of young and sexually active Americans are being infected with high-risk HPV.

M. Gapany, MD

Management of the Clinically Negative Neck in Early-Stage Head and Neck Cancers After Transoral Resection

Rodrigo JP, Shah JP, Silver CE, et al (Hospital Universitario Central de Asturias, Oviedo, Spain; Memorial Sloan-Kettering Cancer Ctr, NY; Albert Einstein College of Medicine, Bronx, NY; et al)
Head Neck 33:1210-1219, 2011

The decision regarding treatment of the clinically negative neck has been debated extensively. This is particularly true with early-stage tumors for which surgery is the treatment of choice, and the tumor has been resected transorally without a cervical incision. Elective neck dissection in this situation is an additional procedure with potential associated morbidity. The alternative strategy for the clinically negative neck is to "wait and watch." Both an elective neck dissection policy and a "watchful waiting" policy have their proponents. The purpose of this article was for us to review the literature about this subject to try to answer the following question: if the tumor has been resected transorally, should an elective treatment of the neck be performed or is a "watchful waiting" policy safe and adequate? We conclude that, currently, the best available evidence suggests that elective neck dissection does not seem to be superior to the policy of observation without neck surgery, with regard to survival and control of neck disease. This review highlights the need for further well-designed prospective studies that will provide more reliable answers to the debatable issue of the management of the clinically negative neck in such cases.

▶ In the era of transoral surgery for early head and neck cancer, the debate of how to manage N0 neck takes on new relevance. Attempts to predict occult metastases based on the thickness of the primary tumor as well as other primary tumor characteristics have not resolved the debate of elective surgery versus watchful waiting. This selected article is an excellent review of available literature on this subject. It reviews the contribution of available diagnostic modalities such as imaging, fine-needle aspiration, biomarkers, and sentinel lymph node biopsy, in the decision-making process on whether to recommend elective neck dissection. The major shortcoming of available literature is the paucity of well-designed, prospective studies. In the absence of convincing evidence one way or another, I personally am very uncomfortable observing a neck with potentially occult metastatic disease. I prefer to accept the added morbidity of an operation (potentially unnecessary) for the sake of peace of mind (potentially fictitious) for both the surgeon and the patient.

M. Gapany, MD

The Increasing Workload in Head and Neck Surgery: An Epidemiologic Analysis
Bhattacharyya N (Brigham and Women's Hosp, Boston, MA)
Laryngoscope 121:111-115, 2011

Objectives/Hypothesis.—Determine if there might be an increase in the workload for head and neck surgery based on an aging population.

Study Design.—Cross-sectional analysis of a national database.

Methods.—The frequency of head and neck surgical procedures (HNSPs) performed in 2006 in the inpatient and outpatient settings in the United States were assessed using the National Hospital Discharge Summary and the National Survey of Ambulatory Surgery, respectively. From US Census Bureau statistics, age-specific HNSP rates were determined and projected to the 2020 population based on census bureau predicted changes in population demographics. The surgical workload burden was assessed in 2006 and projected to 2020 based on the predicted changes in procedure rates and resource-based relative value scale.

Results.—An estimated 366,050 HNSPs (142,397 inpatient vs. 223,653 outpatient) were performed in 2006 requiring a total of 2.49 million physician work relative value units (RVUs). With the expected changes in population demographics in 2020, an estimated 422,183 HNSPs will be performed (163,781 inpatient vs. 258,402 outpatient) requiring 2.88 million work RVUs in head and neck surgery. Both the HNSP rate and projected RVUs increase approximate 15.3%.

Conclusions.—Based on national health statistics and US census data we can anticipate a substantial increase in the workload for head and neck surgeons. Efforts should be directed at assessing manpower requirements in head and neck surgery based on the impact of an aging US population.

▶ This is a very important epidemiologic study that projects a substantial increase in workload for head and neck surgeons. Will we be able to meet this projected growing demand? There is a good reason to worry. Long hours in the operating room, technically difficult operations, sick patients, and high incidence of serious postoperative complications, combined with poor reimbursement (compared with other fields in otolaryngology), make head and neck surgery the least attractive and desirable subspecialty in otolaryngology. The predominant majority of graduates from otolaryngology residency programs who choose to subspecialize elect to do so in pediatric otolaryngology, facial plastic and reconstructive surgery, otology/neuro-otology, rhinology/sinus surgery, laryngology/voice disorders, and, of late, sleep medicine. It is exceptionally rare for a resident who expressed interest in head and neck surgery at the beginning of training to still want to pursue this career pathway at the end of residency. Over the past 18 years in academic otolaryngology, I have trained 72 residents. I can think of only 3 who pursued fellowship training in head and neck surgery: a meager 4%.

So how are we going to deal with this projected increase in demand? In my opinion, definitely not through otolaryngologists in the community, but through designated centers of excellence, with outstanding surgical, radiation oncology, and medical oncology support, which are ready to deliver state-of-the art multidisciplinary care in the most efficient and cost-effective fashion.

M. Gapany, MD

Outcomes

Surgical salvage of the oropharynx after failure of organ-sparing therapy
Nichols AC, Kneuertz PJ, Deschler DG, et al (Univ of Western Ontario, London, Canada; Massachusetts Eye and Ear Infirmary, Boston; et al)
Head Neck 33:516-524, 2011

Background.—The purpose of this study was to evaluate the efficacy of salvage surgery for local recurrences of oropharyngeal squamous cell carcinoma (OPSCC) and identify predictors of survival.

Methods.—The authors reviewed 264 patients with OPSCC treated with radiation or chemoradiation identified retrospectively. Of the 77 patients that experienced recurrences, 37 had local or local and regional recurrences and were considered for salvage surgery.

Results.—Of the 37 patients with local or local and regional recurrence, 5 had unresectable disease whereas 3 refused surgery. The remainder underwent salvage surgery with 2-year and 5-year survival rates of 64.5% and 43.4%, respectively. A history of alcohol abuse and positive surgical margins were the only predictors of poorer overall survival ($p < .05$) after salvage surgery.

Conclusion.—Surgical salvage of locoregional recurrences can be effective if wide resections are performed so that negative margins can be achieved.

▶ Salvage surgery for radiochemotherapy failures is an integral part of organ preservation approach for head and neck cancer. Previous studies from The University of Texas M. D. Anderson Cancer Center have reported relatively good overall survival in patients who underwent salvage surgery for radiochemotherapy in oropharyngeal cancer failures (3-year and 5-year overall survivals of 42% and 28%, respectively). This selected study reports even higher survival rates for salvage surgery in oropharyngeal cancer failures, with 2-year and 5-year survival rates of 64.5% and 43.4%, respectively. It is reported but not emphasized in this study that salvage surgery is associated with very high complication rate (41% in this study and 46% in the study from The University of Texas M. D. Anderson Cancer Center). Major complications included perioperative death (3.4%), myocardial infarction (6.9%), pneumonia (13.8%), wound infections (17.2%), and oropharyngeal fistula (10.3%). While this high complication rate is undoubtedly outweighed by the encouraging survival advantage, it definitely should serve as a deterrent for less experienced head and neck surgeon to perform salvage surgery. Such operations should be relegated to the most experienced head and neck oncologic surgeons who are part of a multidisciplinary head and neck cancer program.

M. Gapany, MD

Comparison of Endoscopic Laser Resection versus Radiation Therapy for the Treatment of Early Glottic Carcinoma

Osborn HA, Hu A, Venkatesan V, et al (Univ of Western Ontario, Ontario, Canada; London Health Sciences Centre, Ontario, Canada)
J Otolaryngol Head Neck Surg 40:200-204, 2011

Objective.—Radiation therapy (RT) and transoral laser microsurgery (TLM) are established treatments for early glottic squamous cell carcinoma (SCC). Similar oncologic outcomes have been reported with both modalities, leading physicians to consider other factors when making clinical recommendations. One such factor is voice-related quality of life. This investigation sought to characterize differences in self-reported voice outcomes in patients undergoing RT or TLM for the treatment of Tis or T1a glottic SCC.

Methods.—A retrospective cohort study was conducted of all individuals who received either RT or TLM for the treatment of Tis or T1a glottic SCC between 2004 and 2009 at the London Regional Cancer Program. The primary outcome measure was voice-related quality of life, as assessed by the Voice-Related Quality of Life questionnaire (V-RQOL). Secondary outcomes included local control, overall survival, and laryngectomy-free survival.

Results.—Fifty-seven patients were eligible for this study; 34 received RT and 23 received TLM. Forty (70.2%) of the 57 patients completed the V-RQOL. No statistically significant difference in total V-RQOL score was observed between the RT and TLM cohorts ($p = .228$). There was, however, a trend toward higher scores (ie, less voice disability) in the physical function domain of the V-RQOL for the RT group (90.0%) compared to the TLM group (80.2%) ($p = .05$). No significant differences were observed in recurrence or overall survival between the two groups.

Conclusion.—Both oncologic outcomes and self-rated voice-related quality of life are similar in patients treated with RT and TLM for early glottic carcinoma.

▶ The oncologic outcomes of treating early cancer of the glottic larynx are equally good regardless of the modality of therapy (radiation or laser microsurgery). The choice of therapy is therefore often determined by the functional outcome (ie, posttherapy voice-related quality of life). Although the common wisdom is that radiotherapy as a rule offers better quality of voice, this has never been consistently shown in studies. The compounding problem is that objective measurements of quality of voice, such as auditory-perceptual analysis and acoustic voice parameters, have been poorly correlating with patient-perceived voice outcomes. Obviously, however, patient-perceived voice outcomes matter the most when assessing the impact of certain therapeutic modality on perceived quality of life. This small study used a self-administered Voice-Related Quality of Life (V-RQOL) questionnaire to assess patient-perceived voice-related outcomes. Not unexpectedly, there were no statistically significant differences in outcomes between radiotherapy and laser microsurgery, resulting in relatively good quality of voice for both therapeutic modalities. So far, most data in the literature have suggested equally good voice outcomes for early glottic cancer with radiotherapy and laser microsurgery.

M. Gapany, MD

Human papillomavirus and survival in patients with base of tongue cancer
Attner P, Du J, Näsman A, et al (Karolinska Univ Hosp, Stockholm, Sweden; Karolinska Institutet, Stockholm, Sweden)
Int J Cancer 128:2892-2897, 2011

The incidence of base of tongue cancer is increasing in Sweden and the proportion of human papillomavirus (HPV) positive cancer has increased in Stockholm, Sweden. Between 2006 and 2007, 84% of base of tongue cancer cases in Stockholm were HPV-positive. The objective of this study was to assess the impact of HPV status on prognosis for base of tongue cancer patients. One-hundred and nine patients were diagnosed with base of tongue cancer between 1998 and 2007 in Stockholm County and 95 paraffin-embedded diagnostic tumor biopsies were obtained and tested for HPV by PCR. Eighty-seven patients had available biopsies, were treated with intention to cure and could be included in the survival analysis. Age, sex, TNM-stage, stage, treatment and survival were recorded from patient charts. Kaplan—Meier curves were used to present survival data. In multivariable analyses, a Cox proportional hazards model was used to adjust for covariates. In total 68 (78%) tumor biopsies from the 87 included patients were HPV DNA positive. Kaplan—Meier estimates showed that the overall survival for patients with HPV-positive cancer was significantly better ($p = 0.0004$), (log-rank test) than that of patients with HPV-negative cancer. Patients with HPV-positive tumors also had significantly better disease-free survival ($p = 0.0008$), (log-rank test) than those with HPV-negative tumors. These results further strengthen the option to consider HPV-status when planning prospective studies on treatment for base of tongue cancer.

▶ Evidence has been mounting that human papillomavirus (HPV) infection constitutes an independent etiologic factor for causing oropharyngeal cancer, and that HPV-associated oropharyngeal cancer has different epidemiologic, biologic, and clinical characteristics from non-HPV cancer. Epidemiologic implications of these findings are of utmost importance, because it is likely that we are witnessing a new form of sexually transmitted disease from changes in sexual behavior. Furthermore, there is ample evidence in the literature that links HPV tumor status with relatively favorable clinical course of tonsillar cancer. This is in part caused by different tumor biology of HPV-positive tumors, compared with HPV-negative, smoking- and alcohol-linked cancers. In part, better outcome could also be associated with improved response to therapy.

This selected article from Stockholm County puts the incidence of HPV-positive tongue base cancer at 84% and confirms what has been documented in tonsillar cancer, namely, that HPV-positive tongue base cancers had a better overall and disease-free survival compared with those that were HPV negative. Chemoradiotherapy was the most commonly used therapeutic modality in this study.

M. Gapany, MD

Transoral Laser Microsurgery as Primary Treatment for Advanced-Stage Oropharyngeal Cancer: A United States Multicenter Study
Haughey BH, Hinni ML, Salassa JR, et al (Washington Univ School of Medicine, St Louis, MO; Mayo Clinic, Scottsdale, AZ; Mayo Clinic, Jacksonville, FL)
Head Neck 33:1683-1694, 2011

Background.—Nonsurgical modalities are sometimes advocated as the standard of care for advanced oropharyngeal tumors. Oncologic and functional results have been modest. The aim of our study was to evaluate outcomes of a minimally invasive approach, using transoral laser microsurgery (TLM) as the primary treatment for advanced oropharyngeal carcinoma.

Methods.—A prospectively assembled database of 204 patients with American Joint Committee on Cancer (AJCC) stages III and IV tonsil or tongue base cancer, treated primarily with TLM during 1996—2006 at 3 centers with minimum 2-year follow-up was analyzed. Survival, locoregional control, and swallowing status were recorded.

Results.—Mean follow-up was 49 months and 79.4% of patients were alive. Three-year overall survival, disease-specific survival, and disease-free survival were 86%, 88%, and 82%, respectively. Local control was 97%, and 87% of patients had normal swallowing or episodic dysphagia.

Conclusions.—TLM as a primary treatment for advanced oropharyngeal malignancy confers excellent survival and swallowing proficiency.

▶ I read this article with great interest. Several fascinating observations emerge from this study. First, authors report 90% positivity for p16 in their series of oropharyngeal cancers, implicating human papillomavirus (HPV) infection in almost all of their treated patients. To my knowledge, this is the highest incidence of HPV infection in oropharyngeal cancers so far reported in the United States and equals to the recent reports from Stockholm County in Sweden. The 90% reduction in risk of death in patients positive for p16 as opposed to those negative for p16 could explain the excellent survival results reported in this study (regardless of the treatment modality).

Another interesting observation emerging from this study is that adjuvant radiotherapy has reduced the risk of death by more than 50% compared with patients treated with surgery only. We learned from the Material and Methods section that the decision on whether to administer adjuvant therapy was based on the operative pathology findings, that is, patients who had clear surgical margins and single metastatic lymph node without extracapsular extension, thus, deemed to be low risk for recurrence, were treated with surgery only, whereas patients with high risk for recurrence were given adjuvant therapy. My conclusion from these findings was 2-fold: first, radiotherapy was highly effective in treating HPV-positive pharyngeal cancer, and second, surgeons have made grave errors in judgment by not giving patients in the so-called "low-risk group" adjuvant radiotherapy, condemning them to more than 50% increase in the risk of death. Based on the presented data, I would recommend that all patients be treated with adjuvant radiotherapy to reduce the risk of death by at least 50%. Furthermore, based on the presented data, I would speculate that radiotherapy was the more effective therapy in this presented group of patients (this, of course, being only a guess). The authors of this article concluded that transoral laser microsurgery was a highly effective primary treatment option for management of advanced-stage oropharyngeal cancer. But of course, their guess was as good as mine.

M. Gapany, MD

Radiotherapy

Radiation-induced hypothyroidism in head and neck cancer patients: A systematic review

Boomsma MJ, Bijl HP, Langendijk JA (Univ Med Ctr Groningen, The Netherlands)
Radiother Oncol 99:1-5, 2011

Purpose.—To review literature on the relationship between the dose distribution in the thyroid gland and the incidence of radiation-induced hypothyroidism in adults.

Material and Methods.—Articles were identified through a search in MEDLINE, EMBASE and the Cochrane Library. Approximately 2449 articles were screened and selected by inclusion- and exclusion criteria. Eventually, there were five papers that fulfilled the eligibility criteria to be included in this review.

Results.—The sample sizes of the reviewed studies vary from 57 to 390 patients. The incidence of hypothyroidism was much higher (23–53%) than would be expected in a non-irradiated cohort. There was a large heterogeneity between the studies regarding study design, estimation of the dose to the thyroid gland and definition of endpoints. In general, the relationship between thyroid gland volume absorbing 10–70 Gy (V10–V70), mean dose (Dmean), minimal dose (Dmin), maximum dose (Dmax) and point doses with hypothyroidism were analysed. An association between dose-volume parameters and hypothyroidism was found in two studies.

Conclusions.—Hypothyroidism is frequently observed after radiation. Although the results suggest that higher radiation doses to the thyroid gland are associated with hypothyroidism, it was not possible to define a clear threshold radiation dose for the thyroid gland.

▶ Hypothyroidism is a common late adverse effect of radiotherapy to the head and neck region. Unfortunately, it is often overlooked and can result in significant clinical symptoms of hypothyroidism before discovered. It is therefore important to incorporate thyroid function testing into the follow-up routine of radiotherapy-treated head and neck cancer patients. The question then arises when to start testing for hypothyroidism, how long to continue such follow-up testing, and who are the patients at the greatest risk to develop hypothyroidism. This systematic literature review set a goal of answering some of these questions. The available data in the literature, however, were inadequate to determine exact dose-volume relationship with the incidence of hypothyroidism. Because the median interval of hypothyroidism after radiotherapy appears to be in the 1.5- to 2-year range, most routine testing should probably be performed during this time interval. It is important to be aware that up to 53% of radiated head and neck cancer patients can develop subclinical hypothyroidism.

M. Gapany, MD

Surgical Technique

Feasibility of submandibular gland preservation in neck dissection: A prospective anatomic-pathologic study

Dhiwakar M, Ronen O, Malone J, et al (Simmons Cancer Inst at Southern Illinois Univ, Springfield, IL; et al)
Head Neck 33:603-609, 2011

Background.—The submandibular gland is commonly removed during neck dissection involving sublevel IB. However, removal reduces basal salivary secretion and therapeutic options for minimizing xerostomia. The purpose of this study was to determine whether all lymph nodes in sublevel IB can be extirpated without removing the submandibular gland.

Methods.—Twenty consecutive patients undergoing 33 neck dissections were prospectively enrolled. Sublevel IB dissection was performed by 3 sequential steps: (1) removal of targeted lymph node groups (preglandular and postglandular, prevascular and postvascular), (2) removal of submandibular gland, and (3) removal of residual lymphoadipose tissue in the surgical bed.

Results.—Complete removal of lymph nodes in sublevel IB was achieved before excising the submandibular gland in all of the 30 eligible neck dissections. The submandibular gland and the surgical bed contained no residual lymph nodes.

Conclusion.—In suitable cases, it is technically feasible to remove all lymph nodes in sublevel IB and preserve the submandibular gland.

▶ Selective neck dissection with preservation of vital structures is a well-established concept in head and neck oncologic surgery. Its oncologic safety has been evaluated in numerous clinical studies. However, the oncologic soundness of submandibular gland preservation in sublevel IB lymphadenectomy for oral cavity cancer as a separate surgical/oncologic issue has not been well investigated. This selected prospective pilot study has addressed this question from both an oncologic and a technical perspective. The results confirm technical and oncologic feasibility of this approach, achieving potential benefit of preserving submandibular salivary flow.

One potential drawback of preserving the submandibular gland is persistent palpable mass in the site of previous lymphadenectomy. Surrounding scar tissue renders this mass quite hard, especially in cases in which postoperative radiotherapy has been used. This mass can be a source of concern for both the patient and the otolaryngologist—head and neck surgeon who follows the patient, leading to repeated needle biopsies, imaging studies, and, on occasion, even removal of the "mass." For this reason, some surgeons insist on routine removal of the submandibular salivary gland, despite oncologic and technical feasibility of preserving it.

M. Gapany, MD

Questionable necessity to remove the submandibular gland in neck dissection
Takes RP, Robbins KT, Woolgar JA, et al (Radboud Univ Nijmegen Med Ctr, The Netherlands; Southern Illinois Univ School of Medicine, Springfield; Univ of Liverpool, UK; et al)
Head Neck 33:743-745, 2011

Saliva is of major importance in taste, speech, swallowing, and protection against dental caries. Neck dissection surgery and/or radiotherapy may impair the function of the submandibular glands. Over the years, there has been a trend toward more conservative approaches to neck dissection. Metastasis to the submandibular gland itself is extremely rare and if removal of the lymph nodes of sublevel IB is imperative, it seems feasible to preserve the submandibular gland, unless it is involved by direct tumor extension of the primary tumor or the adjacent metastatic lymph nodes. Clinical studies to validate this concept are needed.

▶ This review article addresses the question of feasibility of preservation of submandibular salivary gland in cases of selective neck dissection. Oncologically, preservation of submandibular glands in cases in which selective neck dissections are indicated is definitely safe and sound. Technically, the lymphatic compartment of level IB, between the superficial and the deep layers of the cervical fascia, can be easily separated from the parenchyma of the submandibular gland once the submandibular fascia is incised. Incision of the submandibular fascia along the lower aspect of the submandibular gland also facilitates identification and preservation of the mandibular branch of the facial nerve.

I have been preserving the submandibular gland in selective neck dissections since I first learned how to perform a "functional" neck dissection from watching a video recording by the famed Italian surgeon, Dr Ettore Bocca, in the United States. My senior partner, however, insisted in removing the submandibular gland because, in his experience, the preserved submandibular gland often scarred and on follow-up felt like a hard mass in the submandibular trigone, causing concerns for recurrence.

M. Gapany, MD

3 Laryngology

Basic and Clinical Research

Effect of Altered Core Body Temperature On Glottal Closing Force

Wadie M, Li J, Sasaki CT (Yale Univ School of Medicine, New Haven, CT)
Ann Otol Rhinol Laryngol 120:669-673, 2011

Objectives.—A basic function of the larynx is to provide sphincteric protection of the lower airway, initiated by a brain stem—mediated glottal closure reflex. Glottal closing force is defined as the measured pressure generated between the vocal folds during glottal closure. One of the factors thought to affect the glottal closure reflex is a variation in core body temperature.

Methods.—Four adult male Yorkshire pigs were used in this study. The subjects were studied under control conditions (37°C), hyperthermic conditions (38°C to 41°C), and hypothermic conditions (36°C to 34°C).

Results.—We demonstrated that the glottal closing force increased significantly with an increase in core body temperature and also decreased significantly with decreased core body temperature. These results are supported by neurophysiological changes demonstrated by other studies in pups and adult dogs in response to altered core body temperatures. The mechanism for these responses is thought to reside centrally, rather than in the peripheral nervous system.

Conclusions.—We hope that a better understanding of these aspects of glottal closure will alter the care of many patients with postanesthesia hypothermia and many sedated inmates and will also further enhance preventive measures needed to decrease the incidence of sudden infant death syndrome in overheated or febrile infants (Tables 1 and 2).

▶ At its core, the larynx is a sphincter. By denying access to the lower airway, it is able to protect the host from aspiration of bacteria-laden secretions and food during swallowing. This function is life-saving considering that we swallow upwards of 750 times a day, including in our sleep. Like other brainstem-mediated reflexes, the laryngeal adductor reflex can be influenced by core body temperature.

Using a porcine model, the authors tested their hypothesis that the strength of the glottic closing force (GCF) is influenced by core body temperature. They operated on 4 pigs (~50 kg each), severing the internal superior laryngeal nerve (SLN) bilaterally and attaching stimulating electrodes to control eliciting the laryngeal adductor reflex. A pressure transducer between the vocal folds

TABLE 1.—Effects of Hyperthermia on Glottal Closing Force

Animal	Control	38°C	39°C	40°C	41°C
1	283.9 ± 80.0	506.1 ± 81.4	849.3 ± 45.9	891.3 ± 118.5	1,051.8 ± 137.0
2	343.2 ± 80.0	437.0 ± 17.7	641.9 ± 100.7	792.5 ± 94.8	841.9 ± 77.0
3	325.9 ± 65.2	414.8 ± 63.7	661.7 ± 75.5	785.1 ± 71.1	886.4 ± 28.1
4	276.5 ± 34.1	520.9 ± 57.7	679.0 ± 69.6	883.9 ± 28.1	1,064.2 ± 42.9
Mean	307.4 ± 32.3	469.7 ± 51.7*	708.0 ± 95.4[†]	838.2 ± 57.2[†]	961.1 ± 113.4[†]

Data are expressed as mean ± SD in millimeters of mercury.
*$p < 0.05$.
[†]$p < 0.01$.

TABLE 2.—Effects of Hypothermia on Glottal Closing Force

Animal	Control	36°C	35°C	34°C
1	283.9 ± 80.0	282.4 ± 35.5	244.4 ± 34.0	167.9 ± 22.2
2	343.2 ± 80.0	167.9 ± 29.6	86.4 ± 17.7	24.7 ± 7.4
3	325.9 ± 65.2	202.4 ± 54.8	130.8 ± 22.2	69.1 ± 22.2
4	276.5 ± 34.1	234.5 ± 37.0	138.2 ± 28.1	74.0 ± 8.8
Mean	307.4 ± 32.3	222.8 ± 50.3	150.0 ± 67.0*	83.9 ± 60.2[†]

Data are expressed as mean ± SD in millimeters of mercury.
*$p < 0.05$.
[†]$p < 0.01$.

measured the GCF at different electrode stimulus intensity levels of the internal division of the SLN and at different temperatures (37°C was control, 38°C to 41°C was hyperthermic, and 36°C to 34°C was hypothermic). The mean GCF at 37°C was 307 mm Hg (control). At 34°C the closing force was 84 mm Hg, whereas at 41°C, it was 961 mm Hg (Fig 3 in the original article, Tables 1 and 2).

These very large differences in GCF help support the idea that one mechanism for sudden infant death syndrome, an idiopathic deadly condition that kills more than 2000 children a year in the United States, may be elevated core body temperature, leading to a hypersensitive and exaggerated laryngeal adductor reflex. These data also have implications for patients during intentional cooling after brain injury or cardiac procedures because they will tend to protect the airway with less GCF.

R. Franco, MD

Continuous Control of Tracheal Cuff Pressure and Microaspiration of Gastric Contents in Critically Ill Patients

Nseir S, Zerimech F, Fournier C, et al (Univ Hosp of Lille, France)
Am J Respir Crit Care Med 184:1041-1047, 2011

Rationale.—Underinflation of the tracheal cuff frequently occurs in critically ill patients and represents a risk factor for microaspiration of contaminated oropharyngeal secretions and gastric contents that plays a major role in the pathogenesis of ventilator-associated pneumonia (VAP).

Objectives.—To determine the impact of continuous control of tracheal cuff pressure (P_{cuff}) on microaspiration of gastric contents.

Methods.—Prospective randomized controlled trial performed in a single medical intensive care unit. A total of 122 patients expected to receive mechanical ventilation for at least 48 hours through a tracheal tube were randomized to receive continuous control of P_{cuff} using a pneumatic device (intervention group, n = 61) or routine care of P_{cuff} (control group, n = 61).

Measurements and Main Results.—The primary outcome was microaspiration of gastric contents as defined by the presence of pepsin at a significant level in tracheal secretions collected during the 48 hours after randomization. Secondary outcomes included incidence of VAP, tracheobronchial bacterial concentration, and tracheal ischemic lesions. The pneumatic device was efficient in controlling P_{cuff}. Pepsin was measured

TABLE 2.—Patient Characteristics at Randomization and During the 48 Hours After Randomization

| | Continuous Control of P_{cuff} | | |
	Yes n = 61	No n = 61	P Value
At randomization			
Duration of prior intubation, d	1 (0.25–2)	1 (0.5–2)	0.962
Size of tracheal tube	8 (7.5–8)	8 (7.5–8)	0.852
LOD score	4 (1–7)	4 (2–4)	0.538
During the 48 h after randomization			
P_{cuff} cm H_2O	26 (25–27)	22 (20–24)	<0.001
P_{cuff} <20 cm H_2O	2 (3)	34 (55)	<0.001*
P_{cuff} >30 cm H_2O	2 (3)	12 (19)	0.008*
Percentage of P_{cuff} determinations 20–30 cm H_2O, mean ± SD	98 ± 13	74 ± 26	<0.001
Percentage of P_{cuff} determinations <20 cm H_2O, mean ± SD	0.1 ± 12	19 ± 23	0.001
Percentage of P_{cuff} determinations >30 cm H_2O, mean ± SD	0.7 ± 5	5 ± 18	0.003
Head of bed elevation, angle achieved, degrees	40 (36–45)	40 (37–45)	0.637
Quantity of enteral nutrition, ml/d	750 (750–1000)	750 (750–1000)	0.784
Vomiting	10 (16)	5 (8)	0.270
Prokinetic drugs	15 (24)	10 (16)	0.370
Proton pump inhibitor use	21 (34)	15 (24)	0.160
Residual gastric volume, ml/d	80 (30–120)	70 (25–110)	0.546
Sedation	39 (63)	37 (60)	0.853
Ramsay score	4 (2–4)	4 (2–4)	0.537
Paralytic agent use	3 (4)	8 (13)	0.205
Ventilatory mode			0.395
ACV	44 (72)	49 (80)	
PSV	17 (27)	12 (19)	
Positive end-expiratory pressure	5 (5–7.5)	6 (5–8)	0.257
Number of tracheal suctioning/24 h, mean ± SD	8 ± 1	8 ± 1	0.892
Death	2 (3)	1 (1)	>0.999
Unplanned extubation	5 (8)	2 (3)	0.439

Definition of abbreviations: ACV = assist control ventilation; LOD = logistic organ dysfunction; P_{cuff} = cuff pressure; PSV = pressure support ventilation.

Data are n (%) or median (interquartile range) unless otherwise specified.

*Odds ratio (95% confidence interval), 0.02 (0.01–0.12); 0.13 (0.03–0.64).

in 1,205 tracheal aspirates. Percentage of patients with abundant microaspiration (18 vs. 46%; $P = 0.002$; OR [95% confidence interval], 0.25 [0.11−0.59]), bacterial concentration in tracheal aspirates (mean ± SD 1.6 ± 2.4 vs. 3.1 ± 3.7 $\log_{10}$ cfu/ml, $P = 0.014$), and VAP rate (9.8 vs. 26.2%; $P = 0.032$; 0.30 [0.11−0.84]) were significantly lower in the intervention group compared with the control group. However, no significant difference was found in tracheal ischemia score between the two groups.

Conclusions.—Continuous control of P_{cuff} is associated with significantly decreased microaspiration of gastric contents in critically ill patients (Table 2).

▶ Critically ill patients who are intubated for a prolonged time in the intensive care unit (ICU) are at risk for ventilator-associated pneumonia (VAP), microaspiration of gastric contents, and tracheal wall injury from overinflation of the cuff leading to ischemia and eventual stenosis. The authors surmise that constant regulation of cuff pressure in the normal range (not too inflated and not too underinflated) will result in a decrease in microaspiration of gastric contents, VAP, and tracheal wall injuries.

The authors prospectively enrolled 122 patients (Table 2) who were randomly assigned to normal manual cuff pressure regulation and the automated cuff regulation. A total of 1205 tracheal aspirates were obtained with a decrease in the percentage of microaspiration from 46% with manual cuff pressure regulation to 18% when the cuff pressure was automatically regulated. Mean bacterial concentration (Figs 2 and 3 in the original article) decreased from 3.1 log 10 cfu/mL to 1.6 log 10 cfu/mL with VAP rates decreasing from 26.2% down to 9.8%. There was no difference in the tracheal ischemia scores between the 2 groups.

The use of an automated endotracheal cuff pressure regulator decreased the presence of pepsin and bacteria in tracheal aspirates. This in turn decreased the number of VAPs, a substantial cause of ICU-related morbidity for those who are intubated for a prolonged period.

R. Franco, MD

Heat and moisture exchange capacity of the upper respiratory tract and the effect of tracheotomy breathing on endotracheal climate
Scheenstra RJ, Muller SH, Vincent A, et al (The Netherlands Cancer Inst—Antoni van Leeuwenhoek Hosp, Amsterdam)
Head Neck 33:117-124, 2011

Background.—The aim of this study was to assess the heat and moisture exchange (HME) capacity of the upper respiratory tract and the effect of tracheotomy breathing on endotracheal climate in patients with head and neck cancer.

Methods.—We plotted the subglottic temperature and humidity measurements in 10 patients with head and neck cancer with a temporary precautionary tracheotomy during successive 10-minute periods of nose, mouth, and tracheotomy breathing in a randomized sequence.

Results.—End-inspiratory temperatures of nose, mouth, and tracheotomy breathing were 31.1, 31.3, and 28.3°C, respectively. End-inspiratory humidity measurements of nose, mouth, and tracheotomy breathing were 29.3, 28.6, and 21.1 mgH$_2$O/L, respectively. There was a trend toward lower end-inspiratory humidity in patients with radiotherapy or with large surgery-induced oropharyngeal mucosal defects, whereas temperatures were similar.

Conclusion.—This study gives objective information about the HME capacity of the upper respiratory tract in patients with head and neck cancer with precautionary tracheotomy, and thus provides target values for HMEs for laryngectomized and tracheotomized patients (Fig 2).

▶ Of the many functions of the nose, warming and humidifying the air is important because it maintains maximal humidity throughout the airways. Normally, air inspired through the nasal cavities is heated to about 32°C and is 100% saturated with 36 mg H$_2$O/L when it reaches the subglottis. As the air passes further into the airway, it attains body temperature and reaches its point of maximal saturation at 44 mg H$_2$O/L. When the air is not maximally humidified, there is destruction of the airway epithelium and hypersecretion of mucus, as is seen

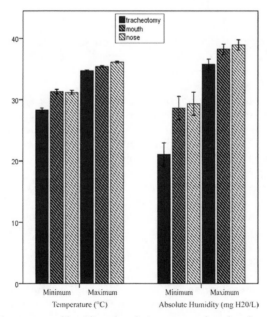

FIGURE 2.—Temperature and humidity values during nose, mouth, and tracheotomy breathing (see Table 2 in the original article). Error bars represent standard errors. (Reprinted from Scheenstra RJ, Muller SH, Vincent A, et al. Heat and moisture exchange capacity of the upper respiratory tract and the effect of tracheotomy breathing on endotracheal climate. *Head Neck.* 2011;33:117-124, and John Wiley and Sons.)

after tracheotomy or laryngectomy. Heat-moisture exchange (HME) devices help to increase the heat and moisture in the airway when the mouth and nose are bypassed, such as when mechanical ventilation is necessary, or after tracheostomy tube placement.

The authors measured the temperature and humidity in the airway in 10 prophylactically tracheotomized patients (Fig 2). They found that the end-inspiratory temperature was 31.1°C for nasal breathing, 31.3°C for mouth breathing, and 28.3°C for tracheostomy tube breathing. The humidity was measured as 29.3 mg H_2O/L for nasal breathing, 28.6 mg H_2O/L for mouth breathing, and 21.1 mg H_2O/L for tracheotomy tube breathing. There is a wide discrepancy between the values obtained with nasal breathing and breathing via the tracheostomy tube that can have an impact on patients' overall health because they become more susceptible to pulmonary infections, mucous plugging, and increasing airway discomfort. Every effort should be made to increase humidification through the use of an HME device and external humidifiers to raise the ambient humidity.

R. Franco, MD

A New Noninvasive Method for Determination of Laryngeal Sensory Function

Bock JM, Blumin JH, Toohill RJ, et al (Med College of Wisconsin, Milwaukee)
Laryngoscope 121:158-163, 2011

Objectives/Hypothesis.—We report a new surface technique for studying sensory conduction in the superior laryngeal nerve (SLN).

Study Design.—Prospective controlled cohort study at an academic tertiary care hospital.

Methods.—Surface stimulation of the vagus nerve 7—10 cm proximal to a surface electrode placed over the cricothyroid muscle was performed in controls and in subjects with needle electromyographic-confirmed laryngeal neuropathy. Cathodal stimulation was applied below the mastoid process behind the sternocleidomastoid muscle. Nerve conduction parameters were determined.

Results.—Noninvasive SLN evoked potential studies were performed on healthy volunteers (n = 28) as well as neuropathic subjects (n = 27). Compared to controls, the neuropathic subjects had statistically significant differences in baselineto-peak amplitude, conduction velocity, and intrasubject side-to-side amplitude ratio (P <.01) of their surface evoked laryngeal sensory action potential (SELSAP).

Conclusions.—Laryngeal sensory nerve conduction can be determined noninvasively by evaluating SELSAP waveform. This study provides a reproducible method for electrophysiologic evaluation of a sensory branch of the SLN.

▶ The larynx is a richly innervated organ that uses its exquisite sensitivity to protect us from the potentially lethal complications of aspiration. Patients with a deficit of the internal branch of the superior laryngeal nerve do not sense food and liquid entering the laryngeal introitus (on that side), making it easier to cross into the subglottis (aspiration) and trachea. Sensory testing typically takes the form of the application of calibrated puffs of air to the laryngeal tissues to elicit the laryngeal adductor reflex. Although this can be a useful clinical test, the calibrated puffs have been found to vary in intensity from puff to puff, the test is relatively invasive because the scope needs to get to the laryngopharynx through the nose, it is difficult to consistently know how far away you are from the tissues, and the intensity of the test puffs decreases dramatically the farther the scope is held from the tissues.

The authors set out to use surface stimulation of the vagus and pick up the laryngeal sensory action potential via surface electrodes over the cricothyroid space. The electromyographic signals (EMG) were compared between a series of normal subjects (n = 28) and patients who had been referred for suspected laryngeal neuropathy (n = 27). The authors found a tiny response they refer to as a surface-evoked laryngeal sensory action potential (SELSAP), which was about 9 mV in normal subjects. The neuropathic patients had lower amplitudes (4.8 mV), lower conduction velocity (51 m/sec vs 41.1 m/sec), and lower intrasubject side-to-side amplitude ratio (0.84 vs 0.59).

Although this noninvasive technique appears promising, the results are still clouded by the nonspecificity of where the signal is originating. This action potential may be a mix of sensory and motor responses. Additional studies will need to be done to correlate the test results with known disease states. The authors have not yet defined the threshold for significance with this technique, making it interesting but not yet useful at this point.

R. Franco, MD

A Murine Model of Airway Granulation and Subglottic Stenosis
Malaisrie N, Ghosh A, Einhorn E, et al (Hosp of the Univ of Pennsylvania, Philadelphia; Veterans Affairs Med Ctr of Philadelphia, PA)
Laryngoscope 121:S174, 2011

Objectives.—The murine model, in which tracheas are transplanted into the subcutaneous tissue of recipient mice and subsequently studied for signs of granulation tissue, has been particularly successful in studying airway disease. Mouse laryngotracheal complexes (LTC's) will undergo airway injury and transplantation into syngeneic recipient mice in order to develop a functional model of airway granulation tissue and subglottic stenosis.

Study Design.—IACUC (Institutional Animal Care and Use Committee) approved animal study.

Methods.—The LTC's of donor mice underwent direct airway injury through mucosal scraping using a wire brush or through application of hydrochloric acid (HCl) solution to the mucosa. A control group did not undergo any airway injury. LTC's were harvested and transplanted heterotopically into the subcutaneous tissue of syngeneic recipient mice and harvested at 3 weeks posttransplantation. Harvested LTC's underwent analysis by standard histochemistry using trichrome staining, specifically to highlight collagen formation and thus to examine degree of granulation tissue in the experimental groups compared to the control group.

Results.—At 3 weeks posttransplantation, trichrome staining showed that direct injury of the airway epithelium, both mechanically using a wire brush and chemically using HCl solution, results in the formation of granulation under the disrupted airway epithelium, with narrowing of the airway lumen and evidence of early fibrosis.

Conclusions.—The development of a murine model of airway granulation tissue is an efficient tool for characterizing the process and for establishing strategies to prevent granulation and subglottic stenosis.

▶ The creation of a model system allows repeated experimentation to study different facets of a disease process. The authors used a mouse model in which laryngotracheal tissue that had been injured chemically or mechanically was transplanted into mice with intact and deficient immune systems. Their purpose was to attempt to elucidate the impact the immune system has on granulation tissue and scar formation in the subglottis.

Mice are easy to manipulate, take up very little room to house, are easy to feed, can be obtained with and without an intact immune system, and are used in many other areas of research, making them ideal animal models. A major drawback is the tiny size of the laryngotracheal complex that requires skill to properly section. A larger animal model, such as the pig or sheep, would have a laryngotracheal complex comparable in size to humans but would also carry with it ethical, financial, and technical/housing dilemmas that are not present with the murine model.

The authors will now be able to test new hypotheses using the same experimental set-up using several variables such as the type of injury (chemical or mechanical) or the length of injury exposure. The resultant granulation tissue can be tested for markers of inflammation and compared with each other. Additionally, therapeutic interventions can be systematically evaluated and the results compared with each other directly.

R. Franco, MD

Evidence of Extraesophageal Reflux in Idiopathic Subglottic Stenosis
Blumin JH, Johnston N (Med College of Wisconsin, Milwaukee)
Laryngoscope 121:1266-1273, 2011

Objectives/Hypothesis.—Idiopathic subglottic stenosis (iSGS) is a disease predominantly of females that, by definition, has no known etiology. Collagen—vascular disease, localized trauma, extraesophageal reflux (EER), and hormonal alterations have all been postulated as potential etiologies of iSGS. It is hypothesized that iSGS is a reflux mediated disease and that evidence of EER exists in affected patients.

Study Design.—Case—control study.

Methods.—Patients with iSGS were identified prospectively over a 2.5-year period (2007—2010). During their endoscopic management, biopsies of the subglottic scar and postcricoid area were evaluated for the presence of pepsin, an indicator of exposure to gastric refluxate. Control patients had similar biopsies while undergoing operative management for disease unrelated to reflux. Charts of both patients and controls were reviewed for clinical history of reflux, pH-metry, and laboratory testing for collagen—vascular disease.

Results.—Twenty-two patients with iSGS were treated. All patients were female. No patient had serology positive for collagen—vascular disease. Thirteen (59%) patients with iSGS had pepsin present in their larynx or trachea. Control patients did not have detectable pepsin in their tissue ($P = .041$). Dual probe 24-hour pH studies were performed in 10 (45%) patients. These studies were positive for EER in seven patients but this did not statistically correlate to the presence of pepsin in their tissue ($P = 1.0$).

Conclusions.—iSGS is a disease almost exclusively of women. EER is implicated in the development of iSGS. Pepsin is detectable in the subglottic scar and larynges of patients with iSGS. Standard pH-metry may be inadequate in predicting degree of EER in patients with iSGS (Fig 1, Table 1).

▶ Idiopathic subglottic stenosis (iSGS) is a clinical entity (Fig 1) without a known cause that seems to affect women exclusively. iSGS can only be diagnosed after known causes of subglottic stenosis such as intubation injury or Wegener disease are ruled out. Proposed causes for iSGS include traumatic

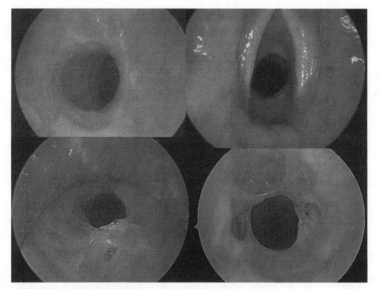

FIGURE 1.—Examples of subglottic stenosis at the cricotracheal junction in four patients with idiopathic disease. Digital photographs were taken at time of endoscopic management with a zero degree laryngeal telescope (Karl Storz Endoscopy, Culver City, CA). Note bridging bands and spiraling of scar. These patients have no history of laryngotracheal trauma, endotracheal intubation, or collagen—vascular disease. (Reprinted from Blumin JH, Johnston N. Evidence of extraesophageal reflux in idiopathic subglottic stenosis. *Laryngoscope.* 2011;121:1266-1273, with permission from The American Laryngological, Rhinological and Otological Society, Inc and John Wiley and Sons (www.interscience.wiley.com).)

TABLE 1.—Patients with iSGS

Patient	Gender	Age	History of GERD	History of LPR	Extent of Stenosis	Dual Probe pH-metry	Pepsin Assay
1	F	53	Yes	Yes	SGS & PGS	upper + lower +	SG + PC +
2	F	68	No	No	SGS	None	SG + PC −
3	F	48	No	No	SGS	None	SG + PC −
4	F	43	No	No	SGS	None	SG + PC −
5	F	28	Yes	Yes	SGS	upper + lower −	SG − PC −
6	F	68	No	Yes	SGS	upper + lower +	SG − PC +
7	F	67	No	No	SGS	None	SG − PC −
8	F	55	Yes	Yes	SGS	None	SG − PC −
9	F	40	No	Yes	SGS	upper − lower −	SG + PC −
10	F	62	Yes	Yes	SGS & PGS	upper + lower +	SG + PC −
11	F	53	Yes	Yes	SGS	None	SG + PC +
12	F	34	Yes	Yes	SGS	upper + lower −	SG + PC −
13	F	44	Yes	Yes	SGS & PGS	None	SG − PC −
14	F	55	Yes	Yes	SGS	upper + lower +	SG − PC +
15	F	82	Yes	Yes	SGS	None	SG − PC +
16	F	56	Yes	Yes	SGS	upper + lower +	SG + PC +
17	F	32	No	Yes	SGS	upper − lower −	SG + PC +
18	F	80	No	No	SGS	None	SG − PC −
19	F	65	Yes	Yes	SGS	None	SG − PC −
20	F	58	Yes	Yes	SGS	None	SG − PC −
21	F	59	No	Yes	SGS	None	SG − PC −
22	F	52	No	Yes	SGS	upper − lower −	SG − PC −

GERD = gastroesophageal reflux disease; LPR = laryngopharyngeal reflux; F = female; SGS = subglottic stenosis; PGS = posterior glottic stenosis; upper = upper probe placed at upper esophageal sphincter; lower = lower probe placed cranial to lower esophageal sphincter; SG = subglottis; PC = posterior commissure.

subluxation of the first tracheal ring inside of the cricoid, scar that is fueled by estrogen, and reflux.

The authors attempt to provide evidence for reflux as the causative factor for iSGS through the detection of the gastric enzyme, pepsin, in the subglottic tissue of patients with iSGS. They prospectively enrolled 5 patients to serve as controls and 22 patients with iSGS (Table 1) who underwent nasolaryngoscopy, cytoplasmic antineutrophil cytoplasmic antibodies and ACE levels to rule out Wegener and sarcoidosis, and biopsy of the stenosis and posterior commissure. Pepsin was detected in 59% (13 of 22) of the subglottic stenoses, but not in any control ($P = .41$). pH testing was performed in 10 of the 22 patients, and extra-esophageal reflux was detected in 7 of the 10 (70%), but this was not statistically significant.

iSGS is a clinically difficult disease to treat with an unknown etiology that affects only women. As clinicians, we would be able to offer directed treatment if we knew the causative forces that fueled the subglottic scarring. The authors found evidence for the presence of pepsin in about 60% (13 of 22) of the stenoses and had positive pH probe tests for extraesophageal reflux in 7 of those 10 patients. Their search for reflux as the underlying cause is to be commended, especially because we now have medications and surgeries that can assist in decreasing reflux, but their study was designed to answer the question, "Is there pepsin in the subglottic tissue?" The authors do not provide us with evidence that this pepsin has directly caused the inflammation or scarring. Pepsin may be an innocent molecular bystander in the 60% who were positive. The authors write that the "aim of this study is to evaluate the relationship of EER [extraesophageal reflux] to iSGS by demonstration of pepsin-related mucosal injury in the upper trachea." The lack of pepsin in 40% of the stenoses does not disprove that pepsin is a causative agent, but conversely, the mere presence of pepsin in 60% does not prove that pepsin is the cause for iSGS. Pepsin is a hearty molecule that can exist in an inactive form until activated by a drop in pH. The authors do not provide evidence, except for the presence of pepsin, that the subglottis sees drops in pH sufficient to activate pepsin.

The authors do not present us with a plausible biochemical mechanism that accounts for the discrete subglottic lesions we see to explain why iSGS affects only women. Presumably men are also capable of refluxing, but why do we not see their subglottic tissue react in this way?

iSGS is a riddle that is worthy of solving. I applaud the authors' efforts and encourage them to continue investigating the relationship between pepsin and iSGS. We may find out in the near future that although reflux may not be the sole cause of iSGS, it does play a role in modulating the severity of disease we see. We need to create a theory that incorporates the clinical signs of inflammation we see with the proper biochemical mechanisms that can be tested to offer robust evidence for the cause of iSGS.

R. Franco, MD

A Large Animal Model of the Fetal Tracheal Stenosis/Atresia Spectrum
Turner CGB, Klein JD, Ahmed A, et al (Harvard Med School, Boston, MA)
J Surg Res 171:164-169, 2011

Background.—Treatment of congenital tracheal stenosis/atresia remains essentially unresolved. Previous models of this disease entity have been restricted to rodents and the chick. We sought to establish the principles of a large, surgical animal model of this spectrum of fetal anomalies.

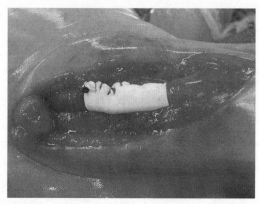

FIGURE 1.—Open cervicotomy on a fetal lamb, with part of the cervical trachea encircled by a biocompatible polytetrafluoroethylene wrap. (Color version of figure is available online.) (Reprinted from The Journal of Surgical Research, Turner CGB, Klein JD, Ahmed A, et al. A large animal model of the fetal tracheal stenosis/atresia spectrum. *J Surg Res*. 2011;171:164-169. © 2011 with permission from Elsevier.)

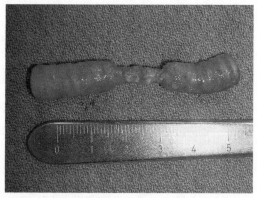

FIGURE 2.—Gross appearance of the manipulated tracheal segment after 41 d of controlled extrinsic compression. (Color version of figure is available online.) (Reprinted from The Journal of Surgical Research, Turner CGB, Klein JD, Ahmed A, et al. A large animal model of the fetal tracheal stenosis/atresia spectrum. *J Surg Res*. 2011;171:164-169. © 2011 with permission from Elsevier.)

Methods.—Fetal lambs (n = 8) underwent open surgery at 90-112 days gestation. Their cervical tracheas were encircled by a biocompatible polytetrafluoroethylene wrap, so as to extrinsically restrict their external diameter by 25%. Survivors (n = 7) were killed at different time points post-operatively before term. The manipulated tracheal segments were compared with their respective proximal portions (controls). Analyses included morphometry, histology and quantitative extracellular matrix measurements.

Results.—At necropsy, the typical gross appearance of tracheal stenosis/atresia was present in all manipulated tracheal segments. Histological

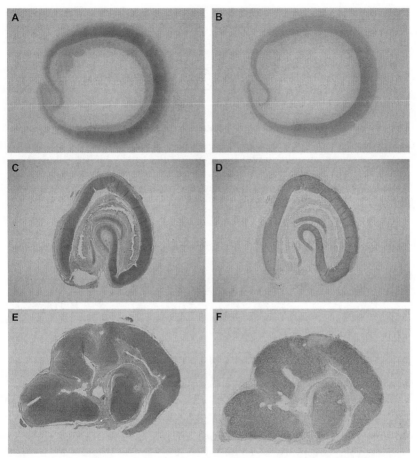

FIGURE 3.—(A), (C), and (E) Hand E stains, and (B), (D), and (F) collagen type-II immunohistochem-istry of fetal ovine tracheas, in cross-section, ×2. (A) and (B) normal; (C) and (D) after 15 d of controlled extrinsic compression; (E) and (F) after 41 d of controlled extrinsic compression. (Color version of figure is available online.) (Reprinted from The Journal of Surgical Research, Turner CGB, Klein JD, Ahmed A, et al. A large animal model of the fetal tracheal stenosis/atresia spectrum. *J Surg Res*. 2011;171:164-169. © 2011 with permission from Elsevier.)

findings included the virtual disappearance of the membranous portion of the trachea, along with infolding, fragmentation, and/or posterior fusion of cartilaginous rings, often with disappearance of the airway mucosa. There were significant decreases in diameter ($P < 0.001$) and total collagen levels ($P = 0.005$) on the manipulated trachea compared with the control portions. No significant differences were observed in overall elastin or glycosaminoglycan contents. A significant time-dependent increase in elastin was noted on the control, but not the experimental side.

Conclusions.—In a surgical ovine model, controlled extrinsic compression of the fetal trachea leads to morphological and biochemical findings compatible with the congenital tracheal stenosis/atresia spectrum. This simple and easily reproducible prenatal model can be instrumental in the development of emerging therapies for these congenital anomalies (Figs 1-3).

▶ The creation of a research model is beneficial to the advancement of the research field because it allows the evaluation of experimental ideas that can be repeated and compared with each other. Small animals such as mice and rabbits are used in tracheal experiments but have the inherent disadvantage of the tiny size of the laryngotracheal complex, which makes it difficult to manipulate.

The current study used a fetal sheep model to simulate tracheal stenosis and atresia by placing a constricting band around the trachea (Figs 1 and 2). The resulting histology is consistent with clinically observed tracheal stenosis in a time-dependent manner, making it useful in recreating varying degrees of stenosis (Fig 3).

The use of a fetal sheep model allows the use of instrumentation that would be used in newborns and experimentation with clinically useful stents and instruments. New therapies can be created and rigorously tested, including the effects of chemical treatments on the stenosis. The authors envision using fetal tissue engineering to create a tracheal construct prior to birth using fetal cells that will be ready for implantation after birth.

R. Franco, MD

A Novel Bioabsorbable Drug-Eluting Tracheal Stent
Zhu GH, Ng AHC, Venkatraman SS, et al (Natl Univ of Singapore; Nanyang Technological Univ, Singapore)
Laryngoscope 121:2234-2239, 2011

Objectives/Hypothesis.—Currently available silicone and metallic stents for tracheal stenosis are associated with problems of granulations, mucus trapping, and difficult removals. Our aim was to develop a novel bioabsorbable tracheal stent with mitomycin C (MMC) drug elution to circumvent such problems.

Study Design.—A randomized animal study.

Methods.—Twenty-five rabbits were randomly assigned into five test groups: 1) controls (without stent), 2) silicone tubular stents (commercially available currently); 3) bioabsorbable helical stents; 4) bioabsorbable tubular stents; and 5) bioabsorbable tubular stents with MMC. Weekly tracheal endoscopy to document granulation, mucus plugging, and extent of tracheal stenosis was performed for 12 weeks. One rabbit was euthanized every 3 weeks for histological analysis of the trachea. In vitro MMC-release profiles in conditions mimicking tracheal conditions were studied.

Results.—The bioabsorbable tubular stents with 0.1 mg MMC drug elution performed the best, with the least mucus trapping and airway obstruction due to tracheal stenosis. Tracheal stenosis was most significant for the bioabsorbable helical stents, followed by the control group without stent, the group of bioabsorbable tubular stents, and then the silicone stents. After 12 weeks, tracheal stenosis for the bioabsorbable tubular stents with MMC was only half that of the silicone stents.

Conclusions.—This study reports on the development of a novel bioabsorbable tracheal stent with sustained MMC drug elution for preventing tracheal stenosis. Further studies are warranted to optimize stent design and drug dosage (Figs 3 and 4).

▶ The trachea is an organ that is easily forgettable until something goes wrong with it. Its role as a conduit for air seems boring to most and makes it seem very simple. Its simplicity ends when what seems like trivial injuries can result in circumferential narrowing of the lumen leading to life-threatening airway distress. These injuries can be the result of external blunt trauma as in high-speed motor vehicle accidents, from inadvertent damage from intubation or bronchoscopy, or due to chemical or thermal injury.

Regardless of the cause, management of the stenosis can be very difficult. Over the years, multiple techniques have been developed to correct the stenosis, including resection and anastomosis of the stenotic segment, tracheoplasty, topical application of various chemicals such as mitomycin C or steroids and stenting. Stenting effectively bypasses the area of stenosis and can be combined with chemicals that retard scar formation and other techniques. A stent that elutes mitomycin C would help decrease the regrowth of scar tissue over the course of weeks to months while maintaining structural tracheal support.

The authors present their work using a bioabsorbable mitomycin C eluting stent and compare it to bioabsorbable stents without medication and a standard silicone stent (Fig 3). They found that the drug-eluting stent performed best, causing the least amount of stenosis after 12 weeks (Fig 4). The amount of stenosis was about 50% less than the standard silicone stent—very encouraging

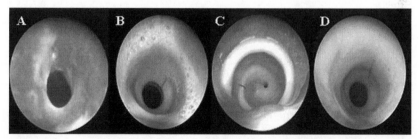

FIGURE 3.—(A) Endoscopic findings in control group 1 with diathermy injury to trachea without stenting 6 weeks after diathermy (40% stenosis). (B) Endoscopic findings in control group 2—commercial silicone tubular-shaped stent at 4 weeks after stent implantation, show mucus trapping throughout the silicone stent narrowing the tracheal airway (45% stenosis). (C) Endoscopic findings in group 3—bioabsorbable helical-shaped stent at 6 weeks after stent implantation. Severe tracheal stenosis (99%) and significant mucus trapping was noted between the helical stent coils (nonstented trachea areas). (D) Endoscopic findings in group 4—bioabsorbable tubular-shaped stent at 6 weeks after stent implantation. Tracheal narrowing was similar to control group 2—commercial silicone tubular-shaped stent, but less than group 3—bioabsorbable helical-shaped stent. [Color figure can be viewed in the online issue, which is available at wileyonlinelibrary.com.] (Reprinted from Zhu GH, Ng AHC, Venkatraman SS, et al. A novel bioabsorbable drug-eluting tracheal stent. *Laryngoscope.* 2011;121:2234-2239, with permission from The American Laryngological, Rhinological and Otological Society, Inc and John Wiley and Sons (www.interscience.wiley.com).)

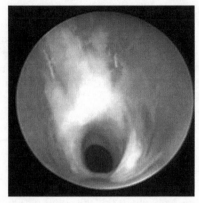

FIGURE 4.—Endoscopic findings in group 5—bioabsorbable tubular-shaped stent with mitomycin C (MMC) at 6 weeks after stent implantation. There was lesser tracheal stenosis compared to silicone and bioabsorbable tubular-shaped stents without MMC. [Color figure can be viewed in the online issue, which is available at wileyonlinelibrary.com.] (Reprinted from Zhu GH, Ng AHC, Venkatraman SS, et al. A novel bioabsorbable drug-eluting tracheal stent. *Laryngoscope*. 2011;121:2234-2239, with permission from The American Laryngological, Rhinological and Otological Society, Inc and John Wiley and Sons (www.interscience.wiley.com).)

results. It will be interesting to see whether varying the amount of mitomycin C that is delivered or adding steroids to the stent can help further decrease the luminal narrowing. As with the success of drug-eluting stents in the gastrointestinal and cardiology realms, airway surgeons will likely be able to add them to their armamentarium in the near future.

R. Franco, MD

Acute Stress to Excised Vocal Fold Epithelium From Reactive Oxygen Species

Alper R, Fu X, Erickson-Levendoski E, et al (Univ of Iowa; Purdue Univ, West Lafayette, IN)
Laryngoscope 121:2180-2184, 2011

Objectives/Hypothesis.—Vocal fold epithelium is exposed to reactive oxygen species from the inhaled environment and from tissue inflammation. The objective of this study was to explore the functional and structural consequences of reactive oxygen species exposure on vocal fold epithelium.

Study Design.—In vitro, prospective study design.

Methods.—Hydrogen peroxide (H_2O_2), a common reactive oxygen species, was utilized in this study. Freshly excised, viable porcine vocal fold epithelia ($N = 32$) were exposed to H_2O_2 or sham challenge for 2 hours. Electrophysiology, western blotting, and light microscopy were used to quantify the functional and structural effects of reactive oxygen species on vocal fold epithelia.

Results.—Exposure to reactive oxygen species did not significantly alter transepithelial resistance. There was a small, nonsignificant trend for

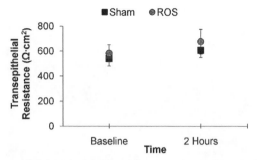

FIGURE 1.—Transepithelial resistance (R_T) in response to reactive oxygen species (ROS) exposure with hydrogen peroxide (H_2O_2). Tissues in sham challenge were exposed to Hanks' balanced salt solution. Two hours of ROS exposure did not significantly change R_T as compared to sham challenge ($P > .05$). Error bars represent standard error of the mean. (Reprinted from Alper R, Fu X, Erickson-Levendoski E, et al. Acute stress to excised vocal fold epithelium from reactive oxygen species. *Laryngoscope.* 2011;121:2180-2184, with permission from The American Laryngological, Rhinological and Otological Society, Inc and John Wiley and Sons (www.interscience.wiley.com).)

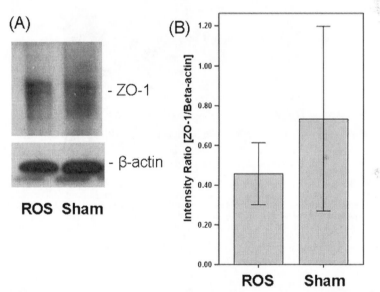

FIGURE 2.—Expression of zona occludens-1 (ZO-1) proteins in vocal fold epithelia following 2 hours of reactive oxygen species (ROS) exposure with hydrogen peroxide (H_2O_2). Tissues in sham challenge were exposed to Hanks' balanced salt solution. (A) Representative western blot. (B) ROS treatment did not significantly alter ZO-1 expression in vocal fold epithelia. Error bars represent standard deviation. (Reprinted from Alper R, Fu X, Erickson-Levendoski E, et al. Acute stress to excised vocal fold epithelium from reactive oxygen species. *Laryngoscope.* 2011;121:2180-2184, with permission from The American Laryngological, Rhinological and Otological Society, Inc and John Wiley and Sons (www.interscience. wiley.com).)

decreased concentration of epithelial junctional complex protein with reactive oxygen species challenge. Minimal changes to the gross structural appearance of vocal fold epithelia were also noted.

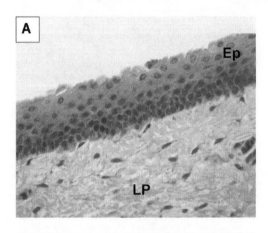

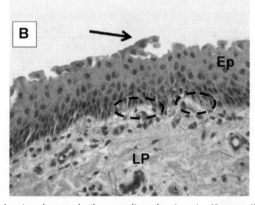

FIGURE 3.—Light microphotographs (hematoxylin and eosin stain, 40× magnification) of representative vocal fold epithelial samples obtained after 2 hours of exposure to (A) sham with Hanks' balanced salt solution and (B) reactive oxygen species (ROS) with hydrogen peroxide H_2O_2. Ep = stratified squamous epithelium; LP = lamina propria; arrowhead = epithelial shedding; dashed oval = sub-basilar edema or vacuolization. (Reprinted from Alper R, Fu X, Erickson-Levendoski E, et al. Acute stress to excised vocal fold epithelium from reactive oxygen species. *Laryngoscope.* 2011;121:2180-2184, with permission from The American Laryngological, Rhinological and Otological Society, Inc and John Wiley and Sons (www.interscience.wiley.com).)

Conclusions.—The stratified squamous epithelia of the vocal folds effectively defend against an acute reactive oxygen species challenge. The current study lays the groundwork for future investigations on the effects of reactive oxygen species on vocal fold epithelia that are compromised from phonotrauma (Figs 1-3).

▶ In this study, porcine true vocal fold epithelium with underlying superficial lamina propria were harvested and exposed to a 3 mM concentration of hydrogen peroxide for 2 hours. Hydrogen peroxide is a commonly encountered reactive oxygen species (ROS) that is inhaled from the environment and would interact with the true vocal fold epithelium. The everyday environment for those of us who live in cities is filled with inhalation of car exhaust, factory fumes, and cigarette smoke, whether from us or others, that can potentially interact and interfere with the barrier function of the epithelium. The aim of this study was to evaluate the barrier function through measurement of the epithelial electrical resistance, amount of ZO-1 (a junctional complex protein that serves as a component of the epithelial cytoskeleton), and gross histology to detect disruption in architecture.

They found that transepithelial resistance was not altered after exposure to 3 mM of hydrogen peroxide for 2 hours (Fig 1). The fact that the barrier protection was intact is encouraging given the amount of reactive oxygen species we breathe each day.

There was a slight decrease in the ZO-1 present after exposure to the hydrogen peroxide, as seen in Fig 2. This difference did not reach statistical significance. The histological changes were also slight with some epithelial disruption, intracellular or intercellular edema, and sub-basilar edema/vacuolization (Fig 3) that did not reach statistical significance.

These results demonstrate the ability of the pseudostratified squamous vocal fold epithelium to resist damage from a prolonged direct assault from a reactive oxygen species. It also makes sense that the true vocal folds, the site of extreme forces seen during phonatory activities could withstand chemical and physical trauma.

R. Franco, MD

Bone Marrow-Derived Mesenchymal Stem Cells Enhance Cryopreserved Trachea Allograft Epithelium Regeneration and Vascular Endothelial Growth Factor Expression

Han Y, Lan N, Pang C, et al (China Med Univ Affiliated Shengjing Hosp, Shenyang; China Med Univ, Shenyang)
Transplantation 92:620-626, 2011

Background.—Epithelium regeneration and revascularization of tracheal implants are challenging issues to be solved in tracheal transplantation research. Bone marrow-derived mesenchymal stem cells (BMSCs) can migrate to the damaged tissue and promote functional restoration. Here, we applied intravenous transplantation of BMSCs combined with a cryopreserved allograft to investigate the role of BMSCs in enhancing implant survival, tracheal epithelium regeneration and revascularization.

Methods.—After transplantation with cryopreserved allografts, PKH-26 labeled 3 to 5 passage BMSCs were injected into recipient rats through the tail vein. Rats in the control groups were injected with a comparable amount of phosphate-buffered saline. We observed the histology of the tracheal allograft and measured vascular endothelial growth factor (VEGF) protein levels in the epithelium to evaluate the effect of BMSCs on epithelium regeneration and revascularization.

Results.—Histologic observation of the rats from the BMSCs injection groups showed that the tracheal lumen was covered by pseudostriated ciliated columnar epithelium. The cartilage structure was intact. There were no signs of denaturation or necrosis. PKH-26 labeled BMSCs migrated to the implant site and exhibited red fluorescence, with the brightest red fluorescence at the anastomotic site. VEGF protein levels in the allograft epithelium of the BMSCs injection group were higher than the levels in the phosphate-buffered saline injection group.

Conclusions.—Our results indicate that given systemic administration, BMSCs may enhance epithelium regeneration and revascularization by upregulating VEGF expression (Figs 1, 2 and 4, Table 1).

▶ One of the greatest challenges to tracheal replacement with tissue-engineered or alloplastic grafts is how to reestablish a viable epithelium. There are other pitfalls, such as how to ensure the graft takes up an adequate blood supply, and how to decrease the immunogenicity of the graft so that it is not rejected and to decrease the need for the recipient to take immunosuppressive drugs.

The authors injected labeled bone marrow—derived stem cells into the tail vein of rats that had been transplanted with cryopreserved allograft tracheas

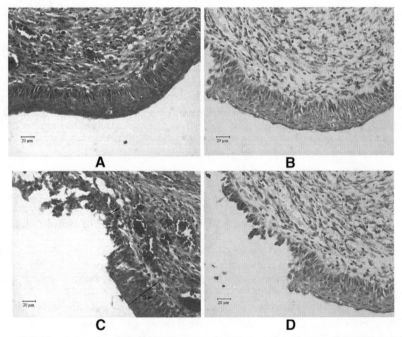

FIGURE 1.—Rat trachea from the bone marrow-derived mesenchymal stem cell (BMSC)-6-week group 4 weeks postsurgery. (A) Normal (recipient) tracheal epithelium (hematoxylin-eosin). (B) Normal tracheal epithelium. Vascular endothelial growth factor (VEGF) immunochemistry. (C) Anastomotic site, recipient normal tracheal epithelia are located at the lower part, thickness = 59 μm, donor tracheal epithelia are located at the upper part, thickness = 26 μm (hematoxylin-eosin). (D) Anastomotic site, VEGF immunochemistry. VEGF-ir levels at the allograft epithelia were higher than those at the normal epithelia. (Reprinted from Han Y, Lan N, Pang C, et al. Bone marrow-derived mesenchymal stem cells enhance cryopreserved trachea allograft epithelium regeneration and vascular endothelial growth factor expression. *Transplantation.* 2011;92:620-626, with permission from Lippincott Williams & Wilkins.)

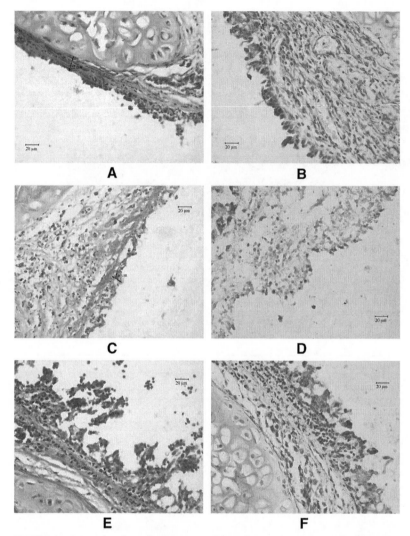

FIGURE 2.—Rat trachea from the bone marrow-derived mesenchymal stem cell (BMSC)-6-week group (A, B), phosphate-buffered saline (PBS)-6-week group (C, D), and BMSC-2-week group (E, F) 4 weeks postsurgery. (A, C, E) (hematoxylin-eosin); (B, D, F) vascular endothelial growth factor (VEGF) immunochemistry. (Reprinted from Han Y, Lan N, Pang C, et al. Bone marrow-derived mesenchymal stem cells enhance cryopreserved trachea allograft epithelium regeneration and vascular endothelial growth factor expression. *Transplantation.* 2011;92:620-626, with permission from Lippincott Williams & Wilkins.)

and observed for tracheal transplant viability, generation of a viable epithelium, and vascular endothelial growth factor (VEGF). The stem cell group had viable tracheal grafts seen at the 1-, 4-, and 8-week time points (Figs 1 and 4). Bone marrow—derived stem cells were identified within the new epithelium, especially concentrated close to the anastomotic sites. The concentration of vascular

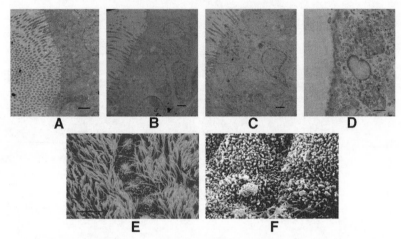

FIGURE 4.—Transmission electron microscope photomicrographs of tracheal epithelia from (A) bone marrow-derived mesenchymal stem cell (BMSC)-6-week group (×4000, scale=2 μm); (B) BMSC-2-week group (×3000, scale=2 μm); (C) phosphate-buffered saline (PBS)-6-week group (×6000, scale=1 μm); (D) PBS-2-week group (×4000, scale=2 μm). Scanning electron microscope photomicrographs for tracheal epithelia from (E) BMSC-6-week group (×5000, scale=5 μm); (F) PBS-2-week group (×15,000, scale= 1 μm). (Reprinted from Han Y, Lan N, Pang C, et al. Bone marrow-derived mesenchymal stem cells enhance cryopreserved trachea allograft epithelium regeneration and vascular endothelial growth factor expression. *Transplantation*. 2011;92:620-626, with permission from Lippincott Williams & Wilkins.)

TABLE 1.—VEGF-ir Levels in Each Experimental Group (Mean ± SD, N=4)

Group	1 wk	4 wk	8 wk
PBS 2 wk	1.5 ± 0.3	N/A	N/A
PBS 6 wk	3.2 ± 0.3	3.0 ± 0.4	N/A
BMSC 2 wk	10.2 ± 0.7^a	10.0 ± 0.8^a	8.8^b
BMSC 6 wk	11.1 ± 0.8^a	11.6 ± 0.6^a	10.7 ± 1.2^a

VEGF-ir, vascular endothelial growth factor immunoreactive; SD, standard deviation; PBS, phosphate-buffered saline; BMSC, bone marrow-derived mesenchymal stem cell; N/A, not applicable.
[a]$P<0.05$, BMSC group >PBS group.
[b]N=1 at this time point.

endothelial growth factor was much higher in the bone marrow stem cell group (Table 1) versus the phosphate buffered saline injection control group (Fig 2).

Bone marrow—derived stem cells lack immunogenicity through a lack of major histocompatibility complex (MHC) class II and very little MHC class I antigens. This makes them ideally suited to work within the body and not cause and immune reaction that could destroy the tracheal grafts. They seem to increase the levels of VEGF, improving the graft's chances of survival.

R. Franco, MD

Vocal fold wound healing after injection of human adipose-derived stem cells in a rabbit model

Hong SJ, Lee SH, Jin SM, et al (Korea Univ College of Medicine, Seoul; Sungkyunkwan Univ School of Medicine, Seoul, Korea)
Acta Otolaryngol 131:1198-1204, 2011

Conclusion.—Injection of injured rabbit vocal folds with human adipose-derived stem cells (hADSCs) led to improved wound healing and fewer signs of scarring as demonstrated by a decreased collagen content in the treated folds compared with the untreated folds. hADSCs remained viable for up to 12 weeks in rabbit vocal folds.

Objective.—The aim of this study was to investigate the morphologic and histologic properties of scarred rabbit vocal folds following injection of hADSCs.

Methods.—This was a randomized, controlled animal study. Twenty-four vocal folds from 12 New Zealand rabbits were scarred using a CO_2 laser and injected with either hADSCs (left vocal fold) or phosphate-buffered saline (right vocal fold). Every 4 weeks for the first 12 weeks after injection, an endoscopic examination was performed to assess the morphology of the vocal folds. Twelve weeks later the animals were euthanized and the tissues were stained for histology.

Results.—In comparison with the right vocal folds, there was significantly less granulation tissue in the hADSCs-injected left vocal folds ($p < 0.05$). Histological examination revealed excessive collagen deposition and perichondral fibrosis in the right vocal folds, whereas the left vocal folds exhibited better wound healing and less collagen deposition

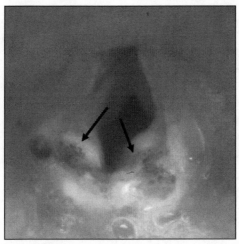

FIGURE 1.—Vocal folds following the scarring procedure using the CO_2 laser (arrow). (Reprinted from Hong SJ, Lee SH, Jin SM, et al. Vocal fold wound healing after injection of human adipose-derived stem cells in a rabbit model. *Acta Otolaryngol.* 2011;131:1198-1204, reprinted by permission of the publisher (Taylor & Francis Group, http://www.informaworld.com).)

($p < 0.05$). Among the 12 specimens injected with hADSCs, 4 specimens demonstrated viable hADSCs under immunofluorescent cytochemistry (Figs 1, 3, and 4, Table 2).

▶ The treatment of dysphonia from vocal fold scarring is considered by many to be the Holy Grail of the phonosurgery community. Vocal scarring is the end result of many processes and can be due to natural phonotrauma from phonation over many years; surgical resection of cancer or nodules, polyps, or cysts; or even secondary to radiation therapy. Some surgical methods have been described that break up the scar, and other methods attempt to augment the vocal fold with off-the-shelf materials such as collagen, calcium hydroxylapatite, and autologous fat. The off-the-shelf items all suffer from lack of permanence but have the advantage of relatively stable decay. Autologous fat has the potential to obtain a blood supply and can theoretically live indefinitely but requires vocal fold overinjection with an unpredictable yield.

The authors formulated an experiment injecting human adipose-derived stem cells into the CO_2 laser—damaged left vocal folds of 12 rabbits and comparing it

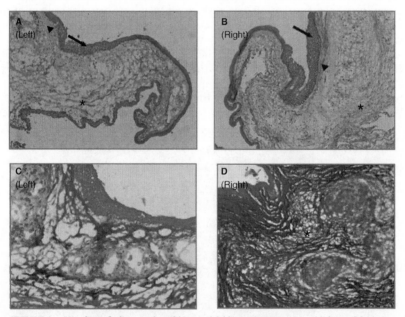

FIGURE 3.—Histologic findings in the rabbit vocal folds. An hADSC-injected left vocal fold (A) and PBS-injected right vocal fold (B) showing intra-epithelial inflammation (arrow), stromal inflammation (arrowhead), and perichondral fibrosis (asterisk) (H&E stain, original × 100). There were no significant differences between the two groups with regard to intra-epithelial inflammation and stromal inflammation. The PBS-injected right vocal folds were found to have significantly more perichondral fibrosis (A, B). Collagen deposition stained blue by Masson's trichrome stain in hADSC-injected left vocal fold (C) and PBS-injected right vocal fold (D) (original × 100). There was significantly more collagen deposition in PBS-injected right vocal fold (D, asterisk). (Reprinted from Hong SJ, Lee SH, Jin SM, et al. Vocal fold wound healing after injection of human adipose-derived stem cells in a rabbit model. *Acta Otolaryngol.* 2011;131:1198-1204, reprinted by permission of the publisher (Taylor & Francis Group, http://www.informaworld.com).)

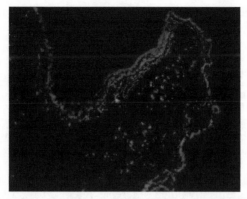

FIGURE 4.—Immunofluorescent staining of rabbit vocal folds after transplantation of hADSCs (green fluorescence, human specific vimentin antibody; red fluorescence, propidium iodide). For interpretation of the references to color in this figure legend, the reader is referred to web version of this article. (Reprinted from Hong SJ, Lee SH, Jin SM, et al. Vocal fold wound healing after injection of human adipose-derived stem cells in a rabbit model. *Acta Otolaryngol.* 2011;131:1198-1204, reprinted by permission of the publisher (Taylor & Francis Group, http://www.informaworld.com).)

TABLE 2.—Average Scoring of the Pathologic Findings of the Vocal Folds After Injection of hADSCs or PBS

Findings	hADSC Group (n = 12)	PBS Group (n = 12)	p Value
Intra-epithelial inflammation	1.17*	1.42	0.320
Stromal inflammation	1.75	1.67	0.721
Perichondral fibrosis	1.42	2.17	0.005[†]
Collagen deposition	1.58	2.58	0.002[†]

hADSCs, human adipose-derived stem cells; PBS, phosphatebuffered saline.
*1, mild; 2, moderate; 3, severe.
[†]Significant difference as determined by the Mann—Whitney U test ($p < 0.05$).

with the CO_2 laser—damaged but untreated right true vocal folds (Fig 1). There was less granulation tissue associated with the human adipose—derived stem cells but no difference with respect to the surface irregularities or atrophic changes. On histological examination, there was a statistically significant reduction in perichondral fibrosis and collagen deposition in the stem cell treated side (Table 2; Fig 3). The authors were able to detect persistence of the stem cells in 4 of the 12 left vocal folds at the 12-week time point (Fig 4).

We need to become more sophisticated with the regulation of these stem cells to support their growth and increase their yield. I think we can be sure that in the years to come, researchers will begin to understand the elements that are necessary to make them useful in vocal fold reconstruction.

R. Franco, MD

Airway epithelial wounds in rhesus monkey generate ionic currents that guide cell migration to promote healing
Sun Y-H, Reid B, Fontaine JH, et al (California Natl Primate Res Ctr, Davis; et al)
J Appl Physiol 111:1031-1041, 2011

Damage to the respiratory epithelium is one of the most critical steps to many lifethreatening diseases, such as acute respiratory distress syndrome and chronic obstructive pulmonary disease. The mechanisms underlying repair of the damaged epithelium have not yet been fully elucidated. Here we provide experimental evidence suggesting a novel mechanism for wound repair: Endogenous electric currents. It is known that the airway epithelium maintains a voltage difference referred to as the transepithelial potential. Using a noninvasive vibrating probe, we demonstrate that wounds in the epithelium of trachea from rhesus monkeys generate significant outward electric currents. A small slit wound produced an outward current (1.59 μA/cm^2), which could be enhanced (nearly doubled) by the ion transport stimulator aminophylline. In addition, inhibiting cystic fibrosis transmembrane conductance regulator (CFTR) with CFTR(Inh)-172 significantly reduced wound currents (0.17 μA/cm^2), implicating an important role of ion transporters in wound induced electric potentials. Time-lapse video microscopy showed that applied electric fields (EFs) induced robust directional migration of primary tracheobronchial epithelial cells from rhesus monkeys, towards the cathode, with a threshold of <23 mV/mm. Reversal of the field polarity induced cell migration towards the new cathode. We further demonstrate that application of an EF promoted wound healing in a monolayer wound healing assay. Our results suggest that endogenous electric currents at sites of tracheal epithelial injury may direct cell migration, which could benefit restitution of damaged airway mucosa. Manipulation of ion transport may lead to novel therapeutic approaches to repair damaged respiratory epithelium.

▶ The airway epithelium serves a very important barrier role, protecting the body from invasion from pathogens. The mechanisms for how the epithelium heals those wounds have not yet been fully elucidated. A full understanding of these steps could allow for manipulation and enhancement of healing in conditions in which there is retarded or lack of healing, as in postradiated tissue. The authors measured the electrical current generated by the intact epithelium using a vibrating probe. They found a current flowing inward of −0.46 μAmp/cm^2. When an incision was made, the current reversed direction and increased in magnitude reaching 1.6 μAmp/cm^2 and flowed in an outward direction. Using various chemicals such as aminophylline and CFTR(inh)-172, they were able to show that this change in current was an active process, not merely the leakage of current due to the epithelial injury.

The authors applied an electric field over epithelial cells and measured the migration over time (Fig 3 in the original article). They found movement in all directions when no field was present, but, when the electric field was applied

(50 mV/mm), there was purposeful movement of most cells to the cathode (about 85%). The speed of migration increased with an increase in the electric field strength (up to 200 mV/mm) (Fig 6 in the original article).

The interplay of electric and chemical signals plays a role in wound healing. As we learn more about the way the body regulates this process, we will be able to create devices and treatment regimens that will exploit these pathways to assist in the healing of wounds that currently heal very slowly or not at all.

R. Franco, MD

Effect of Fibrin Glue on Collagen Deposition After Autologous Fascia Grafting in Rabbit Vocal Folds
Scapini F, da Silva LFF, Tsuji DH, et al (Univ of São Paulo School of Medicine, Brazil)
Ann Otol Rhinol Laryngol 120:663-668, 2011

Objectives.—Fibrin glue (FG) is a reaction product of fibrinogen and thrombin that forms a fibrin clot responsible for tissue adhesion. However, FG and its components may interfere with wound healing by interacting with cytokines such as transforming growth factor–β (TGF-β). The objective of this study was to investigate the effect of FG on collagen deposition after fascia grafting in the vocal folds of rabbits.

Methods.—Eighteen rabbits underwent autologous fascia grafting in both vocal folds, and the left side was fixed with FG. Each animal was painlessly sacrificed after 7, 30, or 90 days. The larynx was removed, and the vocal folds were prepared for histomorphometric analysis by picrosirius red staining to evaluate collagen deposition around the graft.

Results.—There was a significant increase in collagen density around the grafts at 90 days in the vocal folds that were fixed with FG (p = 0.0102) compared with the control vocal folds.

Conclusions.—Application of FG altered collagen deposition around the fascia grafts, leading to significantly increased collagen density after 90 days. Differences found in the composition of the extracellular matrix in later stages of the healing process are a result of changes that occur in the beginning of this process. Therapeutic interventions, such as the use of FG and/or its components, performed in the early stages of wound healing may interfere with the complex interactions of fibroblasts, inflammatory cells, and cytokines (especially TGF-β), thereby modulating the healing process.

▶ Fibrin glue is made by combining fibrinogen with thrombin on the surgical field to create a fibrin clot that can allow 2 surfaces to stick together. This is especially useful where suturing could damage very thin and delicate epithelium, such as with true vocal fold incisions or in areas that are difficult to access, such as deep within the ventricle or along the subcordal aspect of the vocal fold.

There is concern that the use of fibrin glue may have long-lasting effects on the course of wound healing. Healing is a complicated cellular process that involves the cooperation of many types of cells interacting through chemical messengers we call *cytokines*. These cytokines, such as transforming growth factor (TGF)-β, stimulate cells to produce different extracellular matrix products (TGF-β causes fibroblasts to produce collagen) that are useful in wound healing. End products can interact with this delicate process and alter the overall process of wound healing, making it a more fibrotic process.

The authors grafted autologous fascia into the vocal folds of 18 rabbits, using fibrin glue to close the wound on 1 side in each rabbit. The larynges were sectioned after 7, 30, and 90 days of survival to evaluate the degree of collagen deposited (Fig 3 in the original article).

Fig 4 in the original article depicts the mean amount of collagen in the samples taken at the 3 times points. We can see that there is a general trend toward more collagen in the samples with fibrin glue, whereas the natural response to injury is to have a decrease in the collagen over time. There is a statistically significant difference between the amount of collagen at 3 months. Normal voicing is dependent on the proper functioning of the delicate microlayered structure of the vocal folds. Scarring inhibits the independent function of the layers by forcing them to move as one. Surgeons need to be aware of the possible clinical implications of fibrin glue when used on the vocal folds. It may make more sense to use a simple, nonthermal, nonfibrotic, sutureless method to close delicate wounds like photochemical tissue bonding that uses an organic dye (Rose Bengal) and 532-nm laser light to create incredibly strong covalent bonds between the already-present collagen fibers. In a study published in 2011, there was equivalent collagen deposition in a canine vocal fold model after 2 months.

R. Franco, MD

Validity and Efficacy of a Pediatric Airway Foreign Body Training Course in Resident Education
Griffin GR, Hoesli R, Thorne MC (Univ of Michigan Health System, Ann Arbor)
Ann Otol Rhinol Laryngol 120:635-640, 2011

Objectives.—We evaluated the validity and efficacy of a pediatric airway foreign body simulation for otolaryngology resident training.

Methods.—We created a course using a high-fidelity toddler mannequin designed to instruct and evaluate otolaryngology residents in pediatric airway foreign body management. Seven junior and 5 senior residents participated. Their performance was evaluated by 2 observers using an Objective Structured Assessment of Technical Skills (OSATS) instrument.

Results.—By the third trial, all junior and senior residents scored a proficiency level of "independent without errors" or "independent and efficient," and the performance of the junior residents was not different from that of the senior residents. After completing the course, the junior residents self-rated their abilities as commensurate with those of a senior resident, and senior residents rated themselves capable of performing foreign body extraction without supervision. All participants felt that the course and simulator had good overall realism and a realistic feel, demonstrating face validity. Perhaps most importantly, the residents' highest ratings were for "facilitated management of complications" and "facilitated working with the operating room team" — areas difficult to teach during live surgical procedures.

Conclusions.—This pediatric airway foreign body course using a high-fidelity simulator has face and construct validity, and results in statistically improved performance and self-evaluation of all participants.

▶ In the best of circumstances, training a resident to be a competent surgeon can be a difficult task that involves many hours of repetition and time thinking about clinical dilemmas. The desire of the resident to independently execute procedures competes with the patient's interest to be cared for by the most competent person on the team; for the educator, reconciling these competing desires is not easy. Although there is no substitute for actually doing a procedure, medical simulation removes the risks to a live patient during the process of instructing residents in high-risk or rare procedures with the advantage they can repeat their performance until they are deemed competent.

In this study, otolaryngology residents who enrolled in a pediatric airway foreign body simulation were evaluated by 2 observers using an OSATS (Objective Structured Assessment of Technical Skills). They were asked to rate their competence at managing an airway foreign body both prior to their first simulation and after the completion of the simulations. The residents were divided into 2 groups: junior and senior residents.

As with any task, there was a learning curve that is depicted in Fig 1 in the original article. After 3 trials, the gap between the junior and senior residents disappeared. All of the participants felt the exercise was worthwhile and made them feel more prepared for a real patient encounter. Junior residents struggled with assembly of the bronchoscope that improved to the level of the senior residents (from 1.0 to 4.8). One resident performed an esophageal foreign body extraction a week later and felt the simulation experience made a big difference with his comfort in performing the extraction. As with many learning experiences, the new knowledge was used in a related, but novel way with good results. Simulation was able to make these residents into "pretrained novices," hopefully allowing them to take advantage of clinical cases when they present themselves.

R. Franco, MD

Efficacy of Large-Diameter Dilatation in Cricopharyngeal Dysfunction
Clary MS, Daniero JJ, Keith SW, et al (Thomas Jefferson Univ, Philadelphia, PA)
Laryngoscope 121:2521-2525, 2011

Objectives/Hypothesis.—To investigate patient outcomes with large-diameter bougienage in isolated cricopharyngeal dysfunction and understand how esophageal dilatation can be used as an effective diagnostic and therapeutic modality in treating dysphagia.

Study Design.—Retrospective review.

Methods.—A retrospective chart review was performed on 46 patients meeting the criteria for cricopharyngeal dysphagia from 2004 to 2008 presenting in the outpatient setting. Patients were treated with 60 French esophageal dilators. Outcomes were analyzed as a function of symptomatology, manometry, duration of benefit, and safety.

Results.—Over the period reviewed, 59 dilatations were performed on 46 patients with cricopharyngeal dysfunction. Eight patients were dilated more than once. Four patients were lost to follow-up. The average starting Functional Outcome Swallowing Score (FOSS) was 2.07. Of the patients reviewed, 64.29% experienced an improvement in their FOSS with a median duration of 741 days. There were five minor complications and no major complications.

Conclusions.—In the largest series of esophageal dilatation for cricopharyngeal dysfunction in the literature, we found large-bore bougienage to have significant utility due to its efficacy, ease of use, and safety when compared to other modalities such as botulinum injection, balloon dilatation, and cricopharyngeal myotomy.

▶ Of the various conditions laryngologists treat, dysphagia appears to be the least understood and surgically is the least mature branch of our specialty. Patients who have dysphagia from cricopharyngeal hypertonia have access to several effective treatments ranging from Botox injection, bougie or balloon dilation, and cricopharyngeal myotomy.

The authors evaluated 59 dilations in 46 patients performed in the operating room under general anesthesia. Maloney dilators were introduced into the esophagus starting with the 45 F up to the 60 F dilator. They used the FOSS (Functional Outcomes Swallowing Scale) to evaluate the effects of the dilation. They found that 64% of the patients had improvement in the postoperative FOSS with a mean duration of benefit of 741 days. On average, it took about 12 days for the patient to begin to appreciate the benefits of the dilation.

When compared with the other surgical treatment options, dilations are as nearly as quick to perform as Botox injections and quicker than either open or endoscopic cricopharyngeal myotomies. Patients with cricopharyngeal hypertonia typically have comorbid medical conditions that may be made worse with prolonged anesthesia exposure. Morbidity for the dilation is also much lower than for the open or endoscopic procedures with discharge the same day for most patients. There are no consumables, as the Maloney dilators are sterilized, making it the cheapest option. Large bougie dilation (64%) achieves a level of success comparable to that of balloon dilation (58%), Botox (20%–100%), transcervical cricopharngeal myotomy (30%–75%) and endoscopic cricopharyngeal myotomy (22%–78%).

R. Franco, MD

General

"Thumb Sign" of Epiglottitis

Grover C (Stanford Univ Med Ctr and Kaiser Permanente, CA)
N Engl J Med 365:447, 2011

Background.—The "thumb sign" is a radiographic manifestation of an enlarged and edematous epiglottis. Finding this sign suggests a diagnosis of acute infectious epiglottitis.

> *Case Report.*—Man, 58, came to the emergency department with severe throat pain, hoarseness, and fever lasting 2 days. Physical examination revealed no stridor, respiratory distress, or drooling, and oropharyngeal evaluation was unremarkable. A lateral soft-tissue radiograph of the neck demonstrated a thumb sign, and acute infectious epiglottitis was diagnosed. The patient was given intravenous antibiotics. Fiberoptic laryngoscopy confirmed the epiglottis was swollen and inflamed; an apical epiglottic abscess was also found, but was managed medically without being drained. Blood cultures showed no causative organism. The patient was admitted to the intensive care unit for observation, but discharged home once his symptoms diminished with instructions to finish his course of antibiotics.

Conclusions.—When children are routinely immunized for *Haemophilus influenza* serotype b, there is a dramatic reduction in the number of cases of pediatric epiglottitis. Instead cases of infectious epiglottitis are seen in adults.

▶ Acute epiglottitis, or supraglottitis, is a potentially fatal infection that can cause swelling of the epiglottis and the remainder of the supraglottic tissues (aryepiglottic folds, periarytenoid tissue, and false vocal folds) causing airway obstruction. Historically, acute supraglottitis was considered a disease of childhood, with most cases caused by *Haemophilus influenzae*, a gram-negative bacterium. Widespread vaccination with Hib (*Haemophilus influenzae* B vaccine) has nearly eradicated the pediatric form of this disease, leaving just the adult cases. The adult form of the disease is a polymicrobial infection, mostly composed of gram-positive *Streptococcus* species bacteria, few gram negatives, and anaerobes and *Candida* species. In the pediatric form of acute supraglottitis, the epiglottis is typically the only structure that is swollen, whereas nearly all of the supraglottic structures can be swollen in the adult form.

The lateral x-ray (Picture) reveals the classic "thumb sign" of a swollen epiglottis. Regardless of the radiologic findings, the clinical picture dictates the proper course of treatment. As part of the physical examination, the upper airway should be visualized with the aid of a nasolaryngoscope to rule out airway edema and assess the patency of the airway and determine the need for an artificial means to maintain the airway. The presence of stridor is an ominous sign that reveals the

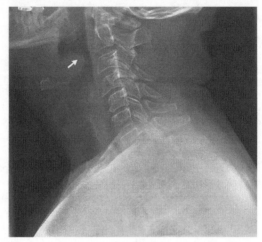

PICTURE.—

presence of supraglottic narrowing. Patients should be empirically started on a second-generation cephalosporin with intravenous corticosteroids to decrease edema. Cultures can help direct antibiotic treatment. These patients need to be placed into a monitored setting until they stabilize.

R. Franco, MD

Acute Supraglottitis in Adults in Finland: Review and Analysis of 308 Cases
Bizaki AJ, Numminen J, Vasama J-P, et al (Tampere Univ and Tampere Univ Hosp, Finland)
Laryngoscope 121:2107-2113, 2011

Objective.—The aim of this article is to study the clinical features, management, and outcome in adult patients with acute supraglottitis.

Study Design.—Retrospective review.

Methods.—We searched the medical records from our database from the years 1989 to 2009 using codes of international statistical classification of diseases and related health problems for acute epiglottitis or supraglottitis. In total, 308 patients were identified.

Results.—Incidence of acute supraglottitis increased from 1.88 (first decade) to 4.73 per 100,000 cases (second decade) ($P=.05$). The mean age of the patients was 49 years old with a slightly male predominance. Sore throat and odynophagia were the most common symptoms. Concomitant disease were common among the patients. Isolated inflammation of epiglottis without involvement of other supraglottic tissue was detected only in 51 patients. Intravenous cephalosporins were the most common empiric antibiotic treatment regimen. Intravenous corticosteroids were administered to half of the cases. *Streptococcus* was the most common organism in throat cultures. In total, 45 patients needed airway intervention. Complications were rare and mortality was 0.6% in our series.

Conclusions.—Acute supraglottitis in adults seems to be a different entity than epiglottitis in children, and inflammation does not usually exclusively involve the epiglottis. Early diagnosis seems to decrease the need for airway intervention and to permit the successful treatment of the patient with intravenous antibiotics and corticosteroids. *Streptococcus* appears as the dominant causative microorganism. However systemic diseases and other local infections that compromise the regional supraglottic immunity may increase the risk for acute supraglottitis (Fig 1, Table 3).

▶ For years until the widespread vaccination of children with the *Haemophilus influenzae* type b vaccine, acute epiglottitis was considered a pediatric entity. Worldwide, the incidence of acute epiglottitis or supraglottitis in children has precipitously decreased, while the adult version of the disease has not. It appears that these 2 entities, despite some common clinical similarities, are very different.

The authors reviewed 308 adults who had acute supraglottitis between 1989 and 2009. There were 177 men and 131 women between the ages of 18 and 92. They found that the incidence increased from 1.88 in 100 000 in the first decade to 4.73 in 100 000 in the years 2000 to 2009. There are also seasonal variations in the distribution of these cases as seen in Fig 1, with the highest incidence between March and August. The mean hospitalization decreased significantly in the second decade from 6.4 nights to 5. The presence of upper airway obstruction from swelling (stridor, tachypnea) and fever were prognostic indicators of

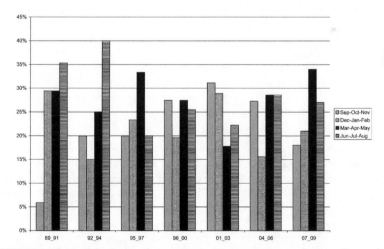

FIGURE 1.—Seasonal distribution of acute supraglottitis cases: percentage of patients diagnosed with acute supraglottitis in association with the time of the calendar year the diagnosis was made. A total studied period of 21 years sorted from oldest to newest in 3-year time intervals. [Color figure can be viewed in the online issue, which is available at wileyonlinelibrary.com.] (Reprinted from Bizaki AJ, Numminen J, Vasama J-P, et al. Acute supraglottitis in adults in Finland: review and analysis of 308 cases. *Laryngoscope.* 2011;121:2107-2113, with permission from The American Laryngological, Rhinological and Otological Society, Inc and John Wiley and Sons (www.interscience.wiley.com).)

TABLE 3.—Microbiology

	No. of Patients		No. of Patients
Blood cultures taken	154	Throat cultures taken	141
Positive Blood culture	16	Positive Throat culture	35
Gram positive	14	Gram positive	29
Streptococci	11	Streptococci	25
Streptococcus pneumoniae	4	Streptococcus pyogenes	14
Streptococcus pyogenes	2	Streptococcus milleri	4
Streptococcus milleri	1	Staphylococci	3
Staphylococci	2		
Gram negative	2	Gram negative	3
Pseudomonas Picketti and Paucimobilis	1	Haemophilus influenzae	1
		Pseudomonas	1
		Fungal—Candida albicans	4

prolonged hospitalization, which in turn is associated with the need for airway intervention.

As would be expected, the most common symptoms were sore throat (94%) and inability to swallow (80%). Frank stridor was rarely encountered (7%). In contradistinction to the pediatric form of the disease, isolated epiglottic swelling was seen in only 225 patients, and 77 patients had supraglottic swelling without involvement of the epiglottis. A swollen epiglottis was associated with the need for intensive care and a prolonged hospital course.

Culturing of the throat revealed a predominately Gram-positive bacterial result (Table 3), mainly with *Streptococci* species. Blood cultures were rarely positive, also reflecting the *Streptococci* infection. Second-generation cephalosporins are the first-line agents, with metronidazole or clindamycin added for anaerobic coverage. Children classically had Gram-negative infections with *H influenzae*. Intravenous corticosteroids are used to help decrease the supraglottic swelling. The presence of stridor, drooling, or hypoxia were possible risk factors for airway intervention and the need for tracheotomy. Obviously, each case is treated on its own merits, but the presence of these advanced signs should alert the clinician that monitoring in the setting of an intensive care unit is necessary.

R. Franco, MD

Classical reflux symptoms, hiatus hernia and overweight independently predict pharyngeal acid exposure in patients with suspected reflux laryngitis
Lien HC, Wang CC, Hsu JY, et al (Taichung Veterans General Hosp, Taiwan; et al)
Aliment Pharmacol Ther 33:89-98, 2011

Background.—Gastro-oesophageal reflux disease (GERD) has been associated with reflux laryngitis.

Aims.—To investigate the risk factors and the predictors of pharyngeal acid reflux (PAR) in Taiwanese patients with suspected reflux laryngitis.

Methods.—With referral from ENT physicians, 104 patients with symptoms and signs suggestive of reflux laryngitis completed a validated symptom questionnaire, an upper endoscopy exam and ambulatory 24-h pH tests with three sensors located at the hypopharynx, proximal and distal oesophagus. Patients with one or more episodes of PAR were considered abnormal.

Results.—Pharyngeal acid reflux was identified in 17% (18/104) of patients. In multivariate logistic regression analysis, PAR was independently associated with classical reflux symptoms [adjusted odds ratio (aOR) = 3.5, 95% confidence interval (CI): 1.0—12.8], hiatus hernia (aOR = 6.7, 95% CI: 1.5—30.2) and overweight (aOR = 3.4, 95% CI: 1.0—11.0). In predicting PAR, classical reflux symptoms had a sensitivity of 78% and hiatus hernia had a specificity of 95%. With all three factors, the positive predictive value for PAR was 80%. Classical reflux symptoms included heartburn, chest pain, dyspepsia and acid regurgitation.

Conclusions.—Classical reflux symptoms, hiatus hernia and overweight are independent risk factors that may predict pharyngeal acid reflux in patients with suspected reflux laryngitis (Figs 1 and 3, Table 1).

▶ As a medical community we continue to struggle with definitively detecting those patients whose complaints of hoarseness, throat clearing, and globus are due to the abnormal acid exposure we call laryngopharyngeal reflux (LPR), pharyngeal acid reflux (PAR), or extraesophageal reflux. The difficulty rests with the ubiquity and the insensitivity of the symptoms and the lack of a true

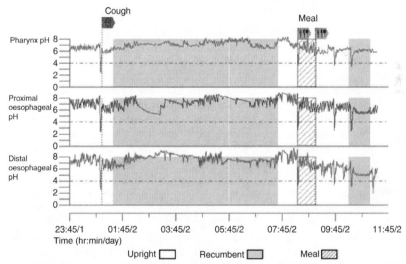

FIGURE 1.—An example of pharyngeal acid reflux demonstrating four events of acid reflux, which reached the pharynx. From the left side to the right side: the first event was temporally associated with cough; the second event was excluded for analysis because it occurred during meal time; the third event occurred with the patient in the upright position; and the fourth event occurred with the patient in the supine position. The 24-h acid exposure in the distal oesophagus was within the normal limit in this particular patient. (Reprinted from Lien HC, Wang CC, Hsu JY, et al. Classical reflux symptoms, hiatus hernia and overweight independently predict pharyngeal acid exposure in patients with suspected reflux laryngitis. *Aliment Pharmacol Ther.* 2011;33:89-98, and John Wiley and Sons (www.interscience.wiley.com).)

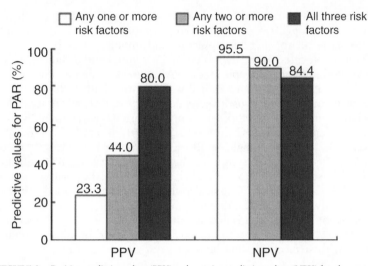

FIGURE 3.—Positive predictive values (PPV) and negative predictive values (NPV) for pharyngeal acid reflux based on any combinations of three risk factors including classical reflux symptoms, hiatus hernia and overweight, where clinical reflux symptoms were defined as RSI score ≥ 3 for the symptoms of heartburn, chest pain, dyspepsia, or acid regurgitation (RSI score $0 =$ no problem, RSI score $5 =$ severe problem), and overweight was defined as BMI ≥ 24 kg/m^2 based on Taiwan's criteria. The positive predictive values increased by increasing the number of risk factors ($P^* = 0.002$ for trend), whereas the negative predictive values were high in all circumstances. *Cochran-Armitage Trend Test. (Reprinted from Lien HC, Wang CC, Hsu JY, et al. Classical reflux symptoms, hiatus hernia and overweight independently predict pharyngeal acid exposure in patients with suspected reflux laryngitis. *Aliment Pharmacol Ther.* 2011;33: 89-98, and John Wiley and Sons (www.interscience.wiley.com).)

gold standard with high specificity and sensitivity. The authors of this study focused on patients who were suspected of having reflux as the cause of their symptoms and used a combination of medical history, upper GI endoscopy, 24-hour triple pH monitoring, and the Reflux Symptom Index to separate the patients with PAR from the greater group of 104 patients. The authors had very stringent inclusion and exclusion criteria, including patients who had the classic symptoms of throat clearing, globus, cough, hoarseness, and signs such as posterior laryngitis, erythema, and edema of the larynx. They had an exhaustive list of exclusion criteria, including any history of exposure to radiation therapy, past smoking, infectious laryngitis in the previous 3 months, excessive voice use, achalasia, chronic nasal symptoms, and even referral from a GI doctor to try to make sure they had as "clean" a study sample as possible, with little contamination from other possible causes for the symptoms.

They defined PAR as a pH drop that occurred below 5, which correlated with a drop in both the upper and lower esophagus, excluding any drops associated with meals (Fig 1). Of the 104 patients, 18 met these criteria. The remaining 86 served as controls for comparison. There were no symptom-free controls in this study. They found no differences in the classic symptoms of hoarseness, throat clearing, globus, or cough between these 2 groups (Table 1). They did find that BMI > 24, the presence of erosive esophagitis (44% vs 14%), and hiatal hernia (33% vs 5%) were significantly associated with PAR. When the 3 risk factors of

TABLE 1.—Comparisons Between Patients With and Without Pharyngeal Acid Reflux by Demography, Clinical Presentations, and Endoscopic Findings

| | Pharyngeal Acid Reflux | | |
	Yes (N = 18)	No (N = 86)	P-Value*
Demography			
Age (years) (mean ± s.d.)	46.2 ± 16.4	48.8 ± 10.7	0.4
Gender (Male), % (n/N)	38.9 (7/18)	57.0 (49/86)	0.2
BMI (kg /m²) (mean ± s.d.)	25.0 ± 4.4	23.3 ± 3.6	0.09
BMI ≥ 24 (kg/m²), % (n/N)	66.7 (12/18)	39.5 (34/86)	0.04
Clinical presentations			
Major complaint of laryngeal symptoms, % (n/N)			
Globus sensation	72.2 (13/18)	65.1 (56/86)	0.6
Sore throat	33.3 (6/18)	36.0 (31/86)	0.8
Hoarseness	55.6 (10/18)	53.5 (46/86)	0.9
Cough	33.3 (6/18)	27.9 (24/86)	0.6
Throat clearing	50.0 (9/18)	44.2 (38/86)	0.7
Duration of laryngeal symptoms, % (n/N)			
3–6 months	33.3 (6/18)	28.0 (23/82)	0.9
7–12	16.7 (3/18)	20.7 (17/82)	0.6
13–24	16.7 (3/18)	19.5 (16/82)	0.7
>24	33.3 (6/18)	31.7 (26/82)	0.8
Refractory postnasal drip, % (n/N)	44.4 (8/18)	42.9 (36/84)	0.9
History of taking anti-reflux medications, % (n/N)	44.4 (8/18)	48.1 (37/77)	0.8
Anti-reflux medication response, % (n/N)	75.0 (6/8)	48.6 (18/37)	0.2
Diabetes mellitus, % (n/N)	11.1 (2/18)	1.2 (1/86)	0.06
Hypertension, % (n/N)	11.1 (2/18)	18.6 (16/86)	0.5
Endoscopic findings			
Erosive oesophagitis, % (n/N)	44.4 (8/18)	14.0 (12/86)	0.005
Hiatus hernia, % (n/N)	33.3 (6/18)	4.7 (4/86)	0.001
Peptic ulcer, % (n/N)	22.2 (4/18)	20.9 (18/86)	0.9
Helicobacter pylori, % (n/N)	28.4 (4/14)	26.9 (18/67)	0.9

BMI, body mass index; s.d., standard deviation.
*t-test for continuous variables; Chi-squared test for categorical variables.

classical reflux symptoms, hiatal hernia, and obesity are combined, there is a positive predictive value of 80% (Fig 3).

Despite these findings and the rigorous exclusion criteria, we are still left with a clinical dilemma concerning those patients who are not frankly positive in a 24-hour pH study. We continue to await a gold standard, possibly a biomarker that acts as a surrogate for the disease that can be easily detected and correlates strongly with symptoms and can predict the response to treatment.

R. Franco, MD

Chronic cough and irritable larynx
Bucca CB, Bugiani M, Culla B, et al (Univ of Turin, Italy; Local Health Agency Turin, Italy)
J Allergy Clin Immunol 127:412-419, 2011

Background.—Perennial rhinitis (PR), chronic rhinosinusitis (CRS), or both, asthma, and gastroesophageal reflux disease (GERD) are the most frequent triggers of chronic cough (CC). Extrathoracic airway receptors might be involved in all 3 conditions because asthma is often associated with PR/CRS and gastroesophageal refluxate might reach the upper airway. We previously found that most patients with rhinosinusitis, postnasal drip, and pharyngolaryngitis show laryngeal hyperresponsiveness (LHR; ie, vocal cord adduction on histamine challenge) that is consistent with an irritable larynx.

Objective.—We sought to evaluate the role of LHR in patients with CC.

Methods.—LHR and bronchial hyperresponsiveness (BHR) to histamine were assessed in 372 patients with CC and in 52 asthmatic control subjects without cough (asthma/CC−). In 172 patients the challenge was repeated after treatment for the underlying cause of cough.

Results.—The primary trigger of CC was PR/CRS in 208 (56%) patients, asthma in 41 (11%) patients (asthma/CC+), GERD in 62 (17%) patients, and unexplained chronic cough (UNEX) in 61 (16%) patients. LHR prevalence was 76% in patients with PR/CRS, 77% in patients with GERD, 66% in patients with UNEX, 93% in asthma/CC+ patients, and 11% in asthma/CC− patients. Upper airway disease was found in most (95%) asthma/CC+ patients and in 6% of asthma/CC− patients. BHR discriminated asthmatic patients and atopy discriminated patients with PR/CRS from patients with GERD and UNEX. Absence of LHR discriminated asthmatic patients without cough. After treatment, LHR resolved in 63% of the patients and improved in 11%, and BHR resolved in 57% and improved in 18%.

Conclusions.—An irritable larynx is common in patients with CC and indicates upper airway involvement, whether from rhinitis/sinusitis, gastric reflux, or idiopathic sensory neuropathy.

▶ The concept of the irritable larynx strengthens the relationship the larynx has with its neighbors, the nasal cavities, nasopharynx, lungs, and esophagus. After pulmonary disease is excluded, for many, the concept of chronic cough is mainly one of controlling reflux. The idea of the unified airway challenges that by claiming that the larynx, as a member of the upper airway, is susceptible to those disease processes that affect the sinuses/nasal cavities and lungs, including perennial rhinitis, allergies, and chronic rhinosinusitis, along with reflux.

The authors used laryngeal and bronchial hyperresponsiveness (LHR and BHR) to a histamine challenge to explore the underlying causes of chronic cough in 372 patients with cough and 52 asthmatics with no history of cough who served as controls. They then divided them into 4 categories—perennial rhinitis (PR), chronic rhinosinusitis (CRS), gastroesophageal reflux disease (reflux), and unexplained chronic cough (UNEX) (unknown cause)—and treated them with H1-antihistamines (PR) for 1 month, nasal saline and intranasal steroids (CRS) for 1 month, omeprazole (GERD) for 3 months, and antihistamines and omeprazole (UNEX) for 1 month.

They found that LHR was very common, present in 76% of the PR/CRS patients, 77% of GERD patients, and 66% of the UNEX patients. Ninety-three percent of the asthma/cough patients and only 11% of the asthmatics without cough had LHR to the histamine challenge. After treatment, LHR resolved in

TABLE V.—Effect of Treatment Within Each Class

	PR/CRS (n=111) Before	After	P Value	GERD (n=14) Before	After	P Value	UNEX (n=47) Before	After	P Value
Cough VAS	3.78 (3.61-3.95)	1.73 (1.57-1.88)	<.0001	4.21 (3.76-4.66)	2.14 (1.62-2.66)	<.0001	3.83 (3.56-4.10)	3.51 (3.18-3.84)	.001
FEV_1 (L)	3.39 (3.22-3.55)	3.41 (3.26-3.58)	NS	3.03 (2.59-3.47)	3.01 (2.56-3.46)	NS	3.19 (2.96-3.41)	3.17 (2.95-3.40)	NS
MEF_{50} (L/s)	4.40 (4.13-4.67)	4.56 (4.30-4.82)	.002	4.06 (3.58-4.54)	4.22 (3.75-4.69)	NS	4.15 (3.84-4.46)	4.10 (3.65-4.56)	NS
MIF_{50} (L/s)	5.16 (4.85-5.48)	5.51 (5.20-5.83)	<.0001	4.75 (3.95-5.55)	5.18 (4.22-6.15)	NS	4.55 (4.10-5.00)	4.52 (4.06-4.99)	NS
$PC_{20}FEV_1$ log (mg/mL)	0.96 (0.87-1.05)	1.23 (1.16-1.30)	<.0001	1.37 (1.23-1.51)	1.50 (1.41-1.59)	<.0001	1.28 (1.18-1.39)	1.31 (1.21-1.41)	NS
$PC_{25}MIF_{50}$ log (mg/mL)	0.44 (0.35-0.54)	1.19 (1.12-1.26)	<.0001	0.64 (0.39-0.89)	1.27 (1.08-1.47)	<.0001	0.75 (0.60-0.89)	0.81 (0.68-0.94)	NS
BHR, % (no.)	43 (48)	17 (19)	<.0001	7 (1)	0 (0)	NS	15 (7)	11 (5)	NS
LHR, % (no.)	89 (99)	19 (21)	<.0001	79 (11)	21 (3)	.01	68 (32)	62 (29)	NS

Values are expressed as means and 95% CIs, where shown.
Note: Patients with UNEX were empirically treated with an H_1-antihistamine plus omeprazole.[1,2]
MEF_{50}, Forced midexpiratory flow; *VAS*, Visual analog scale.
Editor's Note: Please refer to original journal article for full references.

63% and improved in another 11% of patients. BHR also showed a similar improvement with 57% resolution and 11% improvement.

The authors felt the primary trigger of chronic cough was PR/CRS in 56%, GERD in 17%, UNEX in 16%, and asthma in 11% (the asthma with cough patients). When one looks closely at the data, it is clear that the concept of the unified airway is upheld. Table V shows that 48% of the PR/CRS (nasal) subjects had BHR (lung) as well as LHR in 99% of cases. Treatment of the nasal cavities resulted in a decrease of BHR to 19% and LHR to 21% after 1 month. More than anything, this is probably the greatest teaching point—when treating chronic cough, the larynx needs to be seen in its proper context as one part of a larger unified airway.

R. Franco, MD

A Review of Clinical Practice Guidelines for Reflux Disease: Toward Creating a Clinical Protocol for the Otolaryngologist
Altman KW, Prufer N, Vaezi MF (Mount Sinai School of Medicine, NY; Vanderbilt Univ Med Ctr, Nashville, TN)
Laryngoscope 121:717-723, 2011

Objectives.—Reflux disease, including gastroesophageal reflux disease (GERD) and laryngopharyngeal reflux (LPR), is an extremely common condition that is diagnosed and treated routinely in an otolaryngology practice. There is great variability in the methods of both diagnosis and treatment amongst otolaryngologists. Our aim is to review current clinical practice guidelines on reflux disease, to identify areas of agreement and controversy, and to begin to work toward a clinical protocol for reflux disease for the otolaryngologist.

Study Design.—Literature review with discussion.

Methods.—A PubMed search was performed looking for clinical practice guidelines on either GERD or LPR. Five hundred seventy articles were identified and the most clinically relevant practice guidelines were selected.

Results.—Thirteen key articles were identified. Eleven of these come from the gastroenterology literature, and none of them come from the otolaryngology literature. There appears to be a consensus on empiric medication trial as first-line therapy for presumed uncomplicated GERD and on prioritizing early identification of patients with severe disease complications. Areas of controversy include the definition of GERD and LPR, which diagnostic algorithm to use in which patient, and the long-term management of medical therapy.

Conclusions.—Although there are many clinical aspects of reflux disease that still remain a mystery, there is enough literature to support a rudimentary clinical protocol at this time. As further data become available from outcomes measurements, such a protocol may result in improved quality and standardization (Tables 1 and 2).

▶ Reflux diseases, such as gastroesophageal reflux (GERD) and laryngopharyngeal reflux (LPR), show strong prevalence in modern societies, with as much

TABLE 1.—List of Clinical Practice Guidelines on GERD, Specifying Indications for Diagnostic Tests and Interventions

	Lifestyle Changes	Trial of Meds	When to Taper Meds	EGD	BaS	pH Probe/ Impedance Testing	Mano-metry	Nissen Fundoplication	Refer to specialist
Fennerty, 2009	—	First line	To lowest effective dose, intermittently	—	—	—	—	—	—
Kahrilas, 2008 (NEJM)	First line	First line	To lowest effective dose	Odynophagia, dysphagia, GI bleed, anemia		Select patients	Select patients	Failure of therapy	Failure of PPI bid
Kahrilas, 2008 (Gastroenterology)	First line	First line	To lowest effective dose	Troublesome dysphagia, failed PPI bid		Normal EGD and manometry	Normal EGD	Failed or can't tolerate medication	—
Hirano, 2007	—	—	—		—	Normal EGD/ to show causality	—	—	—
Hirota, 2006	—	—	—	Select pts with chronic GERD	—	—	—	—	—
Irwin, 2006	First line	First line	—		If pH probe is normal	Cough patients who fail meds	—	Failure of maximal medical therapy	—
Armstrong, 2005	Not effective	First line	To lowest effective dose	Pts with alarm symptoms	—	Patients who fail medication	—	Failed or cannot tolerate medication	—
DeVault, 2005	First line, but not effective	First line	Should not usually taper	Suspicion of Barrett's or GERD complications	Not recommended	Patients who fail medication	To consider Nissen	Option for maintenance, or for medication failures	—
Katelaris, 2002	First line	First line	To lowest effective dose, intermittently	Alarm symptoms, failed PPI bid	Limited use	Failed meds and normal EGD	To consider Nissen	Failed or cannot tolerate medication	Failure of PPI qd
Moraes-Filho, 2002	First line	First line	4–8 weeks	Age over 40, alarm symptoms	Limited use	Failed meds and normal EGD, or EES	To consider Nissen	Failed or cannot tolerate medication, or young patients who cannot wean off of therapy, or GERD complications	—

(Continued)

TABLE 1.—(*Continued*)

	Lifestyle Changes	Trial of Meds	When to Taper Meds	EGD	BaS	pH Probe/ Impedance Testing	Mano-metry	Nissen Fundoplication	Refer to specialist
SAGES, 1998	—	—	—	Mandatory preoperative evaluation	Some preoperative patients	Select preoperative patients	Mandatory preoperative evaluation	Failed or cannot tolerate medication, or EES, or GERD complications	—

Two of the 13 guidelines were excluded from this table because of their narrow scope.

PPI = proton pump inhibitor; EGD = esophagogastroduodenoscopy; BaS = barium swallow test; EES = extra-esophageal symptoms.

TABLE 2.—Stratification of Disease Complications or Associations, and Possible Alarm Symptoms

Degree of Severity	Clinical Examples	Possible Alarm Symptoms
Mild	Incidental symptoms	None
	Symptomatic nuisance (physiologic reflux)	
	Managed with diet, lifestyle, or intermittent medications	
Moderate	Esophagitis Los Angeles grade A—B	Dysphagia
	Significant hiatal hernia	Odynophagia
	Esophageal/gastric motility disorders	Hematemasis
	Bilious regurgitation	Anemia
	Barrett's metaplasia (may not cause symptoms)	Weight loss
	LPR complications cricopharyngeal spasm, laryngospasm, vocal process granuloma, and other lesions, disabling cough, aspiration pneumonitis, others	Respiratory disturbance
Severe	Esophageal carcinoma	Dysphagia
	Esophagitis Los Angeles grade C—D	Odynophagia
	Massive gastric outlet obstruction	Hematemasis
	Mediastinal mass, esophageal compression	Anemia
	Cardiac etiologies	Weight loss
		Hemoptysis
		Respiratory distress

Note that the *Los Angeles classification system* for reflux esophagitis has been thoroughly tested and validated for both interobserver reliability, as well as high correlation to pH testing, response to PPI, and risk of symptom relapse off of PPI. **Grade A** is a mucosal break (or breaks) less than 5 mm, bounded by two mucosal folds; **grade B** is a mucosal break (or breaks) more than 5 mm, bounded by two mucosal folds; **grade C** is a mucosal break (or breaks) extending beyond two mucosal folds but less than 75% of the circumference; **grade D** is a mucosal break (or breaks) involving at least 75% of the circumference.[42]

Editor's Note: Please refer to original journal article for full references.

as half the population complaining of occasional symptoms. In this era of cost-consciousness, these reflux-associated symptoms translate into major financial expenditures as patients use the medical system to investigate and treat these reflux symptoms. In otolaryngology, there is lack of consensus regarding the true definition of the clinical entity called laryngopharyngeal reflux. It is sometimes difficult to interact with gastroenterologists who do not acknowledge LPR as a distinct entity since we have not yet defined it sufficiently and we do not yet have a test with high specificity and sensitivity to distinguish it from GERD. To this end, the authors reviewed the literature and found 13 clinical practice guidelines that could serve as the genesis of an LPR-specific clinical practice guideline useful to otolaryngologists.

Table 1 summarizes 11 of these clinical practice guidelines. Table 2 stratifies reflux into severity levels, including clinical correlates and possible alarm symptoms.

The reflux issue is one fueled by patient symptoms. The otolaryngology community is left to treat these patients with little empiric evidence as to what is the best regimen. We still debate the differences between GERD and LPR, and some debate whether LPR truly exists as a separate entity. As a specialty, we need access to high-quality data to establish the appropriate duration and dose of medication, when to perform pH testing, and whether impedence testing should be required. We have to calibrate the pH monitor to a level that is significant for LPR and discuss the role of diagnostic testing. What do we do with those who fail an initial regimen? Should we start with a low dose and increase to higher doses or the opposite? It is smart to look into the more well-established field of gastroenterology and learn from experience as we create our own clinical practice guidelines for handling reflux.

R. Franco, MD

Advances in Office-Based Diagnosis and Treatment in Laryngology

Rosen CA, Amin MR, Sulica L, et al (Univ of Pittsburgh School of Medicine, PA; New York Univ of School of Medicine; Weill Cornell Med College, NY; et al)

Laryngoscope 119:S185-S214, 2009

Background.—Historically, laryngology has an office-based, local anesthesia tradition. However, many therapeutic interventions have now moved to the operating room, where the laryngeal surgeon is afforded increased precision and bimanual dexterity. However, moving to the surgical suite has also meant losing the advantages of being able to evaluate and treat patients while they are awake, seated in an upright position, and able to phonate. Voice quality monitoring is an important ability before, during, and after therapeutic interventions. Office-based procedures restore these advantages and add increased patient safety and diminished cost compared to operating room procedures. Office-based diagnostic and therapeutic interventions have been improved by advances in technology, including high-speed imaging, chip-tip flexible endoscopy, ultrathin esophagoscopes, new injection materials, and fiber-based lasers. The possibilities now available for office-based laryngologic procedures were reviewed.

Visualization.—High-quality images of the laryngopharynx are essential to office indirect endoscopy and can be achieved with the technology now available. Continuous light sources paired with standard flexible endoscopic technology allow the hypopharynx to be examined for conditions of the mucosa; pooling in the pyriform sinus, vallecula, and esophageal inlet; and motion in the lateral pharyngeal walls, tongue base, or larynx. Either a Hopkins rod-lens endoscope or a flexible transnasal endoscope or both can be used. One or the other technique is chosen because it provides the needed information. Detailed examination of the vocal fold mucosa and its vibratory characteristics can be achieved using either rigid or flexible instruments. The best combination of light carriers and image transmission is the rigid Hopkins rod-lens endoscope but stroboscopic examination can be performed by other means as well. Experimental techniques to image laryngeal and hypopharyngeal anatomy and function include high-speed cinematography, kymography, and narrow band imaging.

Anesthesia.—Topical anesthesia is appropriate for most endoscopic procedures on the larynx, trachea, and esophagus. Pulse oximetry monitoring is not needed as long as strict guidelines for anesthetic dosing are observed. Adverse reactions are extremely rare.

Evaluation and Treatment.—Several conditions are readily assessed in the office. Among these are cricoarytenoid joint fixation, bilateral vocal fold immobility, paradoxical vocal fold motion disorder, and subglottic and tracheal stenosis. In-office laryngeal laser surgery has flourished because of the new flexible laser systems that can be linked to flexible endoscopic devices. Evidence shows these devices are both safe and effective for various lesions. Each laser has specific physical properties, with none showing an overall advantage for all laryngeal lesions. Time and careful study may allow the development of specific indications and contraindications for laser surgery.

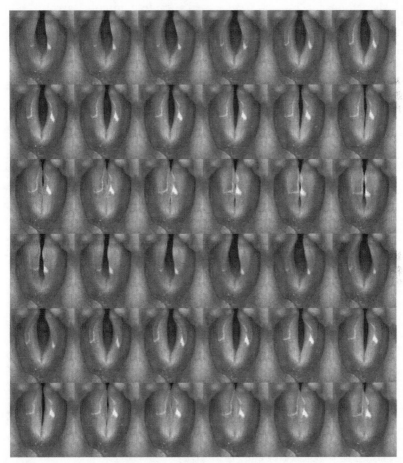

FIGURE 1.—Montage of high-speed imaging from two vibratory cycles. These 36 frames actually represent consecutive images captured during phonation. These were captured at a frame rate of 2,000 images per second. Therefore, these 36 images represent less than 0.002 seconds of phonation. (Image courtesy of Kay Pentax, Lincoln Park, NJ; color high-speed camera, model 9710). (Reprinted from Rosen CA, Amin MR, Sulica L, et al. Advances in office-based diagnosis and treatment in laryngology. *Laryngoscope.* 2009;119:S185-S214, with permission from The American Laryngological, Rhinological and Otological Society, Inc and John Wiley and Sons (www.interscience.wiley.com).)

Vocal Fold Injection.—In-office injection augmentation of the vocal fold may be the most therapeutically useful method done on a daily basis. Injectable materials are evolving. This technique provides a way to administer therapeutic substances such as cidofovir, Botox, and steroids.

Transnasal Esophagoscopy.—In-office transnasal esophagoscopy (TNE) is useful for patients with dysphagia, extraesophageal/gastroesopheal reflux disease, and head and neck cancer. TNE provides results comparable to those achieved with conventional endoscopy, but TNE offers advantages in terms of safety, cost, and patient preference.

Miscellaneous Procedures.—Various laryngeal procedures can be done in the office setting with good results. Included are laryngeal biopsy, secondary tracheoesophageal puncture, superficial vocal fold injection, atypical Botox injections to the larynx, and Botox injection to the false vocal fold.

Conclusions.—Office-based approaches to laryngology include convenience for the patient and surgeon and possibly improved outcomes

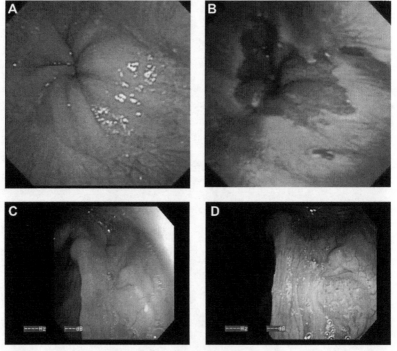

FIGURE 3.—(A) During transnasal esophagoscopy an irregular area of the squamocolumnar junction is seen above the gastroesophageal junction. (B) Narrow band imaging of the same individual clearly shows the area of abnormal epithelium along with 2 small "islands" of abnormal mucosa. (Olympus 280 K 001, Olympus America, Center Valley, PA) (C) View of slight mucosal irregularity in left pyriform sinus when viewed with a halogen light source. (D) View of same left pyriform sinus lesion with narrow band light filter. Punctate vascular pattern is present. On biopsy this was an invasive squamous lesion. (Olympus ENF-V2; Olympus America, Center Valley, PA). (Reprinted from Rosen CA, Amin MR, Sulica L, et al. Advances in office-based diagnosis and treatment in laryngology. *Laryngoscope.* 2009;119:S185-S214, with permission from The American Laryngological, Rhinological and Otological Society, Inc and John Wiley and Sons (www.interscience.wiley.com).)

with respect to the voice. These approaches permit one to monitor voice quality throughout procedures. Issues that need further critical review to determine if they are appropriate for office-based performance include patient selection, technology costs, and insurance and reimbursement. Further inquiry is needed to improved patient care and determine what is best approached in the office and what should be reserved for an operating room (Figs 1 and 3).

▶ This article is a comprehensive review of office-based laryngology diagnostic and therapeutic procedures. From its roots in Manuel Garcia's autovisualization of the larynx, laryngology has been intimately linked and propelled by advances in technology. Although the advent of general anesthesia did offer laryngologists the ability to work in the larynx in ways they could not before with a quiet, stable surgical field, as a specialty we temporarily lost touch with the important advantages of performing procedures in the awake outpatient setting—namely, the ability to monitor the changes to the voice with decreased morbidity and costs.

The authors discuss the technology that allows us to visualize the larynx, from mirrors to fiberoptics, and eventually to distal-chip scopes. High-speed imaging (Fig 1) offers the ability to precisely evaluate the larynx in action but at the expense of having to review too much data. This technology needs to be married to advanced computer algorithms that can detect abnormalities to make it a clinically useful tool in near real time. Narrow-band imaging (NBI), a technique in which the longer wavelength light is filtered out, allowing vessels and abnormal mucosal areas to stand out (Fig 3), appears to be gaining popularity. NBI can help identify those lesions that are nonkeratotic, allowing earlier intervention—and hopefully better patient outcomes.

There is a robust discussion of anesthesia techniques, as well as procedures for palpation of the cricoarytenoid joint, treatment for subglottic stenosis, and the use of various lasers (CO_2, PDL, KTP) to treat laryngeal disease. Injection techniques for augmentation and introduction of Botox, as well as transnasal esophagoscopy, are discussed.

R. Franco, MD

Arytenoid Dislocation: An Analysis of the Contemporary Literature
Norris BK, Schweinfurth JM (Univ of Mississippi, Jackson)
Laryngoscope 121:142-146, 2011

Objectives/Hypothesis.—To discuss the incidence, diagnosis, laryngeal findings, and management of arytenoid dislocation as a separate entity from vocal fold paralysis.

Study Design.—Literature review.

Methods.—A contemporary review of the literature was performed by searching the terms arytenoid cartilage dislocation and subluxation in various combinations. Articles were analyzed and selected based on relevance and content.

Results.—Arytenoid dislocation is described as an uncommon laryngeal finding associated with intubation or blunt laryngeal trauma. The majority of recent publications are case reports or small case series. Diagnosis of arytenoid dislocation with flexible laryngoscopy, helical computed tomography, videostroboscopy, and laryngeal electromyography is recommended. In most reported cases, diagnosis has been made based on the position of the arytenoid at laryngoscopy. Reduction and repositioning of the arytenoid cartilage is reported with limited success noted with delayed diagnosis. Speech therapy may also be a beneficial treatment option.

Conclusions.—Although arytenoid dislocation is reported in the literature, the body of available evidence fails to sufficiently differentiate it as a separate entity from unilateral vocal fold paralysis. Flexible laryngoscopy is inadequate as a standalone procedure to distinguish arytenoid dislocation from laryngeal nerve injury.

▶ The existence of the clinical entity known as arytenoid dislocation is hotly debated by those who are supporters and by nonbelievers. Either external blunt trauma or internal trauma from rough intubation or surgical manipulation causes the arytenoid to dislocate away from the synovial-lined cricoarytenoid joint. The described symptoms are immediate dysphonia, odynophagia, and dysphagia. The diagnosis is made through the synthesis of history, flexible endoscopic evaluation of vocal fold immobility, presence of normal recruitment seen on laryngeal electromyography (EMG) of the immobile side, and possible CT imaging that shows a malpositioned arytenoid.

The authors reviewed the English literature and found a combination of case reports, case series, cadaveric studies, tutorials, and expert reviews. There were some striking differences among the different studies. Video stroboscopy was used in 85% of case series but in only 33% of case reports. CT and EMG were used in 56% and 42% of patients to establish a proper diagnosis. Closed reduction in the operating room was the most commonly used treatment modality (75%), but Botox injection to restore muscular balance to the muscles, speech therapy, or waiting for spontaneous return of function was also described.

The authors conclude that proper diagnosis relies on a combination of a history of appropriate trauma, an endoscopic examination revealing an immobile vocal fold with a laryngeal EMG that shows the immobile vocal fold is innervated, and possibly a CT scan or manual palpation of the arytenoid. Many published cases of arytenoid dislocation do not have enough evidence to differentiate them from neurogenic vocal fold immobility. The controversy continues.

R. Franco, MD

Botulinum Toxin Treatment of Adductor Spasmodic Dysphonia: Longitudinal Functional Outcomes
Novakovic D, Waters HH, D'Elia JB, et al (New York Ctr for Voice and Swallowing Disorders; Cleveland Clinic Head and Neck Inst, OH)
Laryngoscope 121:606-612, 2011

Objectives.—Laryngeal botulinum toxin (BoNT) injection is a well-established symptomatic treatment for adductor spasmodic dysphonia (AdSD). Injections may be followed by a period of muscle weakness characterized by breathiness, voice weakness, and dysphagia for liquids. A recent study described some detriment and limited functional improvement with "good voice" for only one-third of the period between successive injections. Our objective was to examine the longitudinal effect of BoNT treatment for AdSD upon functional outcomes and quality of life when using a patient-specific dosing regimen.

Study Design.—Prospective cohort study.

Methods.—Patients presenting for BoNT treatment of AdSD were asked to complete evaluation of voice function after each injection using the percentage of normal function (PNF) scale (daily for two weeks, then weekly). Other parameters measured included voice handicap index (VHI), duration of effect, and complications.

Results.—A total of 133 patients treated continuously between January 2006 and January 2009 with an individuated regime (dose, pattern, and schedule) were included. Of 1,457 treatments, 50.9% experienced some breathiness. Mean VHI improvement was 9.6%. Mean PNF improvement was 30.3%. There was correlation between the two scales. Dysphagia to liquids was reported after 14.2% of treatments. We describe two distinct types of functional outcome curve. A total of 28.5% of treatments were followed by initial functional decline. Mean time below baseline function was 5.7%. Mean proportion of time in plateau phase was 42.5%.

Conclusions.—It is important to consider longitudinal functional outcomes in BoNT treatment of AdSD. An individuated dosing regimen helps minimize side effects and maximize functional and quality-of-life outcomes (Fig 3, Table 2).

▶ Botulinum toxin injection into the thyroarytenoid muscles is considered the standard of care for treatment of adductor spasmodic dysphonia (ADSD). ADSD is a focal laryngeal dystonia that causes unwanted adduction of the vocal folds during phonation, leading to a pressed and strained voice with audible breaks. Botulinum toxin works by inhibiting presynaptic acetylcholine, effectively disconnecting the nerve from the muscle and quieting the abnormal laryngeal activity.

Although the botulinum toxin injections do improve the voice symptoms, the laryngeal weakness that results from the treatment can lead to vocal breathiness, vocal weakness, and dysphagia, limiting the overall quality of life improvements. The authors prospectively followed 133 patients over the course of 3 years who had individualized botulinum toxin injections. Subjects were asked to rate their function using the PNF (percentage of normal function) daily for the first

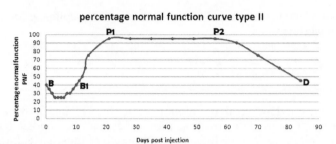

FIGURE 3.—Percentage of normal function (PNF) type 2 curve. (Reprinted from Novakovic D, Waters HH, D'Elia JB, et al. Botulinum toxin treatment of adductor spasmodic dysphonia: longitudinal functional outcomes. *Laryngoscope*. 2011;121:606-612, with permission from The American Laryngological, Rhinological and Otological Society, Inc and John Wiley and Sons (www.interscience.wiley.com).)

TABLE 2.—Treatment Characteristics Botulinum Neurotoxin Type A (BoNT-A) vs. Type B (BoNT-B)

	BoNT-A	BoNT-B	(*P* Value)
Number of treatments	1402 (96.2%)	55 (3.8%)	
Mean dose	1.17 Units	218.6 Units	
Mean breathy days	10	16.8	0.037*
Mean days below baseline function	5.7	0.4	0.000*
Mean time to plateau phase (days)	22.1	11.2	0.001*
Mean plateau phase length (days)	38	31.3	0.15
Mean patient reported benefit (days)	56.8	41.5	0.027*

*Significant results at *P* = 0.05.

2 weeks and then weekly, along with the duration of voice benefit and the voice handicap index.

Of the total 1457 treatments, breathiness was reported after 51% of injections, lasting a mean of 20 days with the longest reported length of breathiness lasting 8 weeks. Dysphagia was reported 14% of the time lasting 1 to 2 weeks. In the botulinum toxin A group (96% of injections), mean dose was 1.17 units, whereas in the botulinum toxin B group, it was 218.6 units. Men time between injections was 15.2 weeks.

In the botulinum toxin A group, higher doses were correlated with breathiness, but not with the duration of that breathiness. This is in contrast to the botulinum toxin B group in which there was correlation between the higher doses and breathiness and higher doses and duration of breathiness.

After botulinum toxin injection, it takes about 22 days to reach the plateau stage in which there is stabilization of the voice. This level of functioning lasts approximately 38 days and then progressively decreases until the next injection (Table 2). It is important to note that there are changes to the level of functioning after injection that need to be discussed with the patients prior to injection (Fig 3).

R. Franco, MD

Comparison of Sonography and Computed Tomography as Imaging Tools for Assessment of Airway Structures

Prasad A, Yu E, Wong DT, et al (Univ Health Network, Toronto, Ontario, Canada)
J Ultrasound Med 30:965-972, 2011

Objectives.—The aim of this study was to compare airway anatomic parameters as measured by sonography and computed tomography (CT).

Methods.—Fifteen adult patients underwent CT followed by sonography of the anterior neck under standard conditions. A radiologist and an anesthesiologist with experience in airway imaging examined the scans and performed measurements of specific airway parameters: distance to the posterior surface of the tongue, thickness of the submental region, hyomental distance, depth of the epiglottis from skin (above and below the hyoid bone), thyrohyoid distance, depth of the arytenoid cartilage from skin, and fat pad thickness at the thyroid cartilage. After performing the measurements, they compared the images by the two modalities for descriptions of the structures. Means and SDs were calculated for the measurements, and a paired t test was performed to determine statistically significant differences in the measurements by sonography and CT.

Results.—The means of all parameters were closely related except hyomental distance (sonography, 5.23 ± 0.58 cm; CT, 3.50 ± 0.42 cm). The paired t test showed that the mean values for depth of the epiglottis below the hyoid (3.89 versus 4.17 cm; $P = .31$), thyrohyoid distance (1.03 versus 1.02 cm; $P = .95$), and depth of the arytenoid cartilage (2.90 versus 2.66 cm; $P = .21$) were not significantly different as measured by sonography and CT, respectively.

Conclusions.—The study shows that sonography can reliably image all of the structures visualized by CT, and in general, infrahyoid parameters agree well between the two modalities, as opposed to suprahyoid parameters, which may be affected by unintentional head extension.

▶ Preoperative assessment of the airway to predict difficulties with intubation is an important part of a presurgical evaluation when endotracheal intubation is anticipated. Physical examination is not sufficient to truly appreciate the anatomic relationships among the tongue base, hyoid, epiglottis, and the preepiglottic fat pad. The typical radiological offerings of CT or MRI have the advantage of being of very high resolution and quality but are expensive, introduce radiation exposure (CT), can be subject to motion artifact (MRI), and are temporally separated from the time of the intervention (intubation). Ultrasonography could allow real-time evaluation of the airway at the time of the intervention that is less expensive and does not expose the patient to radiation. The intervention itself could be visualized as it is happening, allowing it to be used to guide the process.

The authors evaluated the use of ultrasonography by comparing it to the findings on CT scan (Table 1). They found they could identify all of the major structures but had difficulties with the epiglottis. Ultrasound is always difficult when

TABLE 1.—Comparison of Airway Parameters Between Sonography and Computed Tomography

Parameter	n	Sonography	CT	P
Distance to posterior surface of tongue, cm	15	6.27 ± 0.43	6.72 ± 0.62	.007
Thickness of submental region, cm	15	1.18 ± 0.21	1.31 ± 0.21	.06
Hyomental distance, cm	15	5.23 ± 0.58	3.50 ± 0.42	<.001
Thyrohyoid distance, cm	15	1.03 ± 0.44	1.02 ± 0.41	.95
Depth of epiglottis above hyoid bone, cm	15	4.15 ± 0.50	5.48 ± 1.03	<.001
Depth of epiglottis below hyoid bone, cm	15	3.89 ± 0.51	4.17 ± 1.06	.31
Depth of arytenoid cartilage from skin, cm	15	2.90 ± 0.75	2.66 ± 0.52	.21
Fat pad thickness at thyroid cartilage, cm	15	0.40 ± 0.15	0.66 ± 0.26	<.001

Values are mean ± SD. CT indicates computed tomography.

it needs to traverse a tissue-air interface or when it needs to go through a calcified thyroid cartilage (Figs 5 and 6 in the original article). This leads to poor visualization of the posterior pharyngeal wall and at times the paraglottic space and vocal folds.

It is still important to remember that as opposed to the clear and familiar images we obtain from an axial or sagittal CT scan, an ultrasound image is filled with grainy shadows that require skill and knowledge to interpret. The person performing the ultrasound has control of the pressure applied to the tissues and can go back and forth to find an object, giving the operator the advantage when attempting to interpret the findings. Clinicians would be best suited to have some familiarity with the process of performing an ultrasound and interpreting them before attempting to use it to reliably locate airway anatomy.

R. Franco, MD

Outcomes

Impact of a specialized multidisciplinary tracheostomy team on tracheostomy care in critically ill patients
de Mestral C, Iqbal S, Fong N, et al (McGill Univ Health Centre, Montréal, Quebec, Canada)
Can J Surg 54:167-172, 2011

Background.—A multidisciplinary tracheostomy team was created in 2005 to follow critically ill patients who had undergone a tracheostomy until their discharge from hospital. Composed of a surgeon, surgical resident, respiratory therapist, speech language pathologist and clinical nurse specialist, this team has been meeting twice a week for rounds involving patients who transitioned from the intensive care unit (ICU) to the medical and surgical wards. Our objective was to assess the impact of this multidisciplinary team on downsizing and decannulation times, on the incidence of speaking valve placement and on the incidence of tracheostomy-related complications on the ward.

Methods.—This study was conducted at a tertiary care, level-1 trauma centre and teaching hospital and involved all patients who had received a tracheostomy during admission to the ICU from Jan. 1 to Dec. 31, 2004 (preservice group), and from Jan. 1 to Dec. 31, 2006 (postservice group). We compared the outcomes of patients who required tracheostomies in a 12-month period after the team was created with those of patients from a similar time frame before the establishment of the team.

Results.—There were 32 patients in the preservice group and 54 patients in the postservice group. Under the new tracheostomy service, there was a decrease in incidence of tube blockage (5.5% v. 25.0%, $p = 0.016$) and calls for respiratory distress (16.7% v. 37.5%, $p = 0.039$) on the wards. A significantly larger proportion of patients also received speaking valves (67.4% v. 19.4%, $p < 0.001$) after creation of the team. Furthermore, there appeared to be a decreased time to first tube downsizing (26.0 to 9.4 d) and decreased time to decannulation (50.4 to 28.4 d), although this did not reach statistical significance owing to our small sample size.

Conclusion.—Standardized care provided by a specialized multidisciplinary tracheostomy team was associated with fewer tracheostomy-related complications and an increase in the use of a speaking valve (Fig 1, Table 2).

▶ Tracheotomy is a procedure commonly performed in critically ill patients. Because of the popularity of percutaneous tracheotomy performed at the bedside by internal medicine teams, patients who have undergone tracheotomy do not necessarily have follow-up with a surgeon after they leave the critical care unit. In fact, these patients are not followed up even by the surgical teams historically in charge of performing all tracheotomies. This practice can lead to situations in which there are delays in the implementation of capping trials, delays in the initiation of voice with speaking valves, and delays in decannulation.

The authors evaluated the benefits of employing a multidisciplinary team (composed of a general surgeon, a general surgery resident, a clinical nurse

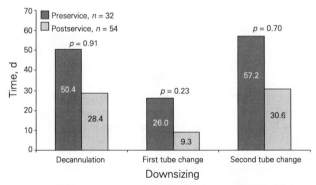

FIGURE 1.—Comparison of downsizing and decannulation times in days between patients before (preservice) and after (postservice) the establishment of the multidisciplinary tracheostomy team. (Reprinted from de Mestral C, Iqbal S, Fong N, et al. Impact of a specialized multidisciplinary tracheostomy team on tracheostomy care in critically ill patients. *Can J Surg.* 2011;54:167-172. © Canadian Medical Association.)

TABLE 2.—Complications Among Patients who Received Tracheostomies Before and After the Establishment of a Multidisciplinary Tracheostomy Team

Complication	Group; % (95% CI)		p Value
	Preservice, $n = 32$	Postservice, $n = 54$	
Calls for respiratory distress	37.50 (22.9–54.8)	16.70 (9.0–28.7)	0.039
Tube blockage	25 (13.3–42.1)	5.50 (1.9–15.1)	0.016
Bleeding	0	5.60 (1.9–15.1)	0.29
Cellulitis or ulceration	3.10 (0.6–15.8)	5.60 (1.9–15.1)	1.00
Respiratory infection	12.50 (5.0–28.0)	13.00 (6.4–24.4)	1.00
Technical complication (displaced, accidental decannulation, cuff rupture)	3.10 (0.6–15.8)	3.70 (1.0–12.5)	1.00
Return to ICU at least once	18.80 (8.9–35.3)	14.80 (7.7–26.6)	0.76
All-cause mortality	19.6 (9.2–36.3)	18.5 (10.4–30.8)	0.88

CI = confidence interval; ICU = intensive care unit.

specialist, a respiratory therapist, and a speech-language pathologist) on the rate of complications and the time to speaking valve placement, decannulation, and discharge from the ICU. The study involved 48 patients who were evaluated prior to the creation of the team and 89 patients who were evaluated after creation of the team.

There was a decrease in tube blockage (5% vs 25%) and calls on the floors for respiratory distress (17% vs 38%) after the creation of the trach team. There were other benefits, including decreased time to decannulation (28 vs 50 days) and decreased time to tube downsizing (26-9 days) (Fig 1). Many more patients received speaking valves after the trach team was established (67% vs 19%) (Table 2).

It seems these benefits were the direct result of having a group actively thinking about managing the tracheotomy tubes and reflecting on whether the patients really still needed the tubes for improvement. In the ICU setting, there are many other important clinical problems that usually draw the ICU team's focus away from optimally managing tracheostomy tubes. It makes complete sense that a dedicated team would be able to make these kinds of improvements. As surgeons, when we place tracheostomy tubes, it is vital that we formulate plans for the eventual removal of those tubes and how they will be managed until the patients can be decannulated. Better yet, we should emulate the authors and create tracheostomy care teams to help improve patient outcomes.

R. Franco, MD

Surgical Technique

Injection Medialization Laryngoplasty in Children
Cohen MS, Mehta DK, Maguire RC, et al (Univ of Pittsburgh School of Medicine, PA)
Arch Otolaryngol Head Neck Surg 137:264-268, 2011

Objective.—To review our experience with vocal fold injection medialization in children.

Design.—Retrospective case series.

Setting.—Tertiary care academic children's hospital.

Patients.—All pediatric patients at our institution who underwent injection laryngoplasty for vocal fold medialization from 2003 to 2009.

Main Outcome Measures.—Age, sex, indication for injection, injection material, surgical and anesthetic technique, outcomes including effect on voice and swallowing, and complications.

Results.—Thirteen patients underwent 27 injections. Mean patient age was 8.0 years (range, 1.3-18.0 years). The causes of glottic insufficiency included prolonged intubation (6 patients, 46%), patent ductus arteriosus ligation (2 patients, 15%), other cardiac surgery (2 patients, 15%), neck surgery or trauma (2 patients, 15%), and postviral status (1 patient, 8%). Eight patients had vocal fold paralysis or paresis; 3 had vocal fold atrophy; and 2 had vocal fold scarring. Indications for surgery included hoarseness (11 patients), aspiration (5 patients), and dysphagia without aspiration (1 patient). Materials injected included Gelfoam (n = 13), Radiesse Voice (n = 10), and Radiesse Voice Gel (n = 4). The average number of injections per patient was 2.1 (range, 1-9). Patients experienced improvement in symptoms (subjective or objective) after injection in 24 of 27 cases (89%); 15 of 16 injections in patients with hoarseness led to improvement (94%); and 11 of 13 injections in patients with dysphagia or aspiration led to improvement (85%). One patient experienced 2 days of inspiratory stridor postoperatively, which resolved spontaneously. There were no other complications.

Conclusions.—This study supports injection laryngoplasty as a safe and effective intervention for children with glottic insufficiency. Further prospective studies are necessary to confirm these findings.

▶ Vocal fold immobility is a common condition in children. The child introduces unique complexity making the typical paradigms used to treat adults less useful. Open medialization is typically performed with the patient awake to evaluate the progress of the surgery and allow the surgeon and patient to work cooperatively to fine-tune the voice, a cooperation that is not possible with most children. Open procedures that require removing a cartilaginous window to place an implant are frowned upon in children because of the possibility of inadvertently disrupting cartilaginous growth centers. Because of this, injection laryngoplasty is a popular technique to correct the dysphonia and dysphagia associated with unilateral vocal fold immobility in children.

The authors review their results in the 13 patients who underwent injection laryngoplasty between 2001 and 2009. These children underwent about 2 procedures each using various injectates including Gelfoam and Radiesse Voice Gel and Radiesse Voice to improve voice and swallowing function. There was improvement in 94% of patients injected for hoarseness (15 of 16), while 11 of 13 had improvement in swallowing (85%). The average duration of improvement for voice was 6 weeks for Gelfoam, 5.6 for Radiesse voice gel, while swallowing improved for 24 weeks after Radiesse and 18 weeks after Gelfoam injection. Of note, there seemed to be a clinical benefit that outlasted the presence of the injectate that may be due to the development of compensatory techniques during the slow resorption of the material. This effect has also been noted in adults who undergo injection with these materials.

R. Franco, MD

A New and Less Invasive Procedure for Arytenoid Adduction Surgery: Endoscopic-Assisted Arytenoid Adduction Surgery
Murata T, Yasuoka Y, Shimada T, et al (Gunma Univ Graduate School of Medicine, Japan)
Laryngoscope 121:1274-1280, 2011

Objectives/Hypothesis.—Arytenoid adduction (AA) is the most effective procedure for improving voice function in patients affected by unilateral vocal fold paralysis (UVFP), but it is often associated with severe complications following airway obstruction. The aim of this study is to describe a new and less invasive AA surgical procedure termed endoscopicassisted AA surgery (EAAS) and to evaluate its voice outcomes.

Study Design.—We demonstrated this method using extirpated larynges from three laryngeal cancer patients. Ten patients with severe UVFP underwent EAAS alone or combined with type I thyroplasty or lipoinjection laryngoplasty.

Methods.—EAAS involves the placement of permanent adducting sutures around the muscular process (MP) of the arytenoid cartilage using two needles, a penetration needle and a loop needle, under endoscopic guidance. To define the anatomic position of the MP for safer needle insertion, the location of the MP was measured relative to three landmarks on computed tomography/X-ray images of the larynges and in resected larynges. For all patients with UVFP, the maximum phonation time, mean airflow rate, and three acoustic analysis parameters were measured before and after EAAS.

Results.—The values of the three variables were similar in all cases. Most patients achieved a maximum phonation time of more than 10 seconds and a mean airflow rate of less than 200 mL/second. All three acoustic analysis parameters were significantly improved after surgery.

Conclusions.—EAAS is a simple and effective arytenoid rotation procedure (Fig 5).

▶ When restoring the voice after unilateral vocal fold immobility (UVFI), it is imperative to think in 3 dimensions because the affected vocal fold may be anterior, lateral, and inferior to the level of the working vocal fold. This is because the arytenoid is perched atop the cricoid, a signet ring, where any movement anterior involves moving lateral and inferior. Clinically, many cases of UVFI have evidence for synkinesis that assists in bringing the vocal fold up the cricoid facet (medial, posterior, and superior). In these cases, a type I thyroplasty as described by Isshiki will be sufficient to close the glottic gap.

Simple medialization is not sufficient in cases in which the vocal fold has drifted into an inferior and anterior location. In that case, the position of the affected arytenoid needs to be addressed either through an adduction arytenopexy or an

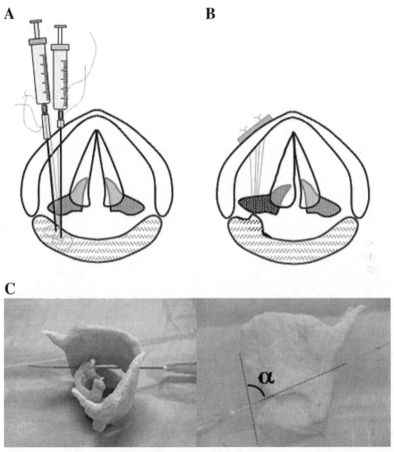

FIGURE 5.—The principle of endoscopicassisted arytenoid adduction surgery. (A) Schematic axial view of the larynx shows that the penetration needle and the loop needle are inserted from the cricothyroid ligament toward the piriform sinus, nearly passing through the muscular process. (B) The retracted nylon threads are tightened with a spacer at the cricothyroid ligament, and the arytenoid cartilage is successfully adducted. (C) A model larynx showing the manner in which the penetration needle should be passed near to the muscular process (left image: posterosuperior view; right image: lateral view; "α" indicates the insertion angle). (Reprinted from Murata T, Yasuoka Y, Shimada T, et al. A new and less invasive procedure for arytenoid adduction surgery: endoscopic-assisted arytenoid adduction surgery. *Laryngoscope.* 2011;121:1274-1280, with permission from The American Laryngological, Rhinological and Otological Society, Inc and John Wiley and Sons (www.interscience.wiley.com).)

arytenoid adduction procedure. In an arytenoid adduction, a suture is passed around the muscular process of the arytenoid to pull it forward, mimicking the action of the lateral cricoarytenoid muscle, whipping the vocal process medially. An adduction arytenopexy directly sutures the arytenoid body in the phonatory position, allowing the bodies to come close together, further increasing laryngeal efficiency.

The typical arytenoid procedures require exposure of the muscular process of the arytenoid. These authors describe a 2-surgeon technique that combines a simultaneous external and endoscopic approach to passing the suture through the muscular process (Fig 5). They first tested it on cadaveric specimen, then enrolled 10 patients with satisfactory results. This technique requires precise knowledge of the anatomy and measurement of the angles and lengths to be successful. The authors feel that they are able to minimize the potential morbidities associated with the standard arytenoid adduction through this technique.

R. Franco, MD

External light guidance for percutaneous dilatational tracheotomy
El-Sayed IH, Ho JE, Eisele DW (Univ of California, San Francisco)
Head Neck 33:1206-1209, 2011

Background.—Percutaneous dilatational tracheotomy (PDT) is considered a safe technique; however, there is still room for improvement. We present our initial experience with an external white light guide to position the endotracheal tube and guide needle placement during PDT.

Methods.—This is a retrospective series of 15 consecutive patients undergoing external light–guided PDT. A white light source was placed on the anterior trachea wall externally and the transmitted light was identified in the tracheal lumen with a bronchoscopic to predict the needle entrance point.

Results.—The transmitted light was rapidly identified in all 15 patients, facilitated endotracheal tube tip placement in the subglottis in approximately 10 seconds in 13 of 15 patients, and predicted needle penetration into the trachea within 1 to 2 mm of the external light in all patients.

Conclusions.—External light guidance facilitates rapid, accurate placement of the needle through the tracheal wall and can reduce surgeon anxiety, especially in teaching situations (Fig 4).

▶ The surgical education of residents and medical students is a delicate balance of protecting the welfare of the patient while simultaneously maximizing the resident's role as surgeon. Teaching residents to perform tracheotomy is fraught with the potential for bleeding from lacerating great vessels lateral to the trachea, longitudinal tracheal injuries, intralaryngeal placement of the trach tube via the cricothyroid membrane, and placement of the trach tube off the midline. Most of these errors are due to not properly identifying the relevant anatomy, such as mistaking the anterior cricoid arch for a tracheal ring.

Procedural enhancements that help reduce placement errors would increase the resident's confidence in successfully performing the procedure and allow the attending to let the resident do more while keeping the patient safe. The authors present a technique that involves shining a light onto the anterior trachea that can be identified intraluminally using a flexible bronchoscope to adjust the position of the tip of the endotracheal tube (Fig 4). They found that this technique allowed retraction of the endotracheal tube to the proper position within 10 seconds and predicted needle placement in the airway to within 2 mm of the tip of the endotracheal tube. The standard dilatational tracheotomy technique

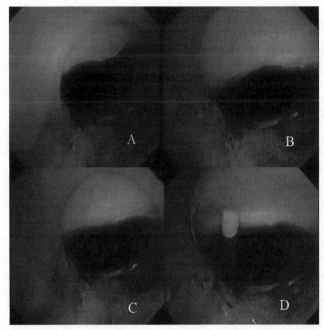

FIGURE 4.—Guiding midline placement of the needle. (A) The light is initially seen on the right lateral wall of the trachea. (B) The light is adjusted to the contralateral side. (C) The light source is positioned in the center of the anterior wall. (D) The needle enters adjacent to the light on the anterior wall. [Color figure can be viewed in the online issue, which is available at wileyonlinelibrary.com.] (Reprinted from El-Sayed IH, Ho JE, Eisele DW. External light guidance for percutaneous dilatational tracheotomy. *Head Neck*. 2011;33:1206-1209, and John Wiley and Sons.)

is then used with the confidence that the procedure is proceeding correctly, with the needle in the proper location (in the midline of the airway) away from the great vessels and close to the upper trachea.

R. Franco, MD

Cervical tracheal resection with cricotracheal anastomosis: experience in adults with grade III–IV tracheal stenosis

El-Fattah AMA, Kamal E, Amer HE, et al (Mansoura Univ, Egypt)
J Laryngol Otol 125:614-619, 2011

Introduction.—Laryngotracheal stenosis is currently one of the most common complications associated with nasal and orotracheal intubation and tracheotomy. Once established, tracheal stenosis can be a complex and difficult problem to manage.

Patients and Methods.—We retrospectively analysed 2004–2010 data for 12 male patients with postintubation cervical tracheal stenosis (grade III–IV) treated in the otolaryngology department, Mansoura University

Hospitals. All patients had a tracheostomy at presentation, and all underwent tracheal resection with primary cricotracheal anastomosis and suprahyoid release.

Results.—Grade III stenosis was present in five patients (41.7 per cent) and grade IV stenosis in seven patients (58.3 per cent). The length of trachea resected ranged from 2 to 4 cm, representing one to four tracheal rings. In all 12 patients, the procedure allowed successful tracheotomy decannulation. Minor complications comprised surgical emphysema ($n = 2$) and wound infection ($n = 1$), and were managed conservatively. Major complications consisted of restenosis ($n = 3$), managed in two patients by repeated dilatation; one patient was lost to follow up.

Conclusion.—Segmental tracheal resection with cricotracheal anastomosis was successful in 11/12 (92 per cent) patients with severe cervical tracheal stenosis. The strategy for treatment of airway stenosis is now well established and success rates are high, with minimal or no sequelae (Table 1).

▶ Postintubation tracheal injury can result in tracheal stenosis and appears to be a major cause of new cases of nontraumatic tracheal stenosis. There is a spectrum of treatment options starting with repeated dilatation of the airway as the patient becomes symptomatic to open resection of the stenotic segment with direct anastomosis. Dilation is not curative and will give relief for a variable amount of time with a quick and relatively morbid-free procedure. There are now examples of centers performing these with balloons in awake patients to further reduce the risks.

Many consider definitive treatment to be resection with anastomosis, and in many cases, it is reserved for those with the greatest degree of stenosis with

TABLE 1.—Upper Tracheal Resection With Primary Cricotracheal Anastomosis: Patient Data Summary

Pt No	Age (y)	Tracheotomy at Surgery?	Stenosis Grade	Trachea Length Resected	Complications	Interventions	Extubated?	Outcome
1	46	Yes	IV	3 rings	Partial stenosis	Repeated dilatation, tracheostomy	Yes	Satisfactory
2	34	Yes	IV	2.5 cm	Surgical emphysema	Conservative	Yes	Satisfactory
3	39	Yes	III	3 cm	–	–	Yes	Excellent
4	29	Yes	IV	2 rings	Wound infection	Antibiotics	Yes	Satisfactory
5	31	Yes	III	3.5 cm	–	–	Yes	Excellent
6	42	Yes	III	2 rings	–	–	Yes	Excellent
7	24	Yes	IV	4 rings	Partial stenosis	Repeated dilatation	Yes	Satisfactory
8	33	Yes	III	2.5 cm	–	–	Yes	Excellent
9	25	Yes	IV	4 cm	Restenosis	Lost to follow up	Unknown	Missing data
10	22	Yes	IV	3 cm	Surgical emphysema	Conservative	Yes	Satisfactory
11	40	Yes	IV	3 rings	–	–	Yes	Excellent
12	27	Yes	III	3 rings	–	–	Yes	Excellent

Pt no = patient number; y = years.

respect to both luminal narrowing and length of stenosis. In this study, 12 male patients with Myer-Cotton grade III (5 patients or 42%) and grade IV (7 patients or 58%) stenoses were retrospectively reviewed. All 12 had tracheostomy tubes in place at the time of presentation, and all underwent tracheal resection for postintubation stenosis with a suprahyoid release and cricotracheal anastomosis.

Anywhere from 2 to 4 cm of trachea was resected, representing 1 to 4 tracheal rings. Patients did not have a chin-to-chest suture, also known as a Grillo stitch, to keep the head in flexion but rather were placed in a hard C-collar. All 12 patients were extubated on the table (8 patients) or 1 day postoperative in the intensive care unit (4 patients) based on surgeon preference.

There were minor complications (Table I) with restenosis in 3 of the patients that required dilations, surgical empyema in 2, and a wound infection in 1 patient. One patient with restenosis was lost to follow-up, giving a 92% (11/12) overall success rate.

Despite the high success that is seen here, it is important to remember that the lower morbidity procedures are still effective for treating those patients in whom higher-risk open tracheal resections are not justified. This procedure should be reserved for those who have severe disease and can tolerate this procedure.

R. Franco, MD

Coblation Removal of Laryngeal Teflon Granulomas
Meslemani D, Benninger MS (Henry Ford Hosp, Detroit, MI; The Cleveland Clinic, OH)
Laryngoscope 120:2018-2021, 2010

Background.—Vocal flow medialization was often accomplished in previous times using Teflon injections. Problems arising from this method include overinjection and delayed granuloma formation, which is relatively common. Techniques to remove these granulomas have included the use of the carbon dioxide (CO_2) laser and an open lateral laryngotomy. These approaches are associated with complications and limitations, including difficulty performing the removal, recurrence of the granuloma, extensive operations, poor voice quality, and destruction of the vocal fold. A new surgical technique using the Procise LW Coblator to help excise Teflon granulomas via a direct microlaryngoscopic approach was described.

Methods.—The larynx is viewed microscopically through a suspension laryngoscope to determine its location and condition. A small cupped forceps is used to obtain a specimen for histopathologic evaluation. The dissection uses a coblator device set at 7 for coblation and 3 for coagulation. The device uses radiofrequency energy directed through a saline medium to create a plasma whose energized particles break the molecular bonds in the tissue. As a result, the tissue dissolves at 40°C to 70°C, which is a relatively low temperature. The target tissue can be removed with minimal damage to surrounding areas. The coblator is used to incise the

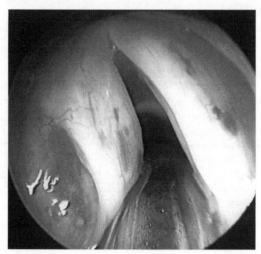

FIGURE 1.—A prominent vocal fold granuloma, obstructing the airway. The larynx of patient from case 1. (Reprinted from Meslemani D, Benninger MS. Coblation removal of laryngeal teflon granulomas. *Laryngoscope.* 2010;120:2018-2021, with permission from The American Laryngological, Rhinological and Otological Society, Inc and John Wiley and Sons (www.interscience.wiley.com).)

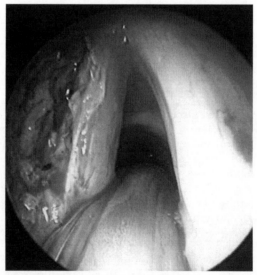

FIGURE 2.—The granuloma was completely excise with minimal soft tissue trauma and preservation of the medial mucosa. The airway became more patent. The larynx from patient in case 1. (Reprinted from Meslemani D, Benninger MS. Coblation removal of laryngeal teflon granulomas. *Laryngoscope.* 2010;120:2018-2021, with permission from The American Laryngological, Rhinological and Otological Society, Inc and John Wiley and Sons (www.interscience.wiley.com).)

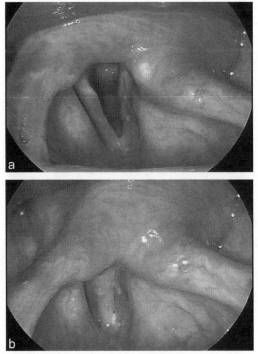

FIGURE 3.—(a) Patient from case 1. Videostrobe >24 months postoperatively. No evidence of granulom formulation. (b) Patient from case1. Videostrobe >24 months postoperatively. No evidence of granuloma formulation. (Reprinted from Meslemani D, Benninger MS. Coblation removal of laryngeal teflon granulomas. *Laryngoscope.* 2010;120:2018-2021, with permission from The American Laryngological, Rhinological and Otological Society, Inc and John Wiley and Sons (www.interscience.wiley.com).)

upper surface of the vocal fold. Dissection is undertaken to ablate the granuloma laterally with the coblation wand, carefully preserving the medial mucosa. Any bleeding sites are controlled using the bipolar cautery from the coblator. Dissection is continued until the left vocal fold appears straight and the airway is enlarged.

Results.—Four patients underwent removal of a Teflon granuloma using the coblator. All short-term results demonstrated substantial subjective improvement of voice quality and statistically significant improvement in quality of life as measured by Vocal Handicap Index (VHI) scores. The degree of postoperative pain was minimal both immediately after surgery and at follow-up 2 to 3 weeks after resection. In two cases, VHI scores were improved up to 2 years postoperatively. No recurrences were reported.

Conclusions.—The coblation device removes Teflon granulomas at low temperature, which prevents significant heat-related damage to the tissues. Superficial bleeding is controlled, with more significant bleeding readily managed using the bipolar cautery on the coblation device. This approach produces precise dissection with minimal to no damage to surrounding tissues and little bleeding while taking minimal time for the operation (Figs 1-3).

▶ Although today Teflon is rarely used as a vocal fold injectate, there was a time when there was a dearth of injectable materials that could medialize a vocal fold, and Teflon was a relatively popular option. Some of those patients now have the formation of Teflon granulomas that can interfere with phonation and require removal to achieve voice improvements. There are open and endoscopic approaches to the paraglottic space to remove these granulomas using cold instruments or the CO_2 laser, with various pros and cons associated with each. The authors present 4 cases of Teflon granuloma treated using an endoscopic approach and a coblator device to make a superior and lateral cordotomy of the true vocal fold (Figs 1-3). Maximal tissue preservation was achieved by coblating the granuloma while preserving the medial mucosa.

When compared with the intense heat generated by a CO_2 laser, the coblator functions in the relatively cool range of 40°C to 70°C. This minimizes the transfer of heat to the surrounding tissues because heat can damage the delicate vocal fold. Cold dissection techniques to remove Teflon granuloma would be the ultimate technique to ensure tissue viability.

R. Franco, MD

4 Otology

Basic and Clinical Research

Speech perception in individuals with auditory dys-synchrony

Kumar UA, Jayaram M (Kasturba Med College (a unit of Manipal Univ), Mangalore; Natl Inst of Mental Health and Neuroscience, Bangalore, India)
J Laryngol Otol 125:236-245, 2011

Objective.—This study aimed to evaluate the effect of lengthening the transition duration of selected speech segments upon the perception of those segments in individuals with auditory dys-synchrony.

Methods.—Thirty individuals with auditory dys-synchrony participated in the study, along with 30 age-matched normal hearing listeners. Eight consonant–vowel syllables were used as auditory stimuli. Two experiments were conducted. Experiment one measured the 'just noticeable difference' time: the smallest prolongation of the speech sound transition duration which was noticeable by the subject. In experiment two, speech sounds were modified by lengthening the transition duration by multiples of the just noticeable difference time, and subjects' speech identification scores for the modified speech sounds were assessed.

Results.—Subjects with auditory dys-synchrony demonstrated poor processing of temporal auditory information. Lengthening of speech sound transition duration improved these subjects' perception of both the placement and voicing features of the speech syllables used.

Conclusion.—These results suggest that innovative speech processing strategies which enhance temporal cues may benefit individuals with auditory dys-synchrony (Figs 2, 3, and 5).

▶ As newborn hearing screening programs have become more widespread, so too has the recognition of auditory dyssynchrony, also known as auditory neuropathy. This affects roughly one out of 200 individuals with sensorineural hearing loss and can be much higher in selected populations. Thus, it is not a rare disorder. As the authors describe in their clear and detailed introduction, traditional hearing amplification strategies are not as beneficial in this disorder as they are with typical sensorineural losses, and cochlear implantation has become an option for treatment. This introduction is well worth reading because it clearly describes the nature of the deficits in speech perception that these individuals suffer. Most importantly, they state that cochlear implantation, although it may be of benefit, is

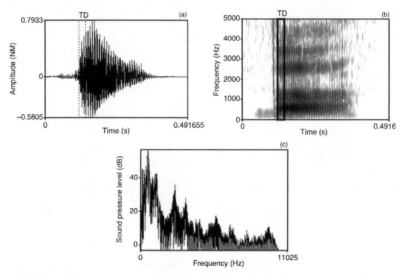

FIGURE 2.—(a) Spectrogram of unmodified speech stimulus /ba/. (b)Waveform of unmodified speech stimulus /ba/; the transition duration (TD) is marked with a rectangle. (c) Frequency spectrum of the unmodified speech stimulus /ba/. (Reprinted from Kumar UA, Jayaram M. Speech perception in individuals with auditory dys-synchrony. *J Laryngol Otol.* 2011;125:236-245, with permission of Cambridge University Press.)

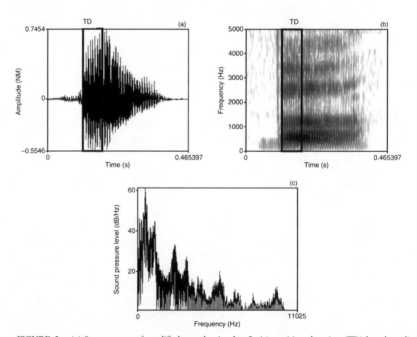

FIGURE 3.—(a) Spectrogram of modified speech stimulus /ba/ (transition duration (TD) lengthened). (b) Waveform of modified speech stimulus /ba/; TD is marked with a rectangle. (c) Frequency spectrum of the modified stimulus /ba/. (Reprinted from Kumar UA, Jayaram M. Speech perception in individuals with auditory dys-synchrony. *J Laryngol Otol.* 2011;125:236-245, with permission of Cambridge University Press.)

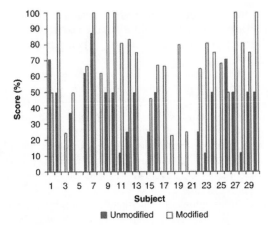

FIGURE 5.—Speech identification scores of individual subjects for both unmodified and modified (i.e. lengthened transition duration) speech stimuli. (Reprinted from Kumar UA, Jayaram M. Speech perception in individuals with auditory dys-synchrony. *J Laryngol Otol.* 2011;125:236-245, with permission of Cambridge University Press.)

not a financially viable option for many in the developing world. Given the increasing focus on rising health care costs and budgets in many countries, exploration of low-tech and cost-conscious alternatives to treatment is both timely and valuable. Another interesting aspect of this study is that it was conducted in adults, the majority of whom had the onset of their disorder in young adulthood rather than infancy. Fig 2 illustrates the unmodified speech pattern used in their investigation, and Fig 3 shows the modified version. Fig 5 demonstrates the effectiveness of the modification in speech pattern presentation with greatly improved speech identification scores. Development of hearing assistive devices that address this temporal processing deficit may lead to more cost-effective methods of treatment than cochlear implantation.

B. J. Balough, Capt, MC, USN

The vascularization of the human cochlea: its historical background
Mudry A, Tange RA (ENT & HNS, Lausanne, Switzerland; Univ Med Ctr Utrecht, The Netherlands)
Acta Otolaryngol Suppl 129:3-16, 2009

The history of vascularization of the human cochlea began with the first anatomical description of the cochlea in the 16th century. Three different periods are recognizable in the development of knowledge concerning this subject: the macroscopic period, with the description of the structure of the cochlea from the 16th to the 19th century; the microscopic period, with the description of the part of the organ of Corti in the 19th century; and the injection period, with the description of the fine vascularization of the cochlea in the 20th century. Various techniques were used during these three periods, which will be presented here, using only original references. This historical study reveals the ingenuity of the researchers in using different aspects of technological progress to enhance their performance in research.

▶ The human cochlea and labyrinth is a complex and marvelous organ. This article provides a tremendous wealth of information regarding the evolution in our understanding of its vascular supply based on the historical discoveries from the 1700s to the present day. The illustrations are magnificent in their detail, and the information was collected from rare book collections. Similarly, the bibliography provides a wealth of information and original citations. Fig 4 in the original article shows the level of complexity that was able to be presented from study with the naked eye alone. The advent of microscopy improved upon this detail, followed by injection contrast as shown in Fig 9 in the original article. By the late 20th century, further refinements of injection techniques and electron microscopy provide enough sufficient detail that a schematic wiring diagram for vascular flow is presented as in Fig 13 in the original article. With this information, the patterns of hearing loss and recovery and their relationship to vestibular insults, as seen in the article by Korres et al,[1] becomes clearer. One further highly significant point is hidden in this very valuable article. From the 1950s through the late 1970s a variety of authors comment on the similarities as well as the differences in the vascular anatomy of the cochlear across species. While the small vessels of the spiral lamina and spiral ligament seem to be preserved, other vascular structures are not, and only primates seem to have vascular anatomy that correlates to the human cochlea. Given the interest in the development of inner ear medical therapy (both transtympanic and oral), it is surprising that this knowledge is not commented on in the animal works that led to human investigations.

B. J. Balough, Capt, MC, USN

Reference

1. Korres S, Stamatiou GA, Gkoritsa E, Riga M, Xenelis J. Prognosis of patients with idiopathic sudden hearing loss: role of vestibular assessment. *J Laryngol Otol.* 2011;125:251-257.

Oxygen consumption by bacteria: a possible cause of negative middle ear pressure in ears with otitis media
Kitaoka K, Kaieda S, Takahashi H, et al (Nagasaki Univ Graduate School of Biomed Sciences, Japan; Nagasaki City General Hosp, Japan)
Acta Otolaryngol 129:63-66, 2009

Conclusions.—Oxygen consumption by bacteria could be a cause of the negative middle ear pressure in ears with otitis media (OM).

Objective.—To determine whether oxygen consumption by bacteria could be a cause for production of negative pressure in ears with OM.

Materials and Methods.—Hermetically sealed bottles containing high dose (group A) and low dose (group B) of Streptococcus pneumoniae

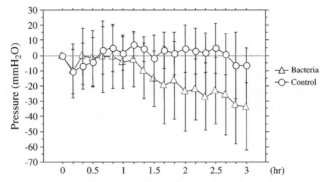

FIGURE 2.—The chronological changes in the mean pressure in the experimental and control bottles in group A. (Reprinted from Kitaoka K, Kaieda S, Takahashi H, et al. Oxygen consumption by bacteria: a possible cause of negative middle ear pressure in ears with otitis media. *Acta Otolaryngol.* 2009;129:63-66, reprinted by permission of the publisher (Taylor & Francis Group, http://www.informaworld.com).)

with air space and maintained at 37°C in a water bath were connected to a microphressure sensor. The chronological pressure changes were monitored in vitro for 3—13 h and were compared with those in the control bottles containing culture medium only.

Results.—The pressure of the group A samples showed significantly lower values than that of controls 3 h later ($p<0.0001$). In group B, the pressure was also significantly lower than that in the control group ($p<0.0001$). The partial pressures of oxygen measured at the beginning and end of the experiment in the six samples in group B showed significant decrease, while that in the control group showed only a slight decrease ($p<0.0019$) (Fig 2).

▶ Why does the tympanic membrane retract and how can it be prevented? The simplistic answer is that in some individuals, the Eustachian tube does not function properly, leading to chronic negative middle ear pressure. Yet even in those with cleft palates where even after repair the function of the eustachian tube is impaired, chronic retraction of the tympanic membrane is not seen after adulthood unless the problem arose in childhood. Other adults will show progressive retraction over time despite otherwise normal function in the opposite ear. Thus, there must be more to the problem than "dysfunction" of the eustachian tube. Here the authors have performed a basic science study to explore an alternative explanation for chronic negative middle ear pressure—namely, oxygen consumption by bacteria. As demonstrated in Fig 2, large negative pressures can be generated in a relatively short period of time when large amounts of bacteria are present, such as an acute infection. Even with the samples with 10 to 100 colony-forming units per milliliter, significant negative pressures were developed and maintained by 10 hours. In chronic middle ear disease, the presence of bacterial biofilms may allow this small number of bacteria to persist, consume oxygen, and lead to chronic negative pressure and formation of cholesteatoma. Thus the genesis of cholesteatoma may be from biofilm. Certainly a great deal more research would need to be done to confirm such a theory.

However, the interesting possibilities that this simple study provokes make it a worthwhile read.

B. J. Balough, Capt, MC, USN

Influence of lipoproteins and fibrinogen on pathogenesis of sudden sensorineural hearing loss
Oreskovic Z, Shejbal D, Bicanic G, et al (Clinical Hosp Ctr Zagreb, Croatia; et al)
J Laryngol Otol 125:258-261, 2011

Aim.—To evaluate the relationship between lipoproteins, fibrinogen and sudden sensorineural hearing loss in a Croatian population. Since pathological derangement of lipoproteins and fibrinogen could be one of the causes of sudden sensorineural hearing loss, we hypothesised that patients with sudden sensorineural hearing loss would have more abnormal fibrinogen and lipoprotein concentrations, compared with subjects with normal hearing.

Methods.—Plasma concentrations of cholesterol, fibrinogen and triglycerides in patients with sudden sensorineural hearing loss were compared with those in a control group (i.e. subjects with normal hearing function).

Results.—Patients with sudden sensorineural hearing loss had significantly higher plasma concentrations of cholesterol and low density lipoprotein cholesterol, compared with controls.

Conclusion.—Higher cholesterol and low density lipoprotein cholesterol concentrations were found in patients with sudden sensorineural hearing loss, within a Croatian population. Cholesterol and low density lipoprotein cholesterol concentrations may be important factors in the pathogenesis of sudden sensorineural hearing loss, and should be assessed during the investigation of patients with this condition (Tables 1 and 2).

▶ The pathophysiology behind sudden hearing loss remains unknown, with the leading theories being viral infection, autoimmunity, membrane rupture, and ischemia/embolic events. In this article, the authors prospectively follow a cohort of patients with sudden hearing loss examining a variety of laboratory values to try to establish a relationship. Similar studies have been done in the past with viral titers. Tables 1 and 2 illustrate the differences between total and low-density lipoprotein (LDL) cholesterol levels. The study represents a 5-year cohort of patients presenting with sudden hearing loss and provides a relatively large

---

TABLE 1.—Plasma Total Cholesterol

Group	X ± SD (mmol/l)	Median (Range) (mmol/l)	p^*
Test	5.9 ± 1.1	6.0 (3.7–8.8)	0.000049
Control	5 ± 1.0	5.2 (2.9–7.2)	

*t-test. X = arithmetic mean; SD = standard deviation.

TABLE 2.—Plasma LDL Cholesterol

Group	X ± SD (mmol/l)	Median (Range) (mmol/l)	*p**
Test	3.7 ± 0.9	3.8 (1.8–5.5)	0.000046
Control	2.9 ± 0.8	2.9 (1.2–5.0)	

*t-test. X = arithmetic mean; SD = standard deviation.

sample for this uncommon disorder. One major limitation of the study is that no table is provided to compare the demographics of the study and control populations. The authors do acknowledge in the discussion an average age difference of 15 years (the study population being older) and the potential impact on this difference in their findings. No explanation, however, is given for why this information was not presented in the results. Despite this flaw, the findings of this study provide a road map for future investigation. If their findings are indeed true, then the widespread use of statins and other drugs to lower total and LDL cholesterol should result in a declining incidence of sudden hearing loss. In fact, populations with better control should have lower rates than those with poor control. Thus, given our limited ability to treat sudden loss when it occurs, the better course may be to address it from a public health perspective and, as with heart disease, reduce the causative factors where we are able. For this potential impact, the article is included in this year's list.

B. J. Balough, Capt, MC, USN

Development of an auditory implant manipulator for minimally invasive surgical insertion of implantable hearing devices

Stieger C, Caversaccio M, Arnold A, et al (Univ of Bern, Switzerland; Univ Dept of ENT, Head and Neck Surgery, Bern, Switzerland; et al)

J Laryngol Otol 125:262-270, 2011

Objective.—To present the auditory implant manipulator, a navigation-controlled mechanical and electronic system which enables minimally invasive ('keyhole') transmastoid access to the tympanic cavity.

Materials and Methods.—The auditory implant manipulator is a miniaturised robotic system with five axes of movement and an integrated drill. It can be mounted on the operating table. We evaluated the surgical work field provided by the system, and the work sequence involved, using an anatomical whole head specimen.

Results.—The work field provided by the auditory implant manipulator is considerably greater than required for conventional mastoidectomy. The work sequence for a keyhole procedure included pre-operative planning, arrangement of equipment, the procedure itself and post-operative analysis.

Conclusion.—Although system improvements are necessary, our preliminary results indicate that the auditory implant manipulator has the

TABLE 1.—Accuracy Study: Translational and Rotational Errors

Error	Axis	Mean ± SD	Min	Max
Translnl (mm)	x	1.2 ± 0.5	0.4	2.7
	y	1.6 ± 0.4	0.8	2.4
Rotnl (°)	x	0.4 ± 0.3	0.1	0.9
	y	0.6 ± 0.7	0.0	3.2

SD = standard deviation; min = minimum; max = maximum; translnl = translational; rotnl = rotational.

potential to perform keyhole insertion of implantable hearing devices (Table 1).

▶ Robotic surgery has become increasingly popular in a variety of surgical disciplines. It seems logical, therefore, that otologic approaches through the mastoid would be a natural application of this technology given the precision and maneuverability that surgical robotics provides. However, as can be seen in this article, it is the approximation of vital structures requiring submillimeter precision that makes robotic development challenging in this location. In their materials and methods, the authors give outstanding detail covering the thought process and engineering steps in the development of such a system. Despite the careful planning and engineering design, Table 1 provides the axis-specific translational and rotational errors. The translational errors of over 1 mm (with maximums exceeding 2) are noteworthy, as these standard errors will be multiplicative as the dissection extends into the temporal bone. It is not surprising, therefore, that an error in excess of 3 mm was encountered leading to dissection into the facial nerve. Considering 3 mm can be the entire depth of the facial recess or middle ear, this degree of error is not acceptable. It is interesting that in their discussion, the comment is made that for drilling the implant bed the robotic system can be removed. It may be that this approach is backwards. The robotics systems may be better suited for drilling implant wells underneath the skin flaps where manual access is limited and for the bulk of the lateral temporal bone work. Here the drilling will be more precise and may speed the operation, leaving the more critical medial drilling around vital structures to be performed under direct human guidance. This may be a less exciting technical challenge but one with a quicker course to implement robotic surgery in otology.

B. J. Balough, Capt, MC, USN

Comparison between bone-conducted ultrasound and audible sound in speech recognition

Yamashita A, Nishimura T, Nagatani Y, et al (Nara Med Univ, Kashihara Nara, Japan)
Acta Otolaryngol 129:34-39, 2009

Conclusion.—This study showed that it is possible to transmit language information using bone-conducted ultrasound (BCU) in normal-hearing subjects. Our results suggest the possibility of a difference in speech recognition between BCU and air-conducted audible sound (ACAS).

Objective.—Ultrasound was audible when delivered by bone conduction. Some profoundly deaf subjects as well as normal-hearing subjects can discriminate BCU whose amplitude is modulated by different speech sounds. These findings suggest the usefulness of developing a bone-conducted ultrasonic hearing aid (BCUHA). However, the characteristics of BCU are still poorly understood. The aim of the present study was to compare BCU and ACAS in terms of their associated speech perception

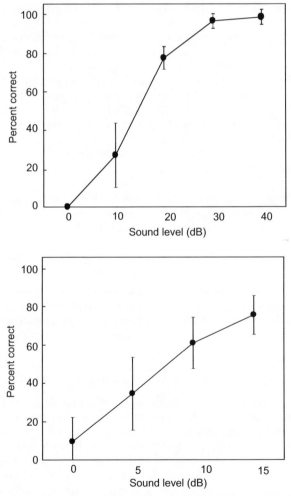

FIGURE 2.—Averaged score of speech discrimination tests with (a) ACAS and (b) BCU. Vertical bars indicate standard deviations. (Reprinted from Yamashita A, Nishimura T, Nagatani Y, et al. Comparison between bone-conducted ultrasound and audible sound in speech recognition. *Acta Otolaryngol.* 2009;129:34-39, reprinted by permission of the publisher (Taylor & Francis Group, http://www.informaworld.com).)

tendency and to investigate the different perceptual characteristics of BCU and ACAS.

Subjects and Methods.—Speech discrimination tests using both BCU and ACAS were performed with normal-hearing subjects. BCU and ACAS were compared for intelligibility and hearing confusion.

Results.—With BCU, the maximum percentage correct totaled about 75%. Our comparison of the hearing confusion with ACAS and BCU according to the individual syllabic nuclear group showed a clear difference in the incorrect rates. In addition, the stimulus nuclear groups were often perceived in other nuclear groups in BCU (Fig 2).

▶ "There is nothing new under the sun" is an often repeated adage. This article shows that this is true in medical science as well. Hearing in the ultrasonic range through 120 kHz, as referenced in the article, was initially described in 1948. The introduction provides a good background of the understanding of this phenomenon and how it interacts with air-conducted audible sound. Most importantly, hearing impaired and even those profoundly deaf can perceive these sounds, as the normal hearing mechanism is not involved. This, as the authors describe, provides an opportunity for new types of hearing rehabilitative devices. Fig 2 illustrates how air-conducted and bone-conducted ultrasound scans compare with regard to speech recognition with increasing signal. Uncomfortable loudness limits the intensity with which the signal can be presented, but in this study, scores of 75% to 80% can be achieved, which may be able to be improved with training. If speech recognition in these levels can be provided to the severe to profoundly deaf, this technology could provide exciting new opportunities for patients who struggle with hearing aids but who may not yet be candidates for cochlear implantation. Thus, for the background information alone, this article is an important read.

B. J. Balough, Capt, MC, USN

Clinical characteristics and audiological significance of spontaneous otoacoustic emissions in tinnitus patients with normal hearing
Kim D-K, Park S-N, Park K-H, et al (The Catholic Univ of Korea, Seoul, South Korea)
J Laryngol Otol 125:246-250, 2011

Objective.—To define the clinical and audiological features of normal-hearing tinnitus patients with spontaneous otoacoustic emissions, and to evaluate the role of spontaneous otoacoustic emissions in tinnitus generation.

Materials and Methods.—Thirty-two patients with spontaneous otoacoustic emissions were compared with 29 patients without spontaneous otoacoustic emissions, regarding clinical and audiological aspects.

Results.—The mean age of the study group subjects was significantly lower, and they experienced the kindling effect less frequently than the control group. The mean tinnitus handicap inventory score of the study group was considerably higher than that of the controls, although the difference was not statistically significant. The study group had significantly quieter tinnitus, and higher transient evoked and distortion product otoacoustic emission responses, compared with the control group.

Conclusions.—Normal-hearing tinnitus patients with spontaneous otoacoustic emissions have different clinical and audiological characteristics, compared with those without spontaneous otoacoustic emissions. Appropriate evaluation and treatment should be considered at an early stage in these patients.

► Tinnitus continues to be one of the most common, and poorly understood, otologic maladies. Here the authors focus on a subgroup of tinnitus patients—those with normal hearing. Mechanistic explanation for tinnitus in those with hearing loss is relatively simple: loss of hearing signal releases inhibitory surround of cortical and brainstem neurons via neural plasticity, and the new, unwanted signal generates the phantom sound. The cause for tinnitus in individuals with normal hearing is more difficult to explain and, as the authors relate, suggests a cochlear source. They provide extensive audiologic and demographic comparisons between those with and without spontaneous otoacoustic emissions (SOAE). Only 2 reach statistical significance, perhaps because of the small numbers in the study. These small numbers also preclude subdivision of the study groups into mild, moderate, and severe tinnitus or by duration of tinnitus, which may have been more revealing. However, despite these limitations, it is the novel way in which they use a conventional audiologic test to explore tinnitus that makes this article a thought-provoking read. The discussion provides additional insights into the theory behind SOAE generation and its relationship to tinnitus.

B. J. Balough, Capt, MC, USN

Abnormal Motion Perception in Vestibular Migraine
Lewis RF, Priesol AJ, Nicoucar K, et al (Harvard Med School, Boston, MA)
Laryngoscope 121:1124-1125, 2011

Background.—Vestibular migraine (VM) is poorly understood, with no specific oculomotor, postural, or perceptual defect and an uncertain pathophysiology. Recent research indicates that the brain uses different mechanisms to generate the perception of head motion and reflexive vestibular-mediated eye movements. This perception appears to depend more on central interactions between semicircular canal cues sensing head rotation and otolith cues that sense gravity and linear acceleration than on eye movements. Quantitative psychophysical methods were used to investigate VM, with the hypothesis that canal-otolith integration may be abnormal in patients with this disorder.

Methods.—Tests were conducted on eight patients with VM, eight migraine patients with no history of vestibular symptoms, and eight normal subjects. These were done at least 2 weeks after the most recent experience of headache or vertigo. None of the patients were taking prophylactic migraine medications. The stimuli were designed to affect the canals and otoliths simultaneously (dynamic roll tilt), the canals only (roll rotation), and the otoliths only (quasistatic roll tilt). Potential nonvestibular motion cues were eliminated by conducting tests in the dark, covering skin surfaces, padding the body, and wearing headphones.

Results.—VM patients had a mean threshold on dynamic roll tilt at 0.1 Hz that was considerably lower than migraine sufferers or normal subjects. Subject group and motion frequency interacted significantly to produce the varying thresholds on the dynamic roll tilt test. Roll rotation thresholds were similar for the VM and normal subjects, and all groups had similar thresholds on the quasistatic roll tilt tests. Vestibulo-ocular reflex (VOR) results were similar for the normal and VM groups. Motion sickness susceptibility was comparable for the three groups of subjects.

Conclusions.—VM patients had a considerable reduction in perceptual motion thresholds compared to normal and migraine subjects who underwent the dynamic roll tilt test. However, other movements did not produce these differences between groups. Thus canal and otolith cues appear to be synthesized differently by persons with VM than by normal persons or migraine sufferers without a vestibular component.

▶ Like most vestibular disorders, vestibular migraine (also known as migraine-associated vertigo) is a clinical diagnosis based on history. These patients are often intolerant of motion stimuli and, in particular, visual stimulation. Normal activity in combination with visual stimulation becomes overwhelming. Here the authors have cleverly designed and evaluated an objective test methodology to confirm what these symptoms represent. For that alone this would be a worthy read. However, just as important is their approach. Most of us like simple tests—easy to perform and easy to interpret. For the complexities of the balance system, which integrates motion, vision, and position sense to give a perception of our place in space and movement, simple tests fall far short of what is truly needed. The explanation of how they arrived at this test and why it is only valid at a lower frequency grants deeper understanding of how balance evaluation can and should be done. Thus, this straightforward study and short article opens a world of possibility for further new examination.

B. J. Balough, Capt, MC, USN

Diagnostics

Comparison of vestibular evoked myogenic potentials elicited by click and short duration tone burst stimuli
Kumar K, Sinha SK, Bharti AK, et al (Univ of Mysore, India)
J Laryngol Otol 125:343-347, 2011

Introduction.—Vestibular evoked myogenic potentials are short latency electrical impulses that are produced in response to higher level acoustic stimuli. They are used clinically to diagnose sacculocollic pathway dysfunction.

Aim.—This study aimed to compare the vestibular evoked myogenic potential responses elicited by click stimuli and short duration tone burst stimuli, in normal hearing individuals.

Method.—Seventeen subjects participated. In all subjects, we assessed vestibular evoked myogenic potentials elicited by click and short duration tone burst stimuli.

Results and Conclusion.—The latency of the vestibular evoked myogenic potential responses (i.e. the p13 and n23 peaks) was longer for tone burst stimuli compared with click stimuli. The amplitude of the p13—n23 waveform was greater for tone burst stimuli than click stimuli. Thus, the click stimulus may be preferable for clinical assessment and identification of abnormalities as this stimulus has less variability, while a low frequency tone burst stimulus may be preferable when assessing the presence or absence of vestibular evoked myogenic potential responses (Figs 2 and 3).

▶ Although increasingly popular for evaluation of a variety of vestibular and otologic disorders since their wider clinical introduction nearly a decade ago, the method used for testing vestibular-evoked myogenic potentials (VEMP) can vary greatly from center to center. In fact, this lack of standardization led to a US Food and Drug Administration action in 2008 against manufacturers of electrophysiologic testing machines for audiology to get them to cease marketing VEMP. This article, then, seeks to better define the variation in response that can be seen between differing signal presentations. To that end, the authors provide a detailed explanation of their testing methodology to include the tonic muscle contraction parameter used for improved standardization of results. This detail is useful for those seeking to establish their own clinical testing or research. Figs 2 and 3 illustrate the significant difference in response that can be found using tone burst or click stimulation. Conclusions are well supported by data and analysis. Thus, the value of this article lies in further establishing that the methodology used for VEMP testing and its

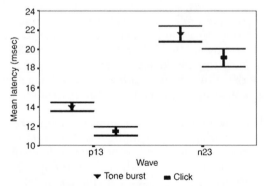

FIGURE 2.—Error bar comparing the mean and standard deviation of P13 and N23 latency of short duration tone burst and click stimuli. (Reprinted from Kumar K, Sinha SK, Bharti AK, et al. Comparison of vestibular evoked myogenic potentials elicited by click and short duration tone burst stimuli. *J Laryngol Otol.* 2011;125:343-347, with permission of Cambridge University Press.)

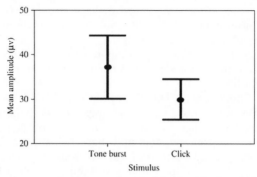

FIGURE 3.—Error bar comparing the mean and standard deviation of peak to peak amplitude (P13-N23) of VEMP evoked by short duration tone burst and click. (Reprinted from Kumar K, Sinha SK, Bharti AK, et al. Comparison of vestibular evoked myogenic potentials elicited by click and short duration tone burst stimuli. *J Laryngol Otol.* 2011;125:343-347, with permission of Cambridge University Press.)

standardization are extremely important in establishing the presence of clinical disease.

B. J. Balough, Capt, MC, USN

External Ear, Middle Ear and Mastoid

Isolated itching of external auditory canal: clinicopathological study with immunohistochemical determination of antimicrobial peptides

Acar B, Simsek GG, Oguztuzun S, et al (Kecioren Training and Res Hosp, Ankara; Kırıkkale Univ, Turkey)

J Laryngol Otol 125:227-230, 2011

Objective.—This study aimed to demonstrate the histological and immunohistological features of skin biopsy specimens from patients complaining of isolated itching of the external auditory canal.

Materials and Methods.—A prospective, case—control study was performed of 24 patients undergoing evaluation for contact dermatitis of the external auditory canal, and 24 controls. Skin biopsies were examined histologically by a single, blinded dermatopathologist, using light microscopy, to determine histopathological characteristics. The immunohistological presence of the antimicrobial peptides human β-defensin-3 and LL-37 cathelicidin was also assessed. Findings for patients and controls were compared.

Results.—There was a statistically significant difference in the degree of inflammation, comparing patients and controls ($p < 0.05$). There was no significant difference in the presence of spongiotic changes, comparing patients and controls ($p > 0.05$). Furthermore, the patients' skin biopsies did not show pronounced expression of human β-defensin-3 or LL-37 cathelicidin.

Conclusion.—Histological and immunohistological examination of skin biopsies from cases of isolated itching of the external auditory canal did not support a diagnosis of dermatitis.

▶ Recurrent or chronic external canal itch is a common presenting complaint to the otolaryngologist. In this study the authors use immunologic stains in an attempt to elucidate the underlying mechanism for this problem. The design, although simple, is well done and the methodology is solid. The authors focus on a series of peptides that, in addition to antimicrobial activity, also stimulate the immune system. This is explained in the introduction and further detailed in the discussion. Although no significance was found from the immunochemistry, the histology revealed an interesting, if unexpected, result—that of increased lymphocytes. As they discuss, the common thought for external canal pruritus is that it is an allergic dermatitis. However, no evidence of this was seen for this. Instead the presence of lymphocytes suggests a resolving infectious cause rather than an acute inflammatory process. As interesting as this may be, it is important to keep in mind that even in the affected group, this was only seen in 37% of the subjects. This may have been because of the prolonged nature of the symptoms with resolution of the peptide and cellular changes. Thus, the cause of external canal pruritus remains a mystery.

B. J. Balough, Capt, MC, USN

Role of mitomycin C in reducing keloid recurrence: patient series and literature review
Gupta M, Narang T (Gian Sagar Med College and Hosp, Punjab, India)
J Laryngol Otol 125:297-300, 2011

Objective.—To study the role of mitomycin C in reducing keloid recurrence.
Study Design.—Prospective, randomised, controlled trial.
Setting.—Tertiary care referral centre.
Patients.—Case series of 20 patients presenting with 26 pinna swellings, mostly following ear piercing.
Interventions.—We used the technique of surgical shave excision combined with topical application of mitomycin C and secondary wound healing, in all 26 pinnae.
Results.—Patients were followed up six to 24 months post-operatively. No recurrences were noted during this period.
Conclusion.—Keloids are fibrotic lesions resulting from abnormal wound healing. The uncontrolled proliferation of normal tissue healing processes results in scarring that enlarges well beyond the original wound margins. Successful treatment of keloids remains a challenge because this disease process has a high propensity for recurrence. Various therapies have previously been reported, and success rates are highly variable. We believe that

shave excision followed by topical mitomycin C application is a promising treatment option for the management of pinna keloids.

▶ Auricular keloids are common, and a wide variety of surgical and nonsurgical treatment methods have been described. Most publications on the topic are short case series with limited objective criteria for success. When multiple options are available, none are clearly superior, each variably lacking in efficacy, simplicity, or some other factor. The method described in this article addresses several of these issues. First, it is a prospective study with an impartial observer grading the results using an objective scale. Second, the method is a simple excision followed by straightforward application of mitomycin C, which in most centers is readily available. Third, as demonstrated in their results, the outcomes are uniformly good to excellent and appear stable 2 years after treatment. There is a good description of the technique used, including duration and concentration of mitomycin C used. There are 2 minor criticisms. The article is listed in the abstract as prospective and randomized; from the methods described, however, it isn't, as there is no control group, nor is there a control in the results. Second, the length of follow-up varies from 6 to 24 months. It does not appear that the longer follow-up leads to poorer results from the data presented. However, the numbers are small, so this may be a consideration. These are minor limitations, though, for what seems to be an elegant and simple method for addressing a difficult problem.

B. J. Balough, Capt, MC, USN

To Pack or Not to Pack? A Contemporary Review of Middle Ear Packing Agents
Shen Y, Teh BM, Friedland PL, et al (The Univ of Western Australia, Perth, Australia)
Laryngoscope 121:1040-1048, 2011

Middle ear packing agents are used in otologic surgery to provide support to the middle ear structures, maintain aeration of the middle ear,

TABLE 1.—Comparison Between Nonabsorbable and Absorbable Middle Ear Packing Agents

Categories	Advantages	Disadvantages	Examples	References
Nonabsorbable MEPAs	Less adhesion and fibrosis; well tolerated	Nonabsorbable; need for a second stage surgery for removal	Silicone products	19—25
			Paraffin	15,16
			Teflon	17
			Polyethylene	17,18
Absorbable MEPAs	Absorbable; no revision surgery for removal required	Some cause fibrosis; insufficient support; generally more expensive; relatively limited availability for some	Gelfoam	8,13,38,50,51
			Gelfilm	6,22,25,57
			Sepragel	53,87
			Seprafilm	11,101
			Merogel	11,54,95

MEPAs = middle ear packing agents.
Editor's Note: Please refer to original journal article for full references.

TABLE 2.—Absorbable Middle Ear Packing Agents

Trade Name	Components	Company	Special Features	Advantages	Disadvantages	References
Gelfoam	Purified porcine skin gelatin	Pharmacia and Upjohn Company, Kalamazoo, MI	Porous sponge/foam	Nontoxicity; nonantigenicity; hemostasis; availability; ease of handling	Adhesion; fibrosis; packing retention; osteoneogenesis	8,13,38,50,51,87
Gelfilm	Purified porcine skin gelatin	Upjohn, Kalamazoo, MI	Thin and transparent; nonporous; cellophane-like sheet/film	Biocompatible; less fibrosis	Rapid absorption; nonexpandable; stiff	6,22,25,57
Carbylan-SX	HA-DTPH-PEGDA	Sentrx Surgical, Inc., Salt Lake City, UT	In situ cross-linked HA; injectable; synthetic	Biocompatible; minimal adhesions; easy to insert	No clinical trials	95,96
Sepragel	HA and CMC	Genzyme Biosurgery Corp., Ridgefield, NJ	Cross-linked HA; injectable; viscoelastic; gel	Biocompatible; nonototoxic; prevent adhesions; easy application; sufficient support	No clinical trials	53, 87
Seprafilm	HA and CMC	Genzyme Corp., Cambridge, MA	Cross-linked HA; film	Biocompatible; nonototoxic; nonimmunogenic; prevent adhesions; easy application	Limited clinical trials	11, 101
Hyaluronic acid foam	HA	Genzyme Corp., Cambridge, MA	Esterified HA; foam	Biocompatible; hemostasis; easy application	Limited clinical trials	9, 79
Merogel	HA	Medtronic Xomed Inc., Jacksonville, FL	Esterified HA; foam	Biocompatible; nonototoxic; expandability; easy application; easily expelled	Difficult to trim; no clinical trials	11, 54, 95
Stammberger Sinu-Foam	CMC	ArthroCare Corp., Sunnyvale, CA	Cellulose; foam	Minimal adhesions; excellent hemostasis	Potential ototoxicity (sensorineural hearing loss)	112
Interceed	ORC	TC7, Johnson and Johnson Medical Inc., Arlington, TX	Cellulose; homologue of Surgicel	Prevent adhesions; biocompatible; nonototoxic	No clinical trials	111
Polylactide	L80/G20 polylacticglycolic acid	W. Lorenz Surgical, Inc., Jacksonville, FL /Bionx, Ltd., Tampere, Finland	Polylactide; L-shaped form or straight cut	Biocompatible; temporary	No clinical trials	109

(Continued)

TABLE 2.—(*Continued*)

Trade Name	Components	Company	Special Features	Advantages	Disadvantages	References
Fibroquel	CPVP	Aspid, S.A. de C.V., DF, Mexico	CPVP sponge	Less chronic inflammatory responses	No clinical trials	110
Nasopore	Synthetic polyurethane	Polyganics, Groningen, The Netherlands	Fragmentable; nasal dressing	Biocompatible; easy application	Poor expandability; tendency to remain; no clinical trials	53

HA-DTPH-PEGDA = hyaluronic acid-3,3-dithiobis/propanoic hydrazide-polyethylene glycoldiacrylate; HA = hyaluronic acid; CMC = carboxymethylcellulose; ORC = oxidized regenerated cellulose; CPVP = collagen-polyvinylpyrrolidone.
Editor's Note: Please refer to original journal article for full references.

and promote hemostasis. However, there is currently a lack of standardization regarding the use of different types of packing agents. The choice of materials and how they are used remain controversial. In fact, some have recently advocated for no packing. In view of this, this review focuses on the types of materials available, a brief historical account of each material, characteristics of an ideal packing agent, and a discussion on the techniques of insertion to optimize surgical outcomes (Tables 1 and 2).

▶ This article provides an overview of middle ear packing materials and attempts to provide a classification scheme. This classification system is found in Table 1 and is further expanded in Table 2 where the manufacturer, materials, advantages, limitations, and references are listed. This provides a comprehensive listing and serves as an excellent reference. The classification scheme is useful, particularly the very interesting theme throughout the article that no agent was specifically developed for middle ear use. Rather, all have been "borrowed" from other surgical fields (ie, Gelfoam from neurosurgery) or other aspects of otolaryngology and, in particular, rhinology. As a result, no agent provides the perfect middle ear packing material combining stability, quick absorption, and lack of reactivity. Given the large number of otologic procedures performed and potentially large market, it is interesting that no agent has been specifically developed for the ear. The authors list their criteria for an ideal material but also question the need for packing through innovation in technique. This is an interesting discussion and concludes an outstanding article that is an important read.

B. J. Balough, Capt, MC, USN

Contributing Factors in the Pathogenesis of Acquired Cholesteatoma: Size Analysis Based on MDCT

Yamashita K, Yoshiura T, Hiwatashi A, et al (Kyushu Univ, Fukuoka, Japan)
AJR Am J Roentgenol 196:1172-1175, 2011

Objective.—The purpose of this article is to explore the factors that contribute to the occurrence of cholesteatoma. We studied the size of the mastoid air cells and the tympanic cavity using high-resolution CT.

Materials and Methods.—Temporal bone CT scans of consecutive patients with unilateral cholesteatoma and healthy control subjects were retrospectively analyzed. We compared the total volume and the greatest cross-sectional area of the cavities of the combined mastoid air cells and tympanic cavity between the affected and unaffected sides in patients with cholesteatoma and in the control subjects. We also compared separately the measured volumes of the cavities of the mastoid air cells and tympanic cavity between the unaffected side of the patients with cholesteatoma and the control subjects.

Results.—One hundred temporal bones of 50 patients with cholesteatoma and 50 control subjects were included. Both the volume and the cross-sectional area of the cavities of the combined mastoid air cells and tympanic cavity in the affected side of the patients with cholesteatoma were significantly smaller than those in the unaffected side ($p < 0.001$). Moreover, both the volume and the cross-sectional area of the cavities of the combined mastoid air cells and tympanic cavity in both affected and unaffected sides of patients with cholesteatoma were significantly smaller than those in control subjects ($p < 0.001$). The volume of the cavities of the mastoid air cells in the unaffected side of patients with cholesteatoma was smaller than that of the control subjects ($p < 0.001$). In contrast, no significant difference was found in the tympanic cavity volume between the unaffected side and the control subjects.

Conclusion.—Our results were consistent with the hypothesized contribution of mastoid air cell underdevelopment to the occurrence of cholesteatoma. A small tympanic cavity is less likely to contribute to the occurrence of cholesteatoma.

▶ This is a straightforward article that provides evidence to support what is commonly encountered in surgery for chronic ear disease and cholesteatoma. Namely, those ears with cholesteatoma have a very constricted mastoid with limited aeration. In performing volumetric analysis, affected ears have one-half the volume of the contralateral unaffected side and are one-quarter the size of those of the control group. The implications are simply stated — if a mastoid cavity needs to be created in the diseased group, it should be very small provided a minimum of normal healthy bone is removed. Often, just the epitympanum and limited air cells beyond the antrum are found and need to be exteriorized without drilling to the sinodural angle and removal of the mastoid tip. Given the information from this data set, that on average should be 1.50 cm^3 and at most 3 cm^3. Thus, the greatest size is less than the average (4.74 cm^3) of the nonaffected side as well as less than the smallest of the control group (3 cm^3). Thus, even with wall-down procedures, a small cavity that is dry and self cleaning can be expected if properly performed. Conversely, in normal ears that do not develop cholesteatoma but where disease is implanted or for some other reason a wall-down cavity is created, a large cavity can be expected. It is in these ears where the most problems occur and, thus, a wall-down cavity is best avoided whenever possible in these situations. Despite these data, no comment can be made if the small mastoid size creates the cholesteatoma or if the cholesteatoma inhibits the aeration of the mastoid. While the data are suggestive, further studies of mastoid development need to be done.

B. J. Balough, Capt, MC, USN

Surgical management of troublesome mastoid cavities
Yung M, Tassone P, Moumoulidis I, et al (The Ipswich Hosp NHS Trust, UK)
J Laryngol Otol 125:221-226, 2011

Objective.—To examine the reasons for discharging mastoid cavities, the operative findings during revision surgery, and the medium-term outcome.

Patients.—One hundred and forty revision mastoidectomies in 131 patients were studied. Post-operatively, patients were followed up at three, six and 12 months and then yearly.

Intervention.—A variety of techniques were performed. Over 80 per cent of ears were treated with mastoid obliteration. Concomitant hearing restorative procedures were carried out in one-third of the ears.

Results.—The mastoid cavities were troublesome because of large cavity size, bony overhang, residual infected mastoid cells, the presence of cholesteatoma or perforations, and/or inadequate meatoplasty. One year after revision mastoidectomy, over 95 per cent of the ears had become completely dry and water-resistant. Overall, 50.9 per cent of the ears had a 12-month post-operative air—bone gap of 20dB or less.

Conclusion.—Revision mastoidectomy has a high success rate in converting troublesome mastoid cavities into dry, water-resistant ears (Tables 5 and 8).

▶ For more than 40 years, the principles of surgery to resolve chronic ear problems have remained the same: to create a safe ear, a dry ear, and an ear that permits hearing restoration. To achieve these ends, the canal wall down mastoidectomy remains a common option for treatment. However, in some cases, this results in an ear with chronic problems. This article represents a marvelous summary of 20 years of experience in dealing with these "difficult" cavities, and it is all the more enhanced by the inclusion of data from regular long-term follow-up (yearly visits with some 82% of cases still available at 5 years). As the senior author relates, these patients are more often than not revisions from primary surgery conducted elsewhere, in patients dissatisfied with the earlier work. In my own practice, the best way to avoid these cavities is to ensure that a minimum of healthy bone is removed as necessary to achieve the smallest cavity that will exteriorize the disease. For those presenting with large and draining cavities, the results presented in Table 5 are truly outstanding. Other tables provide data on the reasons for primary surgical failure and defects encountered during revision surgery. Table 8 compares the data from this series with that of prior series on the subject and provides other valuable references. The primary techniques

TABLE 5.—Ears With Successful Revision Mastoid Surgery, Assessed 6, 12 and 36 Mths Post-op

Parameter of Success	Ears (n (%))		
	6 Mth*	2 Mth[†]	36 Mth[‡]
Dry ear	129 (95)	123 (98)	100 (98)
Intact tympanic membrane	135 (99)	124 (99)	101 (99)
Water resistance	N/A	119 (95)	N/A
No post-op hearing deterioration	N/A	111 (88)	N/A

Not all ears from the original cohort of 140 cases were available for follow-up assessments at six, 12 and 36 months.
*$n = 136$.
[†]$n = 125$.
[‡]$n = 102$. Mth = months; post-op = post-operative; N/A = data not available.

TABLE 8.—Published Studies on Revision Mastoidectomy Outcomes

Study	Case Mix*	Cases (n)	Intervention	FU Period	Outcomes			Hearing Results	Comments
					Dry Ear (%)	Perf (%)	Chol (%)		
Veldman & Braunius[9]	ICW & CWD	348	Tympano ± mastoid ICW or CWD	1–14 yr	90	10	5	62.7% had AC ≤30 dB	Hearing results recalculated by present authors Some ears had >1 op
Sheehy & Robinson[10]	ICW	307 ops in 272 ears	Tympano ± mastoid ICW or CWD	4 mth to 5 yr	NA	NA	NA	80% had ABG ≤20 dB at 1 yr	
Nadol[11]	ICW & CWD	48	CWD ± oblit	1–6 yr	85	NA	NA	NA	
Mills[12]	CWD	54	CWD ± meatoplasty	1–19 yr	59	NA	NA	NA	
Filipo & Maurizio[13]	CWD	24	CWD†	1–2 yr	NA	NA	NA	33% had ABG ≤15 dB; 71% had ABG ≤25 dB	Hearing results included 2-stage tympano
Bercin et al.[14]	ICW & CWD	35	ICW or CWD	3–25 mth	83‡	‡	‡	NA	
Present	Troublesome CWD cavities	140	CWD ± oblit	1, 3 & 5 yr cut-offs	98**	1**	3.7§	50.9% had ABG ≤20 dB at 1 yr	Cut-off analysis for each outcome parameter

FU = follow-up; perf = perforation; chol = cholesteatoma; ICW = intact canal wall procedure; CWD = canal wall down procedure; tympano = tympanoplasty; mastoid = mastoidectomy; AC = air conduction threshold; op = operation; mth = months; NA = data not available; ABG = air-bone gap; oblit = obliteration.
*Previous mastoid surgery.
†With concomitant canal wall reconstruction or obliteration.
‡29/35 dry ears with no cholesteatoma.
**At 1 year.
§At 5 years.

used to achieve these results are detailed in the references and are useful in reducing the overall size of the cavity.[1,2]

B. J. Balough, Capt, MC, USN

References

1. Yung MW. The use of hydroxyapatite granules in mastoid obliteration. *Clin Otolaryngol Allied Sci.* 1996;21:480-484.
2. Yung M, Smith P. Mid-temporal pericranial and inferiorly based periosteal flaps in mastoid obliteration. *Otolaryngol Head Neck Surg.* 2007;137:906-912.

Total Ossiculoplasty in Children: Predictive Factors and Long-Term Follow-up
Nevoux J, Moya-Plana A, Chauvin P, et al (Univ Paris 6, France; Saint Antoine Hosp, Paris, France)
Arch Otolaryngol Head Neck Surg 137:1240-1246, 2011

Objective.—To evaluate the long-term results and predictive factors of a good outcome with the use of a total ossicular replacement prosthesis in children.

Design.—Retrospective case review.

Setting.—Tertiary referral center.

Patients.—The study included 114 children (116 ears).

Interventions.—A total of 116 ears underwent total ossicular chain reconstruction with a titanium prosthesis. Cartilage was always used for tympanic membrane reconstruction.

Main Outcome Measures.—Audiological results were evaluated according to the guidelines of the American Academy of Otolaryngology—Head and Neck Surgery. Predictive factors of audiological results were determined. Logistic regression and χ^2 tests were used for statistical analysis.

Results.—The mean age at surgery was 9.8 years. Ossiculoplasty was performed during second-look surgery in 91 ears (78.4%) and during another stage in 25 ears (21.6%). The first-stage procedure was always performed for cholesteatoma. Audiometric results were available for 116 ears at 1 year, for 89 ears (76.7%) at 2 years, and for 42 ears (36.2%) at 5 years. Closure of the average air-bone gap (ABG) to within 20 dB was achieved in 65 ears (56%) at 1 year. The mean (SD) preoperative and postoperative (at 1 year) ABGs were 41.0 (9.5) dB and 22.4 (12.6) dB, respectively. There were no cases of extrusion, but 17 luxations of the prosthesis were confirmed by computed tomography. Luxation occurred on average at 31.4 months. Only three 4000-Hz degradations of bone conduction were reported, with no dead ears. We examined 3 predictive factors of auditory results: preoperative ABG, footplate status, and postoperative otoscopic findings.

Conclusions.—Total ossiculoplasty is a reliable technique in children. Long-term hearing outcomes are stable and satisfactory, but luxation

TABLE 4.—Review of Pediatric Ossiculoplasty Literature[a]

Variable	Murphy,[11] 2000 (n=55)	Michael et al,[12] 2008 (n=14)	Quesnel et al,[13] 2010 (n=74)	Present Study (n=116)
TORP/PORP	27/28	5/9	47/27	116/0
Age, y	9.3	11	11.3	9.8
COM, %	80	79	88	100
Type of surgery, %	Primary, 71 Revision, 29	Primary, 50 Revision, 50	Primary, 50 Revision, 50	Revision, 100
Type of prosthesis, %	Xomed Brackmann Plasti-pore Richard Black hydroxyapatite	Kurtz titanium, 100	Vario Kurtz titanium, 100	Medtronic Xomed titanium, 52 Spiggle & Theis titanium, 48
Extrusions, No.	2/27	Unknown	2/27	0
Displacements, No.	Unknown	Unknown	5/47 and 2/27	17
Preoperative ABG, dB	TORP, 40.1 PORP, 29.7	TORP, 32.0 PORP, 27.7	TORP, 36.6 PORP, 30.2	TORP, 41.0
Postoperative ABG, dB	TORP, 31.6 PORP, 22.5	TORP, 17.2 PORP, 15.8	TORP, 22.0 PORP, 20.8	TORP, 22.4
Good results, %	TORP, 19 PORP, 43	TORP, 80 PORP, 78	TORP, 51.1 PORP, 53.8	TORP, 56
Sensorineural hearing loss, No.	Unknown	1	1	3
Follow-up, mo	12	12	30	34

Abbreviations: ABG, air-bone gap; COM, chronic otitis media; PORP, partial ossicular replacement prosthesis; TORP, total ossicular replacement prosthesis.
Editor's Note: Please refer to original journal article for full references.
[a]The patients in all studies were children.

can occur at any time. Preoperative ABG and footplate status are negative predictive factors of auditory results (Table 4).

▶ This study provides a large retrospective series on total ossicular reconstruction in children using a single technique and prosthesis type. Their overall excellent (< 10 dB) and good (< 20 dB) results at 51% are similar to other published studies, which are presented in Table 4. Although not stated in the abstract, the authors examined an exhaustive list of preoperative, intraoperative, and postoperative factors to determine which, if any, might have an impact on hearing results. These included age, preoperative air-bone gap, otoscopy, number of prior surgeries, reason for surgery (preoperative); footplate status, tensor tendon, malleus status, experience of surgeon, middle ear inflammation, type of prosthesis, percentage of TM replaced by cartilage (intraoperative); hearing result, effusion, otoscopy, and CT findings (postoperative). Of this list, only 3 factors were found to be predictive. Just as interesting are those that were found not to be predictive, including the experience of the surgeon, number of prior surgeries, malleus status, and middle ear inflammation, among others. The authors discuss one of these, surgical experience, and suggest it was not a predictive factor because of the training in the use of a single uniform technique that all surgeons received. The lack of significance to the malleus status should not be surprising because in their method, a columnella technique, the malleus is not used in the reconstruction. Of the 3 predictive factors, the preoperative air-bone gap is a bit counterintuitive. One would think that a larger gap could be more readily closed. However, their results suggest that the gap may have more factors than the ossicular chain alone. A fair discussion and results are provided on failures. No analysis was provided on the predictive factors and these failures. The number of failures, however, was small, and thus this analysis may not have had sufficient power to be performed. However, this omission in their discussion limits an otherwise fine article on the topic. The literature review serves as a good reference. Given the sample size, references provided, and the fact that the results of this study are similar, this article is a useful read and valuable single reference on the topic.

B. J. Balough, Capt, MC, USN

Facial Nerve and Skull Base

Facial Nerve Decompression Surgery in Patients With Temporal Bone Trauma: Analysis of 66 Cases

Hato N, Nota J, Hakuba N, et al (Ehime Univ School of Medicine, Japan)
J Trauma 71:1789-1793, 2011

Background.—In the treatment of facial nerve paralysis after temporal bone trauma, it is important to appropriately determine whether nerve decompression surgery is indicated. The aim of this study was to examine the efficacy of facial nerve decompression surgery according to fracture location and the ideal time for surgery after trauma by analyzing the therapeutic outcome of traumatic facial nerve paralysis.

Methods.—In total, 66 patients with facial nerve paralysis after temporal bone trauma who were treated at our institution between 1979 and 2009 were studied retrospectively. The patients were divided into five subgroups, according to the fracture location and the period of time between trauma and surgery.

Results.—The number of patients who achieved complete recovery of House-Brackmann (H-B) grade 1 was 31 of 66 (47.0%). There was no difference in therapeutic outcomes among the subgroups classified by fracture location. The rate of good recovery to H-B grade 1 or 2 in patients undergoing decompression surgery within 2 weeks after trauma reached 92.9%, resulting in a significantly better outcome than that of patients undergoing later decompression surgery ($p < 0.01$).

Conclusions.—The results of this study demonstrated that the ideal time for decompression surgery for facial nerve paralysis after temporal bone fracture was the first 2 weeks after trauma in patients with severe, immediate-onset paralysis. Our study also showed that surgery should be performed within 2 months at the latest. These findings provide useful information for patients and help to determine the priority of treatment when concomitant disease exists.

▶ Location, timing, and outcome are important factors to consider in any traumatic injury in which surgical intervention is considered. Nowhere is this more important than with the facial nerve, where poor outcome can be devastating for the patient and extremely difficult to satisfactorily rehabilitate. Furthermore, complete surgical decompression can be a challenging operation with significant risk requiring experience and confidence to be adequately performed. Thus, with many favorable outcomes from observation alone, surgical intervention needs to be carefully studied so that only those standing to receive benefit are subjected to the risk. Similar debate surrounded surgical management of Bell palsy until the excellent study by Gantz.[1] This is provided as a reference, as the pathophysiology is similar in traumatic injury and the concepts are similar.

For traumatic injuries, this article addresses many of those issues of location, timing, and outcome and thus is a very important read for this year. It is interesting that they included House-Brackmann grades 4 and 5 paresis as well as grade 6 paralyses in their surgical cases. Typically, only complete paralysis is considered for surgical intervention. While the authors were surprised that tympanic segment injuries did more poorly than other locations, this makes sense, as this location is a watershed area between the intracranial-extracranial vascularization of the nerve. Thus, this location is much more likely to be susceptible to vascular compromise and variable results depending on individual vascular differences. Lastly, there is an excellent editorial comment at the conclusion of the article, which reinforces the value and impact of this selection.

B. J. Balough, Capt, MC, USN

Reference

1. Gantz BJ, Rubinstein JT, Gidley P, Woodworth GG. Surgical management of Bell's palsy. *Laryngoscope.* 1999;109:1177-1188.

Treatment of Facial Paralysis: Dynamic Reanimation of Spontaneous Facial Expression—Apropos of 655 Patients

Gousheh J, Arasteh E (Shahid Beheshti Univ of Med Sciences, Tehran, Iran)
Plast Reconstr Surg 128:693e-703e, 2011

Background.—Six hundred fifty-five cases of unilateral facial paralysis were treated by different surgical methods to achieve dynamic reanimation of facial muscle movement. In a retrospective study, the recovery of both truly spontaneous smile and facial muscle movement was evaluated independently.

Methods.—The authors performed 505 two-stage gracilis, one rectus abdominis, and 14 single-stage latissimus dorsi microneurovascular muscle transfers, in addition to 28 cross-facial facial nerve neurotization procedures. These procedures were based on neurotization of the paralyzed region by the contralateral healthy facial nerve. Procedures involving motor nerves or muscle beyond the territory of the facial nerve included 73 temporalis muscle transpositions, four lengthening temporalis myoplasty procedures, 26 neurotizations by the hypoglossal nerve, and four neurotizations by the spinal accessory nerve.

Results.—Patients treated by techniques based on the motor function of nerves other than the facial nerve did not recover spontaneous smile. Neurotization by the facial nerve, however, did result in the recovery of spontaneous smile in all satisfactory or better outcomes. Recovery of lip commissure movement based on neurotization by the contralateral healthy facial nerve was better than that of the remaining groups ($p < 0.0001$).

Conclusions.—Temporalis muscle transposition and lengthening myoplasty are acceptable options for patients who are not good candidates for neurotization by the facial nerve. For the restoration of both truly spontaneous smile and facial muscle movement, free microneurovascular muscle transfer neurotized by the contralateral healthy facial nerve has become the authors' first-choice surgical technique.

Clinical Question/Level of Evidence.—Therapeutic, IV (Table 5).

▶ Whether from tumor or trauma, a paralyzed face can be devastating for a patient and a challenging reconstruction for the surgeon. Simple static and cable grafting methods can provide tone and some voluntary motion but do little to restore the dynamic spontaneous facial expressions of emotional response. Previous commentaries have detailed the emotional impact of this disability on patients even after surgically "successful" reconstruction. The lower face in particular is difficult to rehabilitate to normal or near normal function. This excellent article provides a 20-year series on more than 600 cases treated by different methods. The vast majority underwent a 2-stage free muscle transfer procedure in an effort by the authors to push this boundary and provide a more natural facial restoration. The specifics of the procedure are well detailed, as is that of grading the results. Age at time of surgery did not affect the results, with similar outcomes for all age groups. Ninety percent of this group achieved excellent (no asymmetry at rest and more than 2-cm movement at lateral commissure) or good results

TABLE 5.—Final Results of Different Surgical Techniques

	No. of Patients	Excellent (%)	Good (%)	Satisfactory (%)	Bad/Failed (%)	Involuntary Truly Spontaneous Smile Satisfactory or Better (%)
Gracilis muscle transfer	505	71 (14)	384 (76)	40 (8)	10 (2)	495/495 (100)*
Rectus abdominis muscle transfer	1	—	1 (100)	—	—	1/1 (100)*
Latissimus dorsi muscle transfer	14	—	12 (86)	2 (14)	—	14/14 (100)*
Cross-facial grafting	28	—	10 (36)	16 (57)	2 (7)	26/26 (100)*
Temporalis muscle transfer	73	—	22 (30)	43 (59)	8 (11)	0/65 (0)†
Lengthening temporalis myoplasty	4	—	—	4 (100)	—	0/4 (0)†
Neurotization by hypoglossal nerve	26	—	15 (58)	11 (42)	—	0/26 (0)†
Neurotization by spinal accessory nerve	4	—	1 (25)	3 (75)	—	0/4 (0)†

*Neurotization by contralateral facial nerve.
†Motor nerve beyond the territory of the facial nerve.

(mild asymmetry and 1.5- to 2.0-cm movement), and all but the 10 patients (2%) who failed reconstruction regained spontaneous emotional smile expression. The discussion provides the authors' personal journey through the various other methods of facial reanimation, the limitations of each, and how this became their standard. Those results can be found in Table 5, and it is the lack of spontaneous smile that separates the techniques from adequate to better. This discussion is thoughtful and well done and provides an excellent framework for conceptualizing what an excellent result can and should be for this difficult problem. It is only the technical difficulty involved that has limited wider adoption of this as the standard reconstructive option. Articles such as this may help to change that status quo.

B. J. Balough, Capt, MC, USN

Evoked Potential Monitoring Identifies Possible Neurological Injury During Positioning for Craniotomy

Anastasian ZH, Ramnath B, Komotar RJ, et al (Columbia Univ, NY)
Anesth Analg 109:817-821, 2009

Somatosensory-evoked potential (SSEP) monitoring is commonly used to detect changes in nerve conduction and prevent impending nerve injury. We present a case series of two patients who had SSEP monitoring for their surgical craniotomy procedure, and who, upon positioning supine with their head tilted 30°−45°, developed unilateral upper extremity SSEP changes. These SSEP changes were reversed when the patients were repositioned. These cases indicate the clinical usefulness of monitoring SSEPs while positioning the patient and adjusting position accordingly to prevent injury.

▶ Borrowing from lessons learned in aviation to reduce mishaps, surgical care continues to develop a team approach in the operating room to eliminate mistakes and prevent accidents. Prevention of positioning injuries is an excellent example of this team approach in which anesthesia, nursing, and surgeons work collaboratively. This article introduces a new member to that team: the nerve-monitoring technician. In aviation, for crew coordination to be successful, each team member must be willing and able to call attention to potential problems. More importantly, the other team members must be willing to listen, and change their actions based on the information. Thus, to be effective here, the monitoring technician must understand that his or her role begins at the time of positioning, and the other surgical team members must ask for confirmation that monitoring is intact and symmetric before positioning can be considered complete. It is important to note that after repositioning to reverse the monitoring changes, no adverse impact was made regarding the surgical approach. Thus, extremes for positioning—while the surgeon may feel they are necessary—may not in fact add anything to improve exposure. The authors provide a very good review on the topic for a variety of procedures, including their own retrospective data. While their practice is to monitor somatosensory-evoked potentials for all lateral skull base procedures, this is certainly not the universal standard. Certainly, based on this article, it can be considered in high-risk cases, where positioning injury may be more likely and caught early.

B. J. Balough, Capt, MC, USN

Endolympathic hydrops in patients with vestibular schwannoma: visualization by non-contrast-enhanced 3D FLAIR

Naganawa S, Kawai H, Sone M, et al (Nagoya Univ Graduate School of Medicine, Japan; et al)

Neuroradiology 53:1009-1015, 2011

Introduction.—Signal intensity of ipsilateral labyrinthine lymph fluid has been reported to increase in most cases with vestibular schwannoma (VS) on 3D fluid attenuated inversion recovery (FLAIR). The purpose of this study was twofold, (1) to evaluate if endolymphatic space can be recognized in the patients with VS on non-contrast-enhanced 3D-FLAIR images and (2) to know if the vertigo in the patients with VS correlates to vestibular endolymphatic hydrops.

Methods.—From the introduction of 32-channel head coil at 3 T in May 2008 to June 2010, 15 cases with unilateral VS were identified in the radiology report database. The two cases without a significant signal increase on 3D FLAIR were excluded. Resting 13 cases were retrospectively analyzed in regard to the recognition of endolymphatic hydrops in the cochlea and vestibule and to the correlation between the patients' symptoms and endolymphatic hydrops.

Results.—In all cases, vestibular endolymphatic space can be recognized on non-contrast-enhanced 3D FLAIR. Cochlear endolymphatic space can be identified only in one case with significant hydrops. Vestibular hydrops was identified in four cases. Among these four cases, three had vertigo, and one had no vertigo. In those nine cases without hydrops, two had vertigo, and seven did not have vertigo. No significant correlation between vertigo and vestibular hydrops was found.

Conclusions.—Vestibular endolymphatic space can be recognized on non-contrast-enhanced 3D FLAIR. In some patients with VS, vestibular hydrops is seen; however, endolymphatic hydrops in the vestibule might not be the only responsible cause of vertigo in the patients with VS.

▶ The premise of this study is that in some patients, the symptoms of vestibular schwannoma hearing loss, tinnitus, and vertigo may mimic those of endolymphatic hydrops. While on the surface this may be true, very few, if any, patients with vestibular schwannoma have the fluctuating symptoms characteristic of Meniere disease. Thus, it was not for this that the article has been selected for review. Rather, it is to highlight the advances in magnetic resonance imaging and the discussion of the nuances of the various imaging sequences that are often limited in their understanding by otolaryngologists but can add great diagnostic value. Here the 3D fluid inversion recovery sequence is used to examine the endolymphatic space in vivo. This sequence is more sensitive to fluid changes than typical T1 images. This is explained in the introduction and methodology sections of the article. Transtympanic contrast injection can yield similar images, but the method described avoids the need for contrast. Certainly, a method of confirming the anatomic presence of endolymphatic hydrops that avoids invasive injection would be preferable. However, this detail of imaging was obtained on a 3 Tesla magnet; currently that strength is not widely available. However, as technology improves understanding, the abilities of advanced imaging and its role in diagnosis of difficult patients will become increasingly important.

B. J. Balough, Capt, MC, USN

Prediction of Vestibular Schwannoma Growth: A Novel Rule Based on Clinical Symptomatology
Timmer FCA, Artz JCJM, Beynon AJ, et al (Radboud Univ Nijmegen Med Ctr, the Netherlands)
Ann Otol Rhinol Laryngol 120:807-813, 2011

Objectives.—The aim of this study was to formulate a predictive rule for vestibular schwannoma growth during the initial observation period after diagnosis.

Methods.—Logistic regression models were fitted, with tumor growth in the first year as the dependent variable and patient characteristics as the independent variables. Backward selection was used to eliminate superfluous predictors. The area under the receiver operating characteristic curve was taken as a measure of the model's discriminative power.

Results.—Eventually, the model or rule consisted of 4 significant growth predictors: localization (if extrameatal, +1; if intrameatal, 0), sudden sensorineural hearing loss (if present, −1; if absent, 0), balance symptoms (if present, +1; if absent, 0), and complaints of hearing loss for less than 2 years (if present, +1; if absent, or present for more than 2 years, 0). A higher score indicates a higher likelihood of tumor growth during the period of observation after diagnosis. If the total score is 0 or less, the likelihood of tumor growth during the first year after diagnosis is less than 10%. If the score is 3, the likelihood of growth during the first year after diagnosis is more than 70%.

Conclusions.—We were able to create a useful rule to predict vestibular schwannoma growth during the first year after diagnosis.

▶ Having a crystal ball to enable prediction of the future would make medical practice far easier. Knowing which patients will continue to do well without treatment and those who will progress is nowhere more important than in vestibular schwanommas, where many fail to grow and remain indolent with minimal symptoms, while others progress. In this article, the authors attempt to provide us with just such a crystal ball using a series of 240 patients to provide a predictive model based on several characteristics. Importantly, they set out to provide such a predictive rule at the moment of diagnosis, which is when it will be of most use. In addition to tumor size and location at presentation, some 44 other symptoms and audiologic and vestibular tests were used as detailed in their methods for a comprehensive approach. Eventually, 4 factors were found to provide the best combination of predictability and reliability. Fig 2 in the original article illustrates these factors, the scores, and probability for lack of growth based on total score ranging from 100% to 30% chance of no growth. For those with a score of −1 to 0, wait and scan would clearly be the preferable option. For those with a score of 2 to 3, a discussion of treatment becomes more important, particularly to preserve good hearing if it is present. Certainly this retrospectively created model will need validation and refinement via prospective study, but for now it does provide the beginnings of that crystal ball that many patients and surgeons seek. For this it becomes one of the most significant articles in this year's selections.

B. J. Balough, Capt, MC, USN

Clinicopathological factors related to regrowth of vestibular schwannoma after incomplete resection

Fukuda M, Oishi M, Hiraishi T, et al (Univ of Niigata, Japan)
J Neurosurg 114:1224-1231, 2011

Object.—The authors retrospectively analyzed various clinicopathological factors to determine which are related to regrowth during a long-term follow-up period in patients who underwent incomplete vestibular schwannoma (VS) resection.

Methods.—This study involved 74 patients (25 men and 49 women) in whom a VS was treated surgically via the lateral suboccipital approach, and who had postoperative follow-up periods exceeding 5 years. The mean follow-up was 104.1 months (range 60—241 months), and the mean patient age at surgery was 48.1 years (range 19—75 years). The tumors ranged in size from 0 mm (localized within the internal auditory canal) to 56 mm (28.3 ± 12.2 mm [mean ± SD]).

Results.—Gross-total resection (GTR) was performed in 41 (55%) of the 74 patients; subtotal resection ([STR]; 90—99%) in 25 (34%); and partial resection ([PR]; < 90%) in 8 (11%). Regrowth rates in the GTR, STR, and PR groups were 2.4% (1 of 41 cases), 52% (13 of 25), and 62.5% (5 of 8), respectively, and the times to regrowth ranged from 6 to 76 months (median 31.9 months). The regrowth-free survival curves differed significantly between the complete (GTR) and incomplete (STR and PR) resection groups. Eighteen (54.5%) of the 33 patients who underwent incomplete resection showed evidence of regrowth during follow-up. Univariate and multivariate analyses of various factors revealed that both the thickness of the residual tumor, based on MR imaging after surgery, and the MIB-1 index were positively related to residual tumor regrowth. The receiver operating characteristic curves, plotted for both the thickness of the residual tumor and the MIB-1 index, identified the optimal cutoff points for these values as 7.4 mm (sensitivity 83.3%, specificity 86.7%) and 1.6 (sensitivity 83.3%, specificity 66.7%), respectively.

Conclusions.—Greater residual tumor thickness, based on MR imaging after the initial surgery, and a higher MIB-1 index are both important factors related to postoperative tumor regrowth in patients who have undergone incomplete VS resection. These patients require frequent neuroimaging investigation during follow-up to assure early detection of tumor regrowth (Figs 4 and 5).

▶ Complete tumor resection is the ultimate goal for surgery of skull base tumors. However, avoidance of significant cranial neuropathy often takes higher priority, particularly for benign and slow-growing lesions such as vestibular schwannomas. When faced by this dilemma of further tumor removal or nerve preservation, how much is enough to prevent growth? It is this important question that this article attempts to answer. The authors provide a thorough description of their methodology for analysis, and their statistics are sound. The number of tumors studied, however, is small. Although 74 tumors are included in their analysis, less than half of these (33) had subtotal or partial resection. These low numbers may limit the ability to generalize their findings. Although not surprising that greater residual tumor leads to greater rate of recurrence, it is the analysis that tumor thickness greater than 7.4 mm where the likelihood of growth increases that provides guidance to the surgeon on how much tumor needs to be resected for high probability of long-term success. This is best shown in Figs 4 and 5. Larger series in the future will be better able to refine this point. Lastly, although not likely to be significant with respect to these findings, it is important to

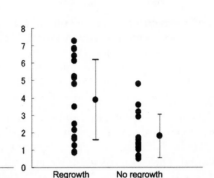

FIGURE 4.—**Left:** Scatterplot comparing residual tumor thickness in patients with and those without recurrence. The residual tumor was significantly thicker in the recurrence group (p < 0.001). **Right:** Scatterplot comparing the MIB-1 index in the recurrence group and the no recurrence group. The MIB-1 index was significantly higher in the recurrence group (p = 0.005). Error bars represent the mean ± SD. (Reprinted from Fukuda M, Oishi M, Hiraishi T, et al. Clinicopathological factors related to regrowth of vestibular schwannoma after incomplete resection. *J Neurosurg*. 2011;114:1224-1231, with permission from American Association for Neurological Surgeons, with Rockwater, Inc.)

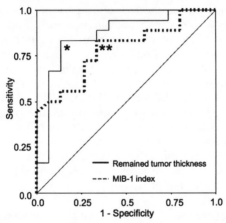

FIGURE 5.—The ROC curves for residual (remained) tumor thickness *(solid line)* and the MIB-1 index *(dotted line)* had areas under the curves of 0.863 and 0.787, respectively. The most discriminative cutoff point for residual tumor thickness *(asterisk)* is 7.4 mm, with a sensitivity of 83.3% and specificity of 86.7%. For the MIB-1 index, the point denoted by *double asterisks* corresponds to a cutoff of 1.6, with a sensitivity of 83.3% and specificity of 66.7%. (Reprinted from Fukuda M, Oishi M, Hiraishi T, et al. Clinicopathological factors related to regrowth of vestibular schwannoma after incomplete resection. *J Neurosurg*. 2011;114:1224-1231, with permission from American Association for Neurological Surgeons, with Rockwater, Inc.)

remember that in this series, only a retrosigmoid/suboccipital approach was used.

B. J. Balough, Capt, MC, USN

Long-term outcomes of vestibular schwannomas treated with fractionated stereotactic radiotherapy: An institutional experience

Kapoor S, Batra S, Carson K, et al (Johns Hopkins Hosp, Baltimore, MD; Johns Hopkins Bloomberg School of Public Health, Baltimore, MD)
Int J Radiat Oncol Biol Phys 81:647-653, 2011

Purpose.—We assessed clinical outcome and long-term tumor control after fractionated stereotactic radiotherapy (FSRT) for unilateral schwannoma.

Methods and Materials.—Between 1995 and 2007, 496 patients were treated with fractionated stereotactic radiotherapy at Johns Hopkins Hospital (Baltimore, MD); 385 patients had radiologic follow-up that met the inclusion criteria. The primary endpoint was treatment failure. Secondary endpoints were radiologic progression and clinical outcome. Logistic regression analysis assessed the association of age, race, tumor side, sex, and pretreatment symptoms.

Results.—In 11 patients (3%) treatment failed, and they required salvage (microsurgical) treatment. Radiologic progression was observed in 116 patients (30.0%), including 35 patients (9%) in whom the treatment volume more than doubled during the follow-up period, although none required surgical resection. Tumors with baseline volumes of less than 1 cm^3 were 18.02 times more likely to progress than those with tumor volumes of 1 cm^3 or greater (odds ratio, 18.02; 95% confidence interval, 4.25−76.32). Treatment-induced neurologic morbidity included 8 patients (1.6%) with new facial weakness, 12 patients (2.8%) with new trigeminal paresthesias, 4 patients (0.9%) with hydrocephalus (1 communicating and 3 obstructive), and 2 patients (0.5%) with possibly radiation-induced neoplasia.

Conclusions.—Although the rate of treatment failure is low (3%), careful follow-up shows that radiologic progression occurs frequently. When reporting outcome, the "no salvage surgery needed" and "no additional treatment needed" criteria for treatment success need to be complemented by the radiologic data (Fig 1).

▶ When comparing various modalities of treatment, measures of effectiveness can vary, and it can be difficult to measure them against each other. This is true in oncologic surgery, where gross total resection with negative margins carries a meaning very different from that of partial or complete response rates resulting from chemotherapy and radiation. In this selection, the authors report their treatment results in nearly 400 patients treated with fractionated stereotactic radiation. They report only a 3% failure rate, which was defined as no further treatment being needed, and only a 4% rate of patients showing new cranial nerve symptoms; both rates compare very favorably with the results of surgery. However, if the definition is failure to progress radiologically, it must be noted that some 30% continued to grow, with 9% more than doubling in size. By this measure of success, this modality does not compare well to surgery where rates of gross total resection average 90% or more. The graphs in Fig 1 illustrate this progression over time. Interestingly, these rates are not much different from previously reported data concerning growth without treatment. What is significant is that the rates of

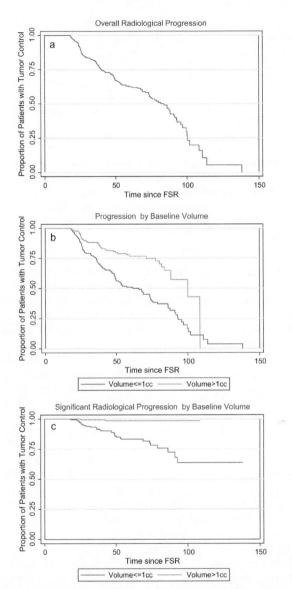

FIGURE 1.—(a) Overall radiologic progression. (b) Progression by baseline volume. (c) Significant radiologic progression by baseline volume. Significant radiologic progression is defined as twice the baseline volume. (FSR = fractionated stereotactic radiotherapy). (Reprinted from the International Journal of Radiation Oncology Biology Physics, Kapoor S, Batra S, Carson K, et al, Long-term outcomes of vestibular schwannomas treated with fractionated stereotactic radiotherapy: an institutional experience. *Int J Radiat Oncol Biol Phys.* 2011;81:647-653. © 2011 with permission from Elsevier Inc.)

continued growth were much higher in tumors less than 1 cm in size. The article's discussion covers this in some detail, citing other studies in which large tumors did not show much tendency to grow, even without treatment, whereas small tumors increased in size. Given these results, observation of tumors less than 1 cm may be the best management. One caveat would be that those with good hearing may wish to opt for treatment, either surgery or radiation, to preserve their hearing rather than take the chance of continued tumor growth. Last, this study reinforces the idea that success rates must be carefully measured against time and that long-term follow-up is necessary, regardless of modality.

B. J. Balough, Capt, MC, USN

Gamma Knife Radiosurgery for Vestibular Schwannomas: Identification of Predictors for Continued Tumor Growth and the Influence of Documented Tumor Growth Preceding Radiation Treatment
Timmer FCA, Mulder JJS, Hanssens PEJ, et al (Radboud Univ Nijmegen Med Ctr, The Netherlands; St. Elisabeth Hosp, Tilburg, The Netherlands)
Laryngoscope 121:1834-1838, 2011

Objectives/Hypothesis.—Gamma knife radiosurgery (GKRS) has become an important treatment modality for vestibular schwannomas. The primary aim of this study was to investigate whether tumor growth at the moment of GKRS has any correlation with the outcome. The secondary aim was to identify clinical predictors of radioresistance in vestibular schwannoma patients treated with GKRS.

Study Design.—One hundred vestibular schwannoma patients, treated with GKRS, were divided into two groups: 1) proven tumor growth preceding GKRS; and 2) previous history of growth unknown. GKRS outcome was defined in two ways. According to the first definition, GKRS was said to have failed when additional treatment had taken place. According to the second one, a volume decrease >20% after 2 years marked successful treatment.

Methods.—Correlations between outcome and growth status were determined with SPSS software. Furthermore, the study assessed how different variables (patient data, history, tumor characteristics, imaging, and audio-vestibular examinations) correlated with the outcome of GKRS.

Results.—No significant difference regarding success and failure of GKRS was found between the two patient groups. The mean reduction in tumor volume after GKRS was less pronounced in patients in whom tumor growth was demonstrated before treatment, but this finding was not significant. No significant predictors ($P < .05$) could be identified in this data set.

Conclusions.—This study found no indication that growth at the moment of GKRS influences therapeutic outcome, nor did it identify any predictors of the outcome after GKRS in vestibular schwannoma patients (Table 2).

▶ This article provides an interesting analysis of radiation-treated vestibular schwannomas. The central premise is that of treatment effectiveness, which is difficult to discern when some 50% to 70% of these tumors continue to grow after presentation. Thus, arrest of continued growth alone may be insufficient to judge the effectiveness of treatment. Moreover, if failure to grow is used as

TABLE 2.—Outcome According to Definition 1

Method 1	GKRS Success	GKRS Failure	Total
Proven tumor growth before GKRS	62	5	67
Previous history of growth unknown	30	3	33

Gamma knife radiosurgery failure is defined as the occurrence of additional treatment.
After Fisher exact test, $P = .78$.
GKRS = gamma knife radiosurgery.

the outcome, is stereotactic radiation less effective in tumors with proven growth? The authors' data, as illustrated in Table 2, demonstrate equal efficacy in treating tumors at initial presentation or after a period of observation with demonstrated growth. Very few require additional treatment. Even with a more rigorous definition of treatment failure—reduction in tumor volume by more than 20%—no difference was found. The authors acknowledge several limitations in their study, the chief being differences in the 2 groups when compared in terms of tumor size and age. However, this seems a minor consideration and is unlikely to change the statistical comparison. Of the 2 outcome measures used, the most important is not requiring additional treatment. In this regard, stereotactic radiation seems to be very effective, even for tumors with demonstrated growth.

B. J. Balough, Capt, MC, USN

Malignancy in Vestibular Schwannoma after Stereotactic Radiotherapy: A Case Report and Review of the Literature
Tanbouzi Husseini S, Piccirillo E, Taibah A, et al (Gruppo Otologico, Piacenza, Italy; et al)
Laryngoscope 121:923-928, 2011

Objectives/Hypothesis.—A relation between conventional radiotherapy and the development of intracranial neoplasma is well known, but radiation-associated tumor following stereotactic radiotherapy of vestibular schwannoma is underestimated.

In this article we will study this relation by doing a complete literature review on all the malignant intracranial tumors that appeared following radiosurgery and adding a case of malignant vestibular schwannoma following stereotactic radiotherapy in a Neurofibromatosis type 2 patient.

Methods.—Literature review and discussion.

Results.—We found 26 cases of malignant brain tumor following stereotactic radiotherapy including our case. In 13 cases the tumor occurred in context of Neurofibromatosis type 2. None of the patients had a tumor size less than 2.5 cm. and the mean latency period between the radiotherapy and malignant tumor development was 5.8 years.

Conclusion.—Patients with vestibular schwannoma should be made aware of the low incidence of the radiation-induced malignant changes and long-term follow-up is mandatory.

▶ Stereotactic radiation for vestibular schwannoma is an attractive option, as it requires no downtime for the patient and has few complications and consistent results. However, the specter of malignant transformation after radiation has remained a concern. This article attempts an exhaustive search of the literature to put that concern into perspective. In just over a decade, they found 26 reports and, though small in number, the rate of malignant transformation is clearly not zero. Of note, one-half of the malignancies identified occurred in patients with neurofibromatosis type 2 (NF2). This is consistent with a survey that is quoted in the article of 1348 NF2 cases in which malignant transformation had a 10% incidence in irradiated patients versus a 0.7% rate in nonirradiated patients.[1] Thus, irradiation in NF2 patients seems to be approached with caution, which is unfortunate, as radiation is useful to have as a treatment modality for these difficult patients. Their discussion of why this may be is valuable. It is also interesting to note that none of the patients with malignant transformation had a tumor less than 2.5 cm in size, thus suggesting the safety of radiation in smaller tumors. Lastly, the authors suggest that the true incidence is unknown and may in fact be underappreciated in the literature, as not all cases are reported.

B. J. Balough, Capt, MC, USN

Reference

1. Baser ME, Evans DG, Jackler RK, Sujansky E, Rubenstein A. Neurofibromatosis 2, radiosurgery and malignant nervous system tumours. *Br J Cancer.* 2000;82:998.

General

Association of age-related macular degeneration with age-related hearing loss

Bozkurt MK, Ozturk BT, Kerimoglu H, et al (Selcuk Univ, Konya, Turkey)
J Laryngol Otol 125:231-235, 2011

Objective.—To assess the association between age-related macular degeneration and age-related hearing loss in Turkish subjects aged 50 years or older.

Study Design and Setting.—Prospective, case—control study within a tertiary university hospital.

Subjects and Methods.—Fifty subjects with age-related macular degeneration and 43 healthy subjects underwent ophthalmological and otolaryngological examination. Statistical analyses were conducted for the poorer eye and ear, comparing age-related hearing loss and pure tone average in the macular degeneration group versus controls.

Results.—Median pure tone average was significantly poorer in the macular degeneration group (35 dBHL) compared with controls (23 dBHL). In the macular degeneration group, hearing loss was significantly greater in dry type (43 dBHL) than wet type (32 dBHL) cases. There was a significant difference between the prevalence of varying degrees of hearing loss in the macular degeneration versus control groups, being respectively: mild, 50 and 35 per cent; moderate, 20 and 5 per cent; and severe, 6 and 0 per cent. There was a weak, but significant correlation between each patient's visual acuity and pure tone average results ($r_s = -0.37, p < 0.001$).

Conclusion.—Age-related hearing loss is more common in patients with age-related macular degeneration. Such patients should be questioned regarding hearing difficulty, and referred to an otolaryngologist if appropriate.

▶ This study provides an interesting epidemiologic correlation between age-related hearing loss and retinal macular degeneration. Though the number of subjects was somewhat small, the design and methodology are well done. Hearing loss represents a large problem in the elderly, leading to social isolation and reduced quality of life. Additional sensory disabilities, like macular degeneration, are all the more disabling when combined. In an age of increased digital visual communication, this is even more important. Studies such as this, however, do not provide causal relationships. Any mechanism behind the relationship remains unknown and the subject for future study, although the authors do suggest a connection to oxidative stress response. It is interesting that a difference was seen between wet and dry types of macular degeneration in terms of hearing loss (dry having worse hearing) despite no difference in visual acuity between the two. A potential limitation in the study is that it involves a relatively homogeneous ethnic population. Coupled with the small sample size, this may limit the applicability of the results to other populations. Still, the message to be aware of these relationships to broaden hearing screening to those at potentially higher risk is valuable.

B. J. Balough, Capt, MC, USN

Prognosis of patients with idiopathic sudden hearing loss: role of vestibular assessment

Korres S, Stamatiou GA, Gkoritsa E, et al (Univ of Athens, Greece; ENT Surgeon, Tripoli, Greece; et al)
J Laryngol Otol 125:251-257, 2011

Objective.—To evaluate the correlation between caloric and vestibular evoked myogenic potential test results, initial audiogram data, and early hearing recovery, in patients with idiopathic sudden hearing loss.

Materials and Methods.—One hundred and four patients with unilateral idiopathic sudden hearing loss underwent complete neurotological evaluation. Results for vestibular evoked myogenic potential and caloric testing were compared with patients' initial and final audiograms.

Results.—Overall, abnormal vestibular evoked myogenic potential responses occurred in 28.8 per cent of patients, whereas abnormal caloric test results occurred in 50 per cent. A statistically significant relationship

TABLE 2.—Hearing Loss Type by Inner Ear Lesion

Hearing Loss (Pts (%))	C	C + S	C + O	C + O + S
High freq*	15.6	20.7	0	30.4
Profound†	11.1	10.3	28.6	52.2

Pts = patients; C = cochlear lesion; S = horizontal semicircular canal lesion; O = otolithic organ lesion.
*$p = 0.29$ (Chi-square).
†$p < 0.01$ (Chi-square).

was found between the type of inner ear lesion and the incidence of profound hearing loss. Moreover, a negative correlation was found between the extent of the inner ear lesion and the likelihood of early recovery.

Conclusion.—In patients with idiopathic sudden hearing loss, the extent of the inner ear lesion tends to correlate with the severity of cochlear damage. Vestibular assessment may be valuable in predicting the final outcome (Table 2).

▶ Although sudden idiopathic hearing loss is named for its hearing effects, many patients also have vestibular symptoms as well, indicating a more global insult to the inner ear. In this study, the authors explore the relationship of injury to those structures supplied by the superior vestibular nerve, the inferior vestibular nerve, or both to hearing injury and recovery. This study represents a large prospective series of more than 100 sudden hearing loss patients collected over 3 years, and all received the same treatment. Of these, approximately one-third complained of balance symptoms. However, half demonstrated injury to the superior nerve structures as evidenced by reduced caloric response, and only slightly more than one-quarter had abnormal results on inferior nerve testing (VEMP). Importantly, all had normal test results on the noninvolved ear. The significance of these testing results is demonstrated in Table 2. Not surprisingly, the greater extent of inner ear involvement, the poorer the prognosis for early recovery. The authors acknowledge the main limitation of their study in that these findings represent early hearing results some 2 weeks after presentation. The real potential value of this study is that it now supports an additional methodology to stratify patients with idiopathic hearing loss. This may be useful in developing studies to examine differences in treatments and response rates and to support power analyses for those studies. It is for that reason that this article is included in this year's review.

B. J. Balough, Capt, MC, USN

Enlarged Vestibular Aqueduct: Review of Controversial Aspects

Gopen Q, Zhou G, Whittemore K, et al (U.C.L.A. Med Ctr; Children's Hosp Boston, MA)
Laryngoscope 121:1971-1978, 2011

Objectives.—To review the controversial aspects of the enlarged vestibular aqueduct syndrome.

Study Design.—Contemporary review.

Methods.—A literature search using the terms "enlarged vestibular aqueduct and large vestibular aqueduct" were used to generate the articles for review in this article.

Results.—The enlarged vestibular aqueduct is a condition causing variable auditory and vestibular dysfunction. Although it has been 32 years since Valvasorri and Clemis recognized the clinical importance of the enlarged vestibular aqueduct, many controversial aspects of the diagnosis remain. The topics reviewed in this discussion are as follows: size criteria for radiographic diagnosis, precipitating factors for hearing loss, corticosteroid treatment and sac surgery, conductive component to hearing loss, natural progression of hearing loss, correlations between aqueduct size and hearing loss, genetics, vestibular symptoms, and theories regarding mechanisms behind the symptoms.

Conclusion.—The enlarged vestibular aqueduct remains a controversial entity with variable presentation, progression, and prognosis (Tables 3 and 4).

▶ This article provides an excellent and systematic review of one of the most commonly encountered inner ear malformations: the enlarged vestibular

TABLE 3.—Hearing Loss—Progression Over Time

Study	Year	Patients	Ears	Stable	Fluctuating	Progressive	f/u Years Mean
Valvassori[38]	1983	15	?	40	0	60	3
Emmet[39]	1985	24	48	83	17*		2 days to 12 years
Jackler[15]	1989	17	33	35	12	53	7.3
Levenson[17]	1989	12	22	27	46	27	4.2
Arcand[16]	1991	13	20	54	46*		4.0
Okumura[18]	1995	13	23	39	61*		1.4
Zalza[14]	1995	15	26	64	36*		3.8
Antonelli[25]	1998	26	42	24	40	36	2.3
Madden[7]	2003	77	144	51	28	21	?
Arjmand[41]	2004	?	?	50	33	17	?
Lai[40]	2004	12	24	67	33*		?
Baerrettini[6]	2005	17	32	30	29	41	?
Colvin[29]	2006	27	50	30	33	37	9.7
Madden[20]	2007	71	119	50	22	28	1.2
Grimmer[31]	2008	32	?	16	29	55	3.6
Reyes[42]	2009	32	64	47	21	32	9.5
Atkin[33]	2009	20	37	50	50*		?
King[43]	2010	83	143	26	37	30	3.7

Editor's Note: Please refer to original journal article for full references.
*Represents combined fluctuating and progressive hearing loss (not delineated separately in these studies).

TABLE 4.—Vestibular Symptoms and Testing

Study	Year	Patients	Vestibular Symptoms	Vestibular Testing
Valvassori[3]	1978	50	10%*	100% patients (6 patients tested) markedly decreased or absent vestibular functions tests
Valvassori[38]	1983	160	4%	vestibular function tests absent or markedly reduced in 80% of patients
Emmett[39]	1985	26	12%	ENG reduced in 53% of patients rotational chair with low-frequency phase lag 100% of patients and 57% of patients had directional preponderance
Jackler[15]	1989	17	29%	ENG in 2 patients one with direction changing nystagmus and normal ENG the other with no response but had no vestibular symptoms
Schessel[83]	1992	3	100%	reduced calorics 67% of patients
Okumura[18]	1995	4	100%	reduced calorics 100% of patients
Okumura[84]	1996	8	80%	none reported
Antonelli[25]	1998	30	43%	none reported
Yetiser[85]	1999	10	30%	90% of patients with ENG reduced or no response
Nakashima[36]	2000	15	33%	VEMP with increased amplitude at reduced threshold in 92% of patients, absent in 8% of patients
Oh[86]	2001	3	100%	1 patient: ENG normal, rotational chair testing normal 1 patient: no testing done 1 patient: ENG normal but rotational chair testing with decreased gain and increased phase lead
Naganawa[78]	2002	7	14%	no testing reported
Madden[7]	2003	77	4%	no testing reported
Sheykholeslami[82]	2004	3	67%	ENG normal (1 patient), VEMP present 2 out of 2 patients tested
Berrettini[6]	2005	17	47%	ENG reduced in 87% of patients
Grimmer[47]	2007	15	47%	no testing reported
Merchant[81]	2007	5	0%	no testing reported
Zhou[87]	2010	25	20%	VEMP with increased amplitude and reduced threshold in 88% of patients, absent in 12% of patients

Editor's Note: Please refer to original journal article for full references.

VEMP = vestibular evoked myogenic potential testing; ENG = electronystagmonography testing.

*In this study, the reported incidence of vestibular symptoms is 10%, but the author goes on to state that "vestibular complaints of inconsequential magnitude could be elicited from many patients."

aqueduct. Numerous studies are cited and several charts and tables collate the findings of the various studies. Among them, Table 3 is particularly useful because hearing loss progression is among the most commonly asked questions after this condition has been discovered. Similarly, Table 4 is helpful in providing data about vestibular symptoms. Both tables show that the numbers vary widely, from few affected patients to many, but taken as a whole, some generalizations emerge. In terms of hearing loss, many (roughly half) will have stable hearing, whereas most of the remaining patients will experience progression of hearing loss. Regarding balance, most will have symptoms, and most will show abnormalities on testing. The review covers many other details, including treatments that have been tried and the various theories concerning causes. Considering how commonly this abnormality is encountered and the great amount of detail provided, this article is recommended reading for all.

B. J. Balough, Capt, MC, USN

Investigation of the Coherence of Definite and Probable Vestibular Migraine as Distinct Clinical Entities

Eggers SDZ, Staab JP, Neff BA, et al (Mayo Clinic, Rochester, MN)
Otol Neurotol 32:1144-1151, 2011

Objectives.—To investigate the following: 1) associations between vestibular symptoms and migraine in a well-characterized cohort of tertiary neurotology patients, 2) effects of comorbidity on clinical presentations, and 3) validity of proposed definitions of definite (dVM) and probable vestibular migraine (pVM).

Study Design.—Retrospective chart review.

Setting.—Tertiary neurotology center.

Patients.—All 228 subjects with headache were selected from a larger investigation of 410 patients with vestibular symptoms who underwent comprehensive medical, surgical, and behavioral neurotologic consultations. Subjects had at least one of 4 diagnoses: dVM/pVM, Ménière's disease, benign paroxysmal positional vertigo, or chronic subjective dizziness.

Interventions.—Subjects were divided into migraine (n = 164) and non-migraine headache (n = 64) groups by International Headache Society criteria, then subdivided by those with vestibular symptoms related or unrelated to headache. Subjects meeting proposed criteria for dVM (n = 46) and pVM (n = 42) were identified. Statistical analyses investigated discriminating features and cohesiveness in each group, with or without comorbidity.

Main Outcome Measures.—Characteristics of dVM and pVM.

Results.—Migraine, particularly migraine with aura, was more often related to vestibular symptoms than nonmigrainous headache. dVM and pVM groups did not differ in demographics, clinical histories, examinations, or vestibular testing. Numerous differences existed between dVM/pVM subjects with and without comorbid Ménière's disease, benign paroxysmal positional vertigo, or chronic subjective dizziness. The pVM group contained 4 subtypes.

Conclusion.—These results support an association between vestibular symptoms and migraine but not proposed distinctions between dVM and pVM. pVM does not appear to be a coherent diagnostic entity. Comorbid conditions are important causes of vestibular symptoms in patients with migraine (Fig 1, Table 1).

▶ Much like patients with endolymphatic hydrops, those with vestibular migraine can often be recognized easily in the office but are extremely difficult to categorize and diagnose definitively. And, if anything, it is a diagnosis that is more common and more difficult to prove. This article, from a large, well-respected, multidisciplinary team, reviews several hundred patients listed in a tertiary-care referral base and are experiencing problems with balance. As represented in Table 1, the proposed diagnostic criteria for vestibular migraine, modeled after the migraine headache criteria, were used to classify the subjects into two categories: definite or probable. Many other comparisons and analyses were then made, the most useful of which are shown in Fig 1. Interestingly, nearly 60% of the patients

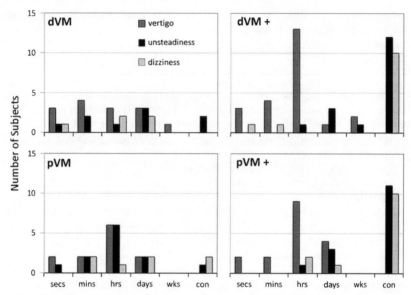

FIGURE 1.—Time distribution of vestibular symptoms in four subgroups of patients with vestibular migraine: dVM as the only neurotologic diagnosis (dVM), dVM + comorbid neurotologic condition(s) (dVM+), pVM as a only diagnosis (pVM), pVM + comorbid neurotologic condition(s) (pVM+). The larger numbers of subjects with vertigo lasting for hours in the 2 comorbidity groups reflect those with coexisting Ménière's disease. The larger numbers with constant (con) unsteadiness or dizziness reflect those with coexisting CSD. (Reprinted from Eggers SDZ, Staab JP, Neff BA, et al. Investigation of the coherence of definite and probable vestibular migraine as distinct clinical entities. *Otol Neurotol.* 2011;32:1144-1151, with permission from Otology & Neurotology, Inc.)

TABLE 1.—Proposed Diagnostic Criteria for Vestibular Migraine (5,9)

Definite vestibular migraine
  A. Recurrent episodic vestibular symptoms of at least moderate severity[a]
  B. Current or previous history of migraine according to ICHD criteria
  C. One of the following migrainous symptoms during at least 2 vertiginous attacks: migrainous headache, photophobia, phonophobia, visual, or other auras
  D. Other causes ruled out by appropriate investigations
Probable vestibular migraine
  A. Recurrent episodic vestibular symptoms of at least moderate severity[a]
  B. One of the following:
    1. Current or previous history of migraine according to ICHD criteria
    2. Migrainous symptoms during ≥2 attacks of vertigo
    3. Migraine precipitants before vertigo in more than 50% of attacks: e.g., food triggers, sleep irregularities, hormonal changes
    4. Response to migraine medications in more than 50% of attacks
  C. Other causes ruled out by appropriate investigations

ICHD indicates International Classification of Headache Disorders (International Headache Society); ICVD, International Classification of Vestibular Disorders (Bárány Society).
Editor's Note: Please refer to original journal article for full references.
[a]Vestibular symptoms as defined by Neuhauser et al. (5) and Neuhauser and Lempert (9) include ICVD (25) vertigo and unsteadiness but not dizziness. Symptoms may be spontaneous, positional, or provoked by head motion. Vestibular symptoms are considered moderate if they interfere with but do not prohibit daily activities and are severe if patients cannot continue daily activities.

diagnosed with vestibular migraine had at least one other comorbid vestibular diagnosis. This subgroup exhibited higher rates of auditory symptoms and abnormalities on testing, further complicating diagnosis. This is further explained in an excellent discussion section. Last, the authors make the point that distinctions between definite and probable vestibular migraine were weak at best and that using headache criteria for this entity may be less useful than approaching it on the basis of the vestibular symptoms, with or without headache. Because migraine-associated vertigo is a problem commonly encountered by the otolaryngologist, this article provides a very good and thoughtful organization of the symptoms encountered in these patients and helps with accurate diagnosis and treatment.

B. J. Balough, Capt, MC, USN

What Is the Effect of Time Between Sequential Cochlear Implantations on Hearing in Adults and Children? A Systematic Review of the Literature
Smulders YE, Rinia AB, Rovers MM, et al (Univ Med Ctr Utrecht, The Netherlands)
Laryngoscope 121:1942-1949, 2011

Objectives/Hypothesis.—Bilateral cochlear implantation is a safe and effective intervention for severe sensorineural hearing loss and is believed to be more effective than unilateral implantation. This review article investigates the effect of time between sequential cochlear implantations on hearing results in both adults and children.

Study Design.—Systematic review of cohort studies.

Methods.—We searched PubMed, Embase, and CINAHL from inception to August 16, 2010, using the terms hearing loss, cochlear implant, delay, and their synonyms.

Results.—Eleven studies evaluating the effect of time between sequential cochlear implantations on hearing performance were included. Although the quality of studies was poor because of a significant risk of bias, all studies reported that auditory performance is better in a bilateral listening situation than with either one cochlear implant activated unilaterally. Five studies discussed postlingually deafened adults. In four, bilateral hearing was not affected by the amount of time between implantations. One study did report a negative effect of delay on speech intelligibility in silence. Seven studies discussed prelingually deafened children. None reported a negative effect of interimplantation delay on sound localization performance. One study reported poorer results after extended intervals on speech intelligibility in silence and two in noise.

Conclusions.—Current evidence suggests that a second implant can be beneficial even after a substantial interval between sequential implantations. The quality of the evidence is, however, rather poor; to confirm this

TABLE 3.—Study Outcome in Adults

Study	Test	Statistical Analysis	Effect of Duration of Interval Between Surgeries
Laske et al., 2009[8]	Speech intelligibility OST quiet (%)	ANOVA, multivariance analysis, multiple linear regression analysis: DOD, interimplantation interval, follow-up	Significant correlation between interval and difference between CI1 and CI2 performance. ($r2 = 55\%$, $P < .001$)
	OST noise (dB SNR)		No effect of interval duration, but there was a trend towards better performance with shorter interval
Zeitler et al., 2008[12]	Speech intelligibility CNC quiet HINT quiet	Pearson product correlation: interimplant delay, age CI2, DOD CI1, DOD CI2	No correlation between interval and absolute or relative improvement in CI2
Ramsden et al., 2005[21]	Speech intelligibility CNC and CUNY in quiet CUNY noise	Post hoc analysis (Tukey)	No correlation between interval and difference between CI1 and CI2 performance in quiet or noise
Nopp et al., 2004[16]	Localization Absolute error (°)	Pearson product correlation: interimplant delay, age onset deafness, DOD	No correlation between interval and localization accuracy
Schleich et al., 2004[17]	Speech intelligibility OST noise (dB SNR)	Correlation: interimplant delay, DOD CI1, DOD CI2	No correlation between interval and binaural advantage

OST = Oldenburger sentence test; ANOVA = analysis of variance; DOD = duration of deafness; CNC = Consonant-Nucleus-Consonant monosyllabic words; HINT = Hearing in Noise Test (sentences); CUNY = City University of New York sentences in silence/noise; SNR = signal-to-noise ratio.
Editor's Note: Please refer to original journal article for full references.

TABLE 5.—Study Outcome in Children

Study	Test	Statistical Analysis	Effect of Duration of Interval Between Surgeries
Grieco-Calub et al., 2010[15]	Localization	Multiple linear regression analysis (age visit, age CI1, age CI2, hearing experience, interimplant delay, BICI experience)	No effect of interval duration on bilateral localization accuracy
Van Deun et al., 2010[14]	Localization	ANCOVA (Age CI1, age CI2 inter implant delay, BICI experience, age onset deafness, HA experience)	No effect
Gordon et al., 2009[6]	Speech intelligiblity Words in quiet	Stepwise linear regression analysis (Age at CI1, DOD, interimplant delay, BICI) experience, test, test condition)	Negative effect of interval duration: 11% of speech perception change relative to CI1 is explained by delay. F = 45.6, P < .0001 0.296±0.04% decrease in speech score per month of delay
	Words in noise	No differences between degree of bilateral benefit in noise across groups with different delays	No effect of interval duration F = 2.6. P > .05
Steffens et al., 2008[11]	Speech intelligiblity OLKI in noise	Correlation between subject characteristics and performance (aetiology, age onset, Age CI1, Age CI2, Interimplant interval, Experience BICI, monaural 1 score, monaural 2 score)	Negative correlation between interval and binaural advantage when speech is presented to CI2. (r = −0.536, P = .027)
	Lateralization		No correlation between interval and lateralization score (r < 0.5 / P > .05)
Zeitler et al., 2008[12]	Speech intelligiblity Words (MLNT, LNT, PBK) and sentences (HINT) in quiet HINT noise	Pearson product correlation: interimplant delay, age CI2, DOD CI1, DOD CI2.	No correlation P > .05
Scherf et al., 2007[13]	Speech intelligiblity Words in quiet Words in noise	Interval - speech recognition graph Interval - speech recognition graph	Significant correlation between interval and CI2 performance (r = −0.514, P < .05) A trend cannot be observed A trend cannot be observed
Kuhn-Inacker et al., 2004[9]	Speech intelligiblity Speech in noise	Linear regression analysis: age at CI1 and interimplant delay.	No effect (F = 0.0001, P = .97)

ANCOVA = analysis of covariance; BICI = bilateral cochlear implantation; HA = hearing aid; DOD = duration of bilateral deafness before CI1; OLKI = Oldenburger Kinder Reimtest: speech and noise presented from +45°; and −45°; MLNT = multisyllabic lexical neighborhood test (words); LNT = lexical neighborhood test (words); PBK = Phonemic Balanced Kindergarten word test; HINT = Hearing in Noise Test (sentences).

Editor's Note: Please refer to original journal article for full references.

postulation, high-quality trials assessing the effectiveness of a second cochlear implant after a time delay should be initiated (Tables 3 and 5).

▶ Two ears are indeed better than one. For those with normal hearing, two ears provide sound localization and improved discrimination in noise. Over recent years, increasing evidence has supported the same effects in those with deafness rehabilitated via bilateral cochlear implantation. However, an unanswered question remains between simultaneous and sequential implantation. For many whose implantation occurred initially several years ago, there are questions about the additional benefits of a second implant in an ear deafened many years earlier. For others contemplating initial surgery, there are considerations regarding the additional operative time and risk. The results of this meta-analysis for adults are summarized in Table 3. As is true for many reviews of cochlear implant data, direct comparisons can be difficult to make because the outcome measures used are not uniform. Yet, despite this limitation, the data suggest that the interval between implantations is not important. For children, as might be expected, it is not the difference in time between implants but the age at second implant that seems to be the most significant factor. These data are presented in Table 5. As with any retrospective study, there are limitations in the conclusions that can be drawn, and the authors acknowledge these in their discussion. Even considering the limitations, this study is an important step in advancing our understanding of bilateral implantations, and supports the practice of sequential implantation, even after significant delay in adults.

B. J. Balough, Capt, MC, USN

Estimation of factors influencing the results of tinnitus retraining therapy
Koizumi T, Nishimura T, Sakaguchi T, et al (Nara Med Univ, Japan)
Acta Otolaryngol 129:40-45, 2009

Conclusion.—The factors of tinnitus loudness and Tinnitus Handicap Inventory (THI) score in tinnitus patients have the potential to relate to therapeutic results of tinnitus retraining therapy (TRT).

Objectives.—To confirm what factors in tinnitus influence the results of TRT.

Patients and Methods.—Twelve factors were investigated in 53 patients with tinnitus, examining the relationship between these factors and the results of TRT. A THI score was determined before and 6 months after TRT introduction (pre- and post-TRT). Moreover, the change of THI score from pre- to post-TRT (ΔTHI) was referred to as the therapeutic effect of TRT. Based on the 12 factors, subjects were respectively divided into two groups, comparing ΔTHI between groups.

Results.—Two groups of greater tinnitus loudness and higher THI score showed significant increases in ΔTHI, indicating that two factors of

TABLE 2.—Changes in THI Score from Pre- to Post-TRT (ΔTHI)

	Group A	THI Score Pre-TRT(A1) (mean±SD)	THI Score Post-TRT(A2)	A Group ΔTHI(A3)	Group B	THI score Pre-TRT(B1) (mean±SD)	THI Score Post-TRT(B2)	B Group ΔTHI(B3)	THI Score Pre-TRT Analysis (A1 vs B1)	ΔTHI Analysis (A3 vs B3)
Age	Under 60 years ($n=26$)	47.3±22.0	33.9±24.0	13.4±17.0	Over 60 years ($n=27$)	47.3±24.6	27.1±19.8	20.3±21.2	NS	NS
Sex	Male ($n=21$)	46.8±21.8	30.9±21.9	15.9±14.1	Female ($n=32$)	47.7±24.3	30.1±22.5	17.6±22.4	NS	NS
Laterality in the ear	Unilateral ($n=33$)	43.5±23.3	26.1±19.7	17.3±21.6	Bilateral ($n=20$)	53.7±21.9	37.5±24.3	16.2±15.5	NS	NS
Period of tinnitus	Under 1 year ($n=26$)	41.3±21.3	28.0±22.7	13.3±16.0	Over 1 year ($n=27$)	53.1±23.6	32.7±21.6	20.4±22.1	NS	NS
Primary disease	Unknown ($n=27$)	41.8±22.4	25.9±18.2	15.9±20.9	Known ($n=26$)	53.1±22.8	35.1±25.0	18.0±18.0	NS	NS
Hearing level	Under 30 dB HL ($n=30$)	47.1±22.8	30.6±23.9	16.5±18.5	Over 30 dB HL ($n=23$)	47.6±24.0	30.2±19.9	17.4±20.9	NS	NS
Recruitment phenomenon	Absent ($n=30$)	50.6±21.4	32.5±24.0	18.1±17.4	Present ($n=23$)	43.0±25.0	27.7±19.4	15.3±22.0	NS	NS
Tinnitus pitch	Under 500 Hz ($n=9$)	51.8±24.1	28.0±30.6	23.8±16.9	Over 2 kHz ($n=44$)	46.4±23.1	30.9±20.3	15.5±19.7	NS	NS
Tinnitus loudness	Under 10 dB SL ($n=16$)	40.4±16.3	31.5±16.1	8.9±9.9	Over 10 dB SL ($n=37$)	50.3±25.1	29.9±24.4	20.4±21.5	NS	$p<0.05$
THI score	Under 50 ($n=31$)	31.1±10.6	21.3±13.8	9.8±14.7	Over 50 ($n=22$)	70.2±15.0	43.3±25.3	26.9±21.1	$p<0.001$	$p<0.001$
Concomitant drug	Absent ($n=16$)	37.5±19.5	22.1±12.9	15.4±15.9	Present ($n=37$)	51.6±23.5	34.0±24.2	17.6±20.9	$p<0.05$	NS
Number of consulting doctors	Under 1 ($n=28$)	45.1±23.5	32.5±22.3	12.6±14.5	Over 2 ($n=25$)	49.8±22.9	28.1±22.0	21.8±23.0	NS	NS

tinnitus loudness and THI score were related to the therapeutic effect of TRT (Table 2).

▶ Tinnitus retraining therapy (TRT), while effective, is resource and time intensive for both practitioner and patient alike. Given this requirement and the limited number of sites where TRT is available, this study becomes important in helping stratify which patients may benefit the most from this particular form of therapy. Table 2 shows the results for all the various parameters measured. Unfortunately, only 2 factors emerge, and one of those, tinnitus handicap inventory, is relatively unhelpful as a screening method, as only those most severely affected will seek TRT. However, tinnitus loudness did emerge, and given the modest improvement in the less than 10 dB group, this may be useful in steering these patients away from TRT as a primary therapeutic option. Like most studies on tinnitus, this one suffers from small numbers. However, given the relatively large standard deviations and similar averages in each of the parameters measured, increased numbers likely would not have impacted these results. In reviewing the data, this would seem to be from the overall high positive benefit of TRT with an average decline of more than 15 points in tinnitus handicap index. In all, this article is a valuable read for those referring patients for TRT.

B. J. Balough, Capt, MC, USN

Systematic Review and Meta-Analyses of Randomized Controlled Trials Examining Tinnitus Management
Hoare DJ, Kowalkowski VL, Kang S, et al (Univ of Nottingham, UK)
Laryngoscope 121:1555-1564, 2011

Objectives/Hypothesis.—To evaluate the existing level of evidence for tinnitus management strategies identified in the UK Department of Health's Good Practice Guideline.

Study Design.—Systematic review of peer-reviewed literature and meta-analyses.

Methods.—Searches were conducted in PubMed, Cambridge Scientific Abstracts, Web of Science, and EMBASE (earliest to August 2010), supplemented by hand searches in October 2010. Only randomized controlled trials that used validated questionnaire measures of symptoms (i.e., measures of tinnitus distress, anxiety, depression) were included.

Results.—Twenty-eight randomized controlled trials met our inclusion criteria, most of which provide moderate levels of evidence for the effects they reported. Levels of evidence were generally limited by the lack of blinding, lack of power calculations, and incomplete data reporting in these studies. Only studies examining cognitive behavioral therapy were numerous and similar enough to perform meta-analysis, from which the efficacy of cognitive behavioral therapy (moderate effect size) appears to be reasonably established. Antidepressants were the only drug class to show any evidence of potential benefit.

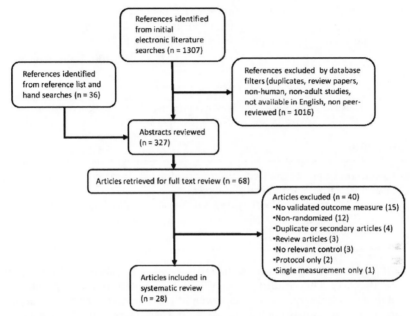

FIGURE 1.—Summary of the systematic literature search. (Reprinted from Hoare DJ, Kowalkowski VL, Kang S, et al. Systematic review and meta-analyses of randomized controlled trials examining tinnitus management. *Laryngoscope*. 2011;121:1555-1564, with permission from The American Laryngological, Rhinological and Otological Society, Inc and John Wiley and Sons (www.interscience.wiley.com).)

Conclusions.—The efficacy of most interventions for tinnitus benefit remains to be demonstrated conclusively. In particular, high-level assessment of the benefit derived from those interventions most commonly used in practice, namely hearing aids, maskers, and tinnitus retraining therapy needs to be performed (Fig 1).

▶ This study comes from the United Kingdom as a meta-analysis of the levels of evidence to support the tinnitus management recommendations found in their national good clinical practice guidelines. The methodology for their meta-analysis is solid and well described in great detail. This serves as an excellent review on the various therapies used for tinnitus treatment and is well organized with an extensive bibliography. While this is extremely valuable, there is another aspect of this article that makes it worthy of review. More than 1300 articles were identified in their initial data search on tinnitus therapies. Of this number, only one-quarter met the criteria for their abstracts to be reviewed for inclusion. Some 68 underwent full-text review, and of these, only 28 were included in this systematic review. This process is illustrated in Fig 1. In the discussion and conclusion, this low number of high-quality studies receives comment. Frequently encountered issues were the lack of power and incomplete reporting of data. This leads to only limited bits of evidence in support of widely recommended treatments for a very common problem. A similar review was done more than a decade ago by Dobie,[1] and although some progress has been made in consensus outcome measures, there continues to be an issue with inadequate sample sizes. Hopefully, this will be addressed by improved studies in the coming decade.

B. J. Balough, Capt, MC, USN

Reference

1. Dobie RA. A review of randomized clinical trials in tinnitus. *Laryngoscope.* 1999; 109:1202-1211.

Outcomes

Surgical Treatment of the Periocular Complex and Improvement of Quality of Life in Patients With Facial Paralysis
Henstrom DK, Lindsay RW, Cheney ML, et al (Massachusetts Eye and Ear Infirmary, Boston; Bethesda Naval Med Ctr, Baltimore, MD)
Arch Facial Plast Surg 13:125-128, 2011

Objective.—A devastating sequela of facial paralysis is the inability to close the eye. The resulting loss of corneal protection can potentially lead to severe consequences. Eyelid weight placement, lower eyelid suspension, and brow ptosis correction are frequently performed to protect the eye. We sought to measure and report the change in quality of life (QOL) after surgical treatment of the periocular complex, using the validated Facial Clinimetric Evaluation (FaCE) QOL instrument.

Methods.—From March 2009 to May 2010, 49 patients presenting to the Facial Nerve Center with paralytic lagophthalmos requiring intervention were treated with static periocular reanimation. Thirty-seven of the patients completed preoperative and postoperative FaCE surveys.

Results.—Overall QOL, measured by the FaCE instrument, significantly improved following static periocular treatment. Mean FaCE scores increased from 44.1 to 52.7 ($P < .001$). Patients also reported a significant decrease in the amount of time their eye felt dry, irritated, or scratchy ($P < .001$). The amount of artificial tears and/or ointment also significantly decreased ($P = .03$). There were 2 cases of localized cellulitis with 1 eyelid weight extrusion.

Conclusions.—We report the first series of postoperative QOL changes following static periocular treatment for paralytic lagophthalmos. Patients report a notable improvement in periocular comfort and overall QOL.

▶ Medical necessity and objective measurement typically define the metrics of most publications. In this regard, we are mostly treating ourselves in preventing complications from disease or convincing ourselves that one form of treatment is somehow equal or superior. Patients, however, want to know how their lives will be improved when making informed decisions and evaluating risks. For cancer or infection, the metrics for treatment of disease are straightforward. But in the area of rehabilitation from physical disability and, in particular, surgical rehabilitation, outcome studies such as this are far more useful. Certainly in the care of the eye in the patient with facial paralysis, many options exist from low-tech options such as patching, moisture shields, and ocular lubricants to surgical interventions of varying complexity for the upper lid, lower lid, and brow. Interestingly, while the scores improved similarly for upper lid rehabilitation and upper lid, lower lid, and brow procedures, scores for combined upper lid and lower lid procedures did not improve as much. As health care costs become increasingly scrutinized and patients become more savvy consumers, studies such as this will help define how our recommended care provides benefit.

B. J. Balough, Capt, MC, USN

Taste disturbance after stapes surgery—clinical and experimental study
Miuchi S, Sakagami M, Tsuzuki K, et al (Hyogo College of Medicine, Nishinomiya, Japan)
Acta Otolaryngol Suppl 129:71-78, 2009

Conclusion.—Most of the clinical cases experienced taste disturbance after stapes surgery, and in a few cases this disturbance persisted for a long time. The animal experiment suggested the role of geniculate ganglion (GG) cells in nerve generation.

Objectives.—To clinically examine taste disorder and its recovery after stapes surgery and experimentally demonstrate a role of GG.

Patients and Methods.—Taste function after preservation of chorda tympani nerve (CTN) in stapes surgery was prospectively investigated with a questionnaire and electrogustometry (EGM). Further, expression of neurotrophic factors in GG after injury of CTN was examined by in situ hybridization histochemistry (ISSH) and RT-PCR.

Results.—Among the cases, 15/18 (83.3%) were associated with taste disturbance and 6/18 (33.3%) were associated with tongue numbness 2 weeks after surgery; however, the symptoms ceased in 14/18 cases (77.8%). Two weeks after surgery, the EGM threshold was found to be elevated in 15/18 cases (83.3%), while in 10/18 cases (55.6%), it did not decrease until 1 year after surgery. Expression of ISSH and amplified bands of BDNF and GFR increased at 7 and 14 days after nerve injury in ipsilateral GGs and also increased at 7 days on the contralateral side (Fig 3).

▶ This article actually represents 2 studies, 1 clinical and 1 animal, intended to improve understanding of recovery of taste function after stapes surgery. As the authors note in their introduction, this has been a frequently studied topic. Several references are provided that are useful for those interested in the subject. There are two unique aspects to this study that make it noteworthy. First, the authors detail the time course of recovery through 2 years and compare symptomatic recovery with electrogustometry. Second, they demonstrate that symptomatic recovery occurs prior to return to electrical baseline. The high correlation at 1 month in which 15 of 18 cases had both taste disturbance and abnormal electrical responses reinforces that this response is in fact from the chorda tympani nerve and not the trigeminal enervation to the tongue.

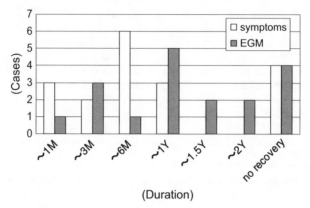

(Duration)

FIGURE 3.—Duration of persistence of postoperative symptoms and elevation of the EGM threshold. (Reprinted from Miuchi S, Sakagami M, Tsuzuki K, et al. Taste disturbance after stapes surgery — clinical and experimental study. *Acta Otolaryngol.* 2009;129:71-78, reprinted by permission of the publisher (Taylor & Francis Group, http://www.informaworld.com).)

Thus, when symptomatic recovery occurs prior to electrical, it helps confirm that taste sensation is replaced by the other side and the whole mouth and is interpreted centrally rather than restored. Similarly when neither taste sensation nor electrical baseline is recovered by 2 years, the injury may be considered permanent. This relationship is best seen in Fig 3. Although many will recover within 3 months, some may take as long as 1 year. Symptoms that are still present after 1 year are unlikely to improve. For its contribution to understanding the timing of recovery, this article has been included.

B. J. Balough, Capt, MC, USN

Effect of Type I Tympanoplasty on the Quality of Life of Children
Habesoglu TE, Habesoglu M, Deveci I, et al (Haydarpassa Numune Education and Res Hosp, Istanbul, Turkey)
Ann Otol Rhinol Laryngol 120:326-330, 2011

Objectives.—Quality-of-life issues related to chronic otitis media (COM) include physical symptoms, emotional symptoms, hearing loss, speech symptoms, social symptoms, and parents' emotional symptoms. In this study we evaluated the effects of tympanoplasty on the quality of life of pediatric patients.

Methods.—In a questionnaire-based outcome study, we reviewed 56 of 78 pediatric patients with COM who were treated with type I tympanoplasty at our institution between December 2008 and February 2010. All patients were asked to fill out the COM-5 questionnaire with their parents, before operation and 6 months after operation. Preoperative and postoperative total ear scores, preoperative and postoperative ear scores with an intact tympanic membrane, preoperative and postoperative ear scores with a perforated tympanic membrane, and preoperative and postoperative audiological results were assessed.

Results.—After type I tympanoplasty, 45 patients (80.3%) had successful closure of the tympanic membrane, but 11 patients (19.7%) had unsuccessful closure of the tympanic membrane. There was a significant decrease in physical suffering, hearing loss, emotional distress, activity limitations, and caregiver's concerns scores in patients with intact tympanic membranes after operation (p < 0.01).

Conclusions.—Children with COM had a significant increase in their quality of life after successful tympanoplasty. Our results also suggested that tympanoplasty was successful in pediatric patients with COM (Fig 2).

▶ The majority of medical literature focuses on statistical improvements between one set and another. Success is measured in rates of tympanic membrane closure, reductions in air-bone gaps, recurrence, or disease-free intervals. All this becomes very physician-centric as we try to convince each other and ourselves of what we should be doing, which is all well and good. However, for the patient and his or her family, the outcome of treatment is "will I be better" and, if so, how much? This is quite a different yardstick of success and requires a different approach. And while it may seem intuitive to us that their lives will be improved (or worse illness prevented), the new economic realities of medicine require we have this quality-of-life data at our disposal in addition to our traditional metrics of success. Copays and other out-of-pocket expenses related to surgery are significant costs and, as with any other economic decision faced by the public, they must determine if the value received is worth the expense, particularly for non—life-threatening conditions. Further, as insurers and government attempt to rein in health care costs, the value received for treatment must go beyond simple success

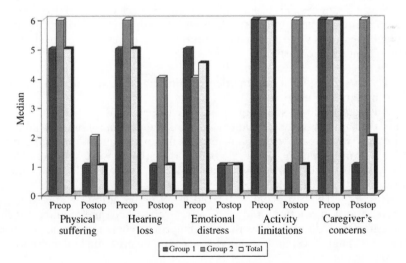

FIGURE 2.—Distribution of COM-5 survey scores before and after tympanoplasty in children. (Reprinted from Habesoglu TE, Habesoglu M, Deveci I, et al. Effect of type I tympanoplasty on the quality of life of children. *Ann Otol Rhinol Laryngol.* 2011;120:326-330. © Annals Publishing Company.)

rates or abstract measures of success and focus on real societal benefits. It is in this light that the data from this article become so significant. As illustrated in Fig 2, physical suffering, hearing loss, and emotional distress are all greatly improved by surgery, even in the group in which closure of the tympanic membrane was not achieved. Thus, the act of surgery in and of itself to remove disease provides benefit and is sorely dependent on the outcome. This is similar to my own experience in underserved communities as referenced.[1] Preoperative counseling can now include this information as well as the traditional metrics for families to have a better understanding of the potential benefits of surgery for chronic ear disease.

B. J. Balough, Capt, MC, USN

Reference

1. Horlbeck D, Boston M, Balough B, et al. Humanitarian otologic missions: long-term surgical results. *Otolaryngol Head Neck Surg.* 2009;140:559-565.

Surgical Technique

Outcome of the Bone-Anchored Hearing Aid Procedure Without Skin Thinning: A Prospective Clinical Trial

Hultcrantz M (Karolinska Univ Hosp, Stockholm, Sweden)
Otol Neurotol 32:1134-1139, 2011

Objective.—To evaluate the outcome of Bone-Anchored Hearing Aid surgery without skin thinning, a test group with direct implantation without such thinning was compared with a control group that underwent the traditional procedure.

Study Design.—This was a single-center, prospective clinical trial designed to evaluate a novel approach to Bone-Anchored Hearing Aid implantation. Eligible patients were enrolled consecutively in the test group or selected to be age-matched controls.

Setting.—University Hospital.

Patients.—Eighteen adult patients, suffering from hearing loss, suitable for implantable hearing aid.

Methods.—Single-step surgery was performed on 18 patients under local anesthesia. In 9 of these, a linear incision was made, a hole was punched through the skin above the bone-anchored implant, and a longer abutment (8.5–12 mm) was introduced, whereas the other 9 were subjected to the standard protocol, using a dermatome and skin thinning. All of the patients were followed for 12 months.

Results.—The test group exhibited good preservation of the tissue, no increasing skin reactions and no adverse events. The time required for this surgery was reduced, as was their healing time. These patients also experienced less numbness and pain in the surrounding area and had an improved cosmetic outcome.

Main Outcome and Conclusion.—This clinical trial indicates that introduction of the abutment to the osseointegrated screw directly through the skin, without skin thinning, could be beneficial. This approach had fewer negative effects than the conventional procedure during the 12-month follow-up period.

▶ Since its introduction, the surgical method for bone-anchored hearing devices has undergone several changes. Initially, a 2-staged approach was used. This was followed by a thin pedicled skin flap using a dermatome and later a single vertical incision, followed by wide thinning of the skin. Unfortunately, despite these modifications, skin infections remain common short- and long-term complications. Additionally, the skin thinning can leave an unsightly scar and depression even if the abutment is later removed. Here the authors provide a further simplified alternative method of implantation without skin thinning in a prospective study. Although this study included a small sample size, the procedure demonstrated fewer complications and more rapid healing. Most importantly, over the 1-year period of follow-up, the local skin infection rate was reduced from greater than 40% to 14%. Although the authors compare the procedure with the skin flap technique, the 40% rate in their control group is comparable to other published series for both skin flap and single-incision methods, and if the 14% number is confirmed in larger series, this would be a great improvement. No analysis of hearing results or of whether the lack of skin thinning led to decreased effectiveness was made. This is a limitation of the study, but it can be inferred that this was not the case because all subjects were still participating at 1-year of follow-up. Two other studies with similar results are referenced in the article. Thus, the era of skin thinning for this procedure may be at an end.

B. J. Balough, Capt, MC, USN

Hyaluronic Acid Fat Graft Myringoplasty: An Office-Based Technique Adapted to Children
Saliba I, Froehlich P (Montreal Univ, Quebec, Canada)
Arch Otolaryngol Head Neck Surg 137:1203-1209, 2011

Objectives.—To evaluate hyaluronic acid fat graft myringoplasty (HAFGM) for different tympanic membrane perforation (TMP) sizes and to compare its success rate with that of the underlay and overlay techniques.
Design.—Prospective study.
Setting.—Tertiary care pediatric center.
Patients.—Two hundred eight children aged 4 to 16 years (mean age, 11.84 years) with TMPs.
Interventions.—The HAFGM is a new technique for TMP repair in an outpatient pediatric population using local anesthesia. All the patients in groups 1 (underlay) and 2 (overlay) were operated on using general anesthesia, whereas group 3 (HAFGM) was operated on at the outpatient office using local anesthesia.
Main Outcome Measures.—Postoperative status of the eardrum, hearing improvement, and incidence of complications.

Results.—Patients with TMP were divided into 3 groups: group 1 had 75 patients; group 2, 65; and group 3, 73. The global success rate was 87% in group 3, with no difference with the remaining 2 groups. Successful closure of different TMP sizes was the same for the 3 groups. Postoperatively, air-bone gap improvement was better for group 3. No bone conduction threshold worsening was noted. The mean duration of the operative procedure was 65, 74, and 18 minutes for groups 1, 2, and 3, respectively ($P = .02$). Mean postoperative follow-up was 20.7, 17.5, and 14.6 months for groups 1, 2, and 3, respectively. Identification of the anterior perforation rim is mandatory to perform HAFGM.

Conclusions.—The HAFGM did not require hospitalization for pediatric patients. It had the advantage of being feasible in children using local anesthesia. Its success rate was comparable with that of conventional techniques.

▶ As health care costs rise, there is a growing trend toward office-based procedures. Both rhinology with balloon sinoplasty and laryngology with transnasal esophagoscopy and a host of other procedures have led the way. Other than pressure equalization tubes and transtympanic administration of medications, otology has relatively few office-based procedures. This study presents data to support the expansion of tympanic membrane repair to an office-based procedure. The scientific basis to support the use of fat as a graft material and the benefits of hyalaronic acid are well discussed. The data presented make a compelling argument that once this technique is acquired, the results equal those of more traditional methods. In fact, the reduction in air-bone gap may be better. A better description of their local anesthetic method is needed, as that is likely the most challenging aspect in the younger child. Injection anesthesia of the external ear may be the main limitation of this technique for these patients. However, roughly one-third of their subjects were younger than 11 years, with the average age between 11 and 12 years. Further explanation of the technique is provided in the reference by Saliba.[1] Advancements such as this to promote office-based otology will be increasingly important in coming years.

B. J. Balough, Capt, MC, USN

Reference

1. Saliba I. Hyaluronic acid fat graft myringoplasty: how we do it. *Clin Otolaryngol.* 2008;33:610-614.

5 Pediatric Otolaryngology

Airway

Bronchoscopy versus multi-detector computed tomography in the diagnosis of congenital vascular ring

Gaafar AH, El-Noueam KI (Alexandria Univ, Egypt)
J Laryngol Otol 125:301-308, 2011

Background.—Vascular rings are congenital vascular anomalies of the aortic arch complex which cause compression of the trachea and/or oesophagus. A variety of investigations may lead to diagnosis of these anomalies, including bronchoscopy and computed tomography. During the latter, image acquisition and processing use the multi-detector row technique and new reconstruction algorithms, producing high-resolution images which can be visualised as complex, three-dimensional renditions.

Objective.—This study aimed to assess and compare the roles of bronchoscopy and multi-detector row computed tomography in the diagnosis of congenital vascular ring.

Patients and Methods.—We included infants and children below the age of 16 years who presented with congenital vascular ring. All patients underwent rigid bronchoscopy under general anaesthesia, with spontaneous respiration. All computed tomography scans were obtained using a 16 multi-detector row computed tomography system, followed by data reconstruction on a three-dimensional workstation.

Results.—Ten patients with congenital vascular ring were identified (six boys and four girls). Fifty per cent of cases presented within the first year of life. Double aortic arch was the most common anomaly (40 per cent). Bronchoscopy detected external tracheal compression in nine cases (90 per cent). Associated airway lesions were detected endoscopically in three cases. In contrast, multi-detector row computed tomography detected the vascular ring in all cases, with accurate detection of the compressing vessel; however, it did not detect any associated airway lesions.

Conclusion.—Bronchoscopy and radiological evaluation are essential for the diagnosis and pre-operative evaluation of congenital vascular ring. Multi-detector row computed tomography can provide more information about the nature of the disease, and can facilitate better communication between clinicians, compared with conventional computed tomography.

▶ Vascular rings are congenital vascular anomalies of the aortic arch complex. These rare lesions cause compression of the trachea and/or esophagus. This case series is a good summary of the roles of bronchoscopy and imaging in the diagnosis of the underlying lesion. These lesions often manifest with airway compromise because of extrinsic tracheal compression or, less commonly, with feeding problems secondary to esophageal compression. Patients with airway symptoms usually present earlier, whereas those with esophageal symptoms present later in childhood after they start taking solids. This study of 10 children is aimed to assess and compare the roles of bronchoscopy and multidetector-row CT in the diagnosis of congenital vascular ring. Persistent cough was the most common presenting symptom (6 of 10), followed by stridor (3 of 10) and recurrent cyanotic episodes (3 of 10). Other reported symptoms consisted of recurrent asthma (2 patients), recurrent pneumonia (1 patient), recurrent choking (1 patient), and recurrent dysphagia (1 patient). The types of congenital vascular ring detected in this series comprised a double aortic arch in 4 cases (40%), innominate artery compression in 3 cases (30%), right aortic arch in 2 cases (20%), and aberrant subclavian artery in 1 case (10%). The diagnosis of a vascular ring requires a heightened index of clinical suspicion. Once the diagnosis has been made, it is important to obtain different imaging studies to confirm and further delineate the anatomical arrangement. Bronchoscopy is superior at assessing the endoluminal airway and the vocal cords and in diagnosing associated airway lesions. Computed tomography can precisely delineate the exact anatomy of the compressing vessel, enabling optimal surgical intervention. Multidetector row provides better visualization. Throughout this article, there are great figures with amazing detail of congenital vascular rings/anomalies. The study does not compare CT to MRI. With increasing concern about radiation exposure in children with CT scan, the role of CT versus MRI may need to be revisited.

R. B. Mitchell, MD

Common and uncommon vascular rings and slings: a multi-modality review
Dillman JR, Attili AK, Agarwal PP, et al (Univ of Michigan Health System, Ann Arbor; Univ of Kentucky College of Medicine, Lexington)
Pediatr Radiol 41:1440-1454, 2011

Vascular rings and pulmonary slings are congenital anomalies of the aortic arch/great vessels and pulmonary arteries, respectively, that commonly present early during infancy and childhood with respiratory and/or feeding difficulties. The diagnosis of these conditions frequently utilizes a multi-modality radiological approach, commonly utilizing some combination of radiography, esophagography, CT angiography and MR angiography. The purpose of this pictorial review is to illustrate the radiological findings of *common* and *uncommon* vascular rings and pulmonary slings in children using a state-of-the-art multi-modality imaging approach.

▶ A vascular ring is defined as an abnormal encircling of the trachea and esophagus by the aortic arch and its branches, whereas a pulmonary sling is present when the left pulmonary artery arises anomalously from the right pulmonary artery. When symptomatic, these conditions most commonly present with respiratory and feeding difficulties early in life. A double aortic arch is the most commonly detected symptomatic vascular ring, followed by a right aortic arch with an aberrant left subclavian artery (with intact ligamentum arteriosum). A pulmonary sling is diagnosed when the left pulmonary artery arises anomalously from the right pulmonary artery, passing over the right main bronchus and coursing between the trachea and esophagus to reach the left pulmonary hilum. Pulmonary slings most commonly present in the first year of life with respiratory symptoms, such as stridor, wheezing, or recurrent pneumonia. This is an excellent review with excellent illustrations and radiological images of uncommon and rare lesions including a discussion of the role of CT and MR angiography in the diagnosis of these lesions.

R. B. Mitchell, MD

Basic and Clinical Research

A placental chorionic villous mesenchymal core cellular origin for infantile haemangioma

Itinteang T, Tan ST, Guthrie S, et al (Victoria Univ of Wellington, New Zealand; et al)
J Clin Pathol 64:870-874, 2011

Aims.—To investigate the expression of the placental cell-specific associated proteins in infantile haemangioma (IH).

Methods.—Immunohistochemical staining was used to investigate the expression of human chorionic gonadotrophin (hCG), human placental lactogen (hPL), human leucocyte antigen-G (HLA-G), cytokeratin 7 (CK7) and smooth muscle actin in paraffin-embedded sections of proliferating and involuted IHs.

Results.—The proteins hCG and hPL were expressed by the endothelium but not the pericyte layer of proliferating IH, but these proteins were not detected in involuted lesions. There was no expression of CK7 and HLA-G in IH.

Conclusions.—The expression of hCG and hPL, but not CK7 or HLA-G, by the endothelium of proliferating IH supports a placental chorionic villous mesenchymal core cellular origin for IH rather than a trophoblast origin.

▶ This report is from a group of investigators who have reported on the origins of infantile hemangioma (IH) in several previous studies. IH is considered a primary tumor of the microvasculature; however, recent data support a primitive mesoderm-derived hemogenic endothelium phenotype for the microvessels of proliferating IH. This is further substantiated by the observation that cells from proliferating IH have the ability to undergo erythropoietic and mesenchymal differentiation. The demonstration of embryonic stem cell associated proteins in proliferating IH suggests that this lesion contains cells with an early embryonic origin (trophoblasts) and is more consistent with the notion that IH is a developmental anomaly rather than simply an aberrant proliferation of immature endothelial cells (extraembryonic primitive mesoderm). Using immunohistochemical staining of infantile hemangioma, the investigators demonstrate expression of human chorionic gonadotrophin and human placental lactogen, but not cytokeratin 7 or human leucocyte antigen-G, by the endothelium of proliferating IH. This supports a placental chorionic villous mesenchymal core cellular origin for IH. The study explains previous observations of the unique similarities between IH and placental tissue. Additionally, the authors propose an explanation to account for the origin of segmental and focal IH.

R. B. Mitchell, MD

General

Acute otitis media—induced petrous apicitis presenting as the Gradenigo syndrome: successfully treated by ventilation tube insertion
Kong S-K, Lee I-W, Goh E-K, et al (Pusan Natl Univ, Busan, Korea)
Am J Otolaryngol 32:445-447, 2011

Petrous apicitis has traditionally been treated with aggressive surgical methods. However, recent reports describe good results with more conservative medical treatment and minimal surgical intervention. We report a case of petrous apicitis presenting as the Gradenigo syndrome treated by ventilation tube insertion. We recommend aggressive surgical intervention for patients who failed to respond to conservative therapy including ventilation tube insertion.

▶ The incidence of acute petrous apicitis is reported to be approximately 2 per 100 000 children with acute otitis media. Petrositis caused by acute otitis media was common at the beginning of the 20th century and is seen less frequently because of widespread use of antibiotics. Petrous apex pneumatization is not essential for the spread of infection, and petrous apicitis might be the result of direct extension due to bone destruction or spread via venous channels. The infection may spread outside of the petrous apex to affect the meninges and cranial nerves and may be the cause of encephalitis or brain abscess formation. Temporal petrositis may present with the triad of otorrhea, pain in the distribution of the fifth cranial nerve, and abducens palsy, classically known as Gradenigo syndrome. The management of this condition has classically been surgical decompression with a high associated morbidity. In this report, a 10-year-old child with clinical and radiologic findings of petrous apicitis was treated effectively with intravenous antibiotics and a ventilation tube. The authors argue and summarize recent reports that describe good results with more conservative medical treatment and minimal surgical intervention. They recommend aggressive surgical intervention for patients who did not respond to conservative therapy, including ventilation tube insertion. This is an interesting report and an approach that may become more commonplace as a first-stage approach to management of this challenging but rare condition.

R. B. Mitchell, MD

Ophthalmic complications of otitis media in children
Pollock TJ, Kim P, Sargent MA, et al (Univ of British Columbia, Vancouver, Canada)
J AAPOS 15:272-275, 2011

Purpose.—To evaluate the outcome of ophthalmic complications in children with otitis media.

Methods.—The records of children with ophthalmic complications arising from otitis media who presented to the British Columbia Children's Hospital between August 2006 and March 2008 were reviewed retrospectively.

Results.—Of 1,400 patients presenting to the emergency department for otitis media during the study period, 7 with ophthalmic complications were identified (age range, 1-11 years). All patients had abducens nerve palsy on presentation. Other notable ophthalmic complications included papilledema, Horner syndrome, and proptosis. Extracranial and intracranial complications included mastoiditis, petrositis, parapharyngeal abscess, hydrocephalus, epidural abscess, and cerebral venous thrombosis, including cavernous sinus thrombosis in 2. Of the 7 patients, 6 were treated with surgery, including myringotomy and tube placement (6 patients) and mastoidectomy (3 patients). All patients were initially anticoagulated and received intravenous antibiotics. Satisfactory final visual outcomes and stereopsis ranging from 40 to 100 seconds were achieved in all patients.

Conclusions.—Ophthalmic complications of otitis media in children are likely to include abducens palsy. All patients in our series required anticoagulation and intravenous antibiotics. Most required otolaryngologic surgery, but none required strabismus surgery, and all patients had satisfactory visual and ocular motility outcomes.

▶ The purpose of this study was to identify the ophthalmic, extracranial, and intracranial complications that may occur secondary to otitis media in an era of presumably reduced antibiotic use. Approximately 1400 patients presented to the British Columbia Children's Hospital Emergency Department with otitis media during the study period, and 7 had ophthalmic complication. These complications included abducens nerve palsy or Gradenigo syndrome (7 patients [100%]), papilledema (otitic hydrocephalus, 4 patients [57%]), proptosis (2 patients [29%]), and Horner syndrome (1 patient [14%]). It is possible that more patients developed milder ophthalmological complications of otitis media but were not referred because of relatively subtle findings. Regardless of this, there is a low rate of significant complications. No conclusive evidence links an increased incidence of otitis media complications with reduced or judicious use of antibiotics based on this study. The authors suggest that clinicians maintain a high level of suspicion in patients with recurrent or persistent otologic disease, especially those with symptoms of headache, blurred vision, or diplopia. Clinicians should be particularly vigilant regarding the development of orbital symptoms, which in this series were associated with a high incidence of potentially life-threatening cavernous sinus thrombosis.

R. B. Mitchell, MD

Otitis media with effusion with or without atopy: audiological findings on primary schoolchildren
Martines F, Martines E, Sciacca V, et al (Università degli Studi di Palermo, Via del Vespro, Italy; Università degli Studi di Palermo, Via Archirafi, Palermo Italy)
Am J Otolaryngol 32:601-606, 2011

Objective.—The objective of the study was to evaluate the role of atopy in otitis media with effusion (OME) in children attending primary school, focusing on the audiometric and tympanometric measurements among atopic and nonatopic subjects suffering from OME.

Materials and Methods.—Three hundred ten children (5—6 years old) were screened in Western Sicily by skin tests and divided into atopics (G1) and nonatopics (G2). The samples were evaluated for OME by pneumatic otoscopy, tympanogram, and acoustic reflex tests. The parameters considered were as follows: documented persistent middle ear effusion by otoscopic examination for a minimum of 3 months, presence of B or C tympanogram, absence of ipsilateral acoustic reflex, and a conductive hearing loss greater than 25 dB at any one of the frequencies from 250 Hz through 4 kHz.

Results.—The overall prevalence rate of OME was 12.9% (42.85% for G1 and 6.30% for G2, odds ratio = 11.16); OME was bilateral in 28 children (70%). B tympanogram was evidenced in 48 ears (70.59%), with a significative difference between G1 and G2 ($P < .001$). The analysis of mean air conduction pure tone (31.97 dB for G1 and 29.8 dB for G2) and of tympanometric measurements such as ear canal volume, tympanometric peak pressure, and static compliance by analysis of variance test showed a significative difference between G1 and G2 ($P < .05$).

Conclusions.—The higher prevalence of OME in atopic children and the statistically significant differences in audiometric and tympanometric measurements among atopic and nonatopic subjects suffering from OME suggest the important role of allergy in the genesis and recurrence of OME.

▶ The involvement of immunoglobulin E—mediated allergic reactions in the pathogenesis of otitis media with effusion (OME) has been suggested by clinical observations of a high prevalence of OME among patients with allergies. In fact, several studies reported that 40% to 50% of children with OME aged older than 3 years had nasal allergy, and 21% of allergic children have OME. This study compared children with and without positive skin-prick tests using a variety of clinical and audiological measures of OME. The study supports the hypothesis that allergic inflammation may have a role in the genesis and recurrence of OME. The results show a prevalence rate of OME among primary schoolchildren aged 5 to 6 years of 12.9%. The incidence of OME was higher in atopics (42%) than the nonatopic subjects (6%). Moreover, the results show a clear difference in audiometric and tympanometric measurements between atopic and nonatopic populations. The data support the use of antiallergic medication as a first-line treatment of children with OME.

R. B. Mitchell, MD

Do-it-yourself grommets
Maung KH, Tun T, Stafford ND (Castle Hill Hosp, Cottingham, UK; Yangon Ear, Nose and Throat Hosp, Myanmar)
J Laryngol Otol 125:1268-1269, 2011

In the absence of a healthcare budget enabling the import of ready-made aural grommets, Myanmar ENT surgeons have devised an ingenious 'home-grown' solution. We describe how grommets are made from raw materials bought from the local market (Figs 1-4).

▶ This is an interesting report that highlights the adaptability of otolaryngologists under difficult circumstances. In Myanmar (Burma), annual per capita health care spending is US$394 (2.8% of gross domestic product) compared with multiples of this in the United States. As such, ear tubes (grommets) are unavailable. As a result, Myanmar clinicians have used their ingenuity to create solutions to commonly encountered health care problems. Below are diagrams illustrating how otolaryngologists in Myanmar have devised a quick, cheap, and very effective method of producing their own grommets (Figs 1—4). The

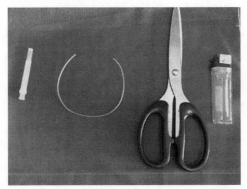

FIGURE 1.—Materials required for grommets. (Reprinted from Maung KH, Tun T, Stafford ND. Do-it-yourself grommets. *J Laryngol Otol.* 2011;125:1268-1269, with permission of Cambridge University Press.)

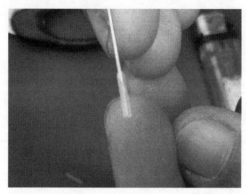

FIGURE 2.—The polythene tube section is mounted on the tip of a 21 gauge green needle. (Reprinted from Maung KH, Tun T, Stafford ND. Do-it-yourself grommets. *J Laryngol Otol.* 2011;125:1268-1269, with permission of Cambridge University Press.)

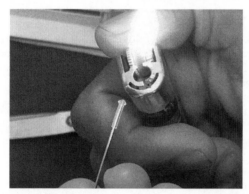

FIGURE 3.—The cigarette lighter flame is used to partially melt and roll the free edge of the tube section. (Reprinted from Maung KH, Tun T, Stafford ND. Do-it-yourself grommets. *J Laryngol Otol.* 2011;125:1268-1269, with permission of Cambridge University Press.)

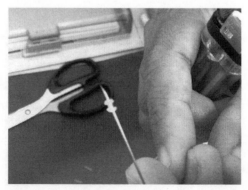

FIGURE 4.—The process is repeated at the other end of the tube, producing a grommet. (Reprinted from Maung KH, Tun T, Stafford ND. Do-it-yourself grommets. *J Laryngol Otol.* 2011;125:1268-1269, with permission of Cambridge University Press.)

average in situ life of a grommet ranges from 6 to 10 months. Local audit data indicate that the incidences of otorrhoea and persistent perforation after grommet extrusion are 5% and 3%, respectively.

R. B. Mitchell, MD

Dexamethasone and Postoperative Bleeding Risk After Adenotonsillectomy in Children
Ahmed KA, Dreher ME, King RF, et al (Mayo Clinic, Rochester, MN; Mayo School of Health Sciences, Rochester, MN)
Laryngoscope 121:1060-1061, 2011

Background.—Reports on the general risk of bleeding after adenotonsillectomy have cited rates between 5.4% and 6.75%. A recent study by Czarnetzki et al noted a dose-dependent increase in the rate to as much as 24% when 0.5 mg/kg dexamethasone was used to prevent postoperative nausea and vomiting. A retrospective review of data from an unpublished trial was conducted to determine if these high rates could be duplicated.

Methods.—The efficacy of low-dose ketamine to manage the postoperative pain of adenotonsillectomy was evaluated in 122 pediatric patients (age 3 to 12 years) who underwent outpatient procedures. Patients were randomly assigned to receive 0.1 mg/kg ketamine or normal saline solution, but all received 0.5 mg/kg dexamethasone (maximum dose 10 mg) immediately after anesthesia induction. Follow-up data were obtained via telephone 1, 3, and 5 days postoperatively and at a 30-day postoperative visit.

Results.—Seven patients (5.7% incidence) reported bleeding episodes. One occurred at some time before the 30-day visit and did not require emergency department evaluation. Six occurred a mean of 6.7 days postoperatively. Five were minor and required no cauterization, but one required operative cauterization of the left and right inferior tonsillar poles.

Conclusions.—The increased risk of bleeding associated with dexamethasone to manage nausea and vomiting reported in the Czarnetzki et al study could not be reproduced. It would be premature to recommend not using dexamethasone during pediatric adenotonsillectomy because of the risk of bleeding.

▶ This is a rapid communication to alleviate concerns from a previous study that linked use of dexamethasone with a high rate of bleeding after adenotonsillectomy. A recent study in pediatric patients studied by Czarnetzki et al[1] reported a dose-dependent increase in the rate of postoperative bleeding with the use of dexamethasone for preventing postoperative nausea and vomiting. The reported rates were 12% (6 of 50 patients) with 0.05 mg/kg dexamethasone, 3.9% (2 of 51) with 0.15 mg/kg dexamethasone, and 24% (12 of 50) with 0.5 mg/kg dexamethasone, compared with 3.8% (2 of 53) with placebo. This is an alarming result, particularly because many otolaryngologists have used dexamethasone at doses higher than 0.5 mg/kg to prevent postoperative nausea and vomiting or swelling. The authors report data from an unpublished trial (Dreher et al) designed to evaluate the efficacy of low-dose ketamine for the treatment of postoperative adenotonsillectomy pain, with 122 children aged 3 to 12 years who all received dexamethasone 0.5 mg/kg (maximum dose, 10 mg). Patients in this study experienced a far lower postoperative bleeding rate of 5.7%. These results correspond well with previously published reports on the general risk of bleeding after adenotonsillectomy, with rates ranging from 5.4% to 6.75%. Although the results of the study by Czarnetzki et al are concerning, the current study suggests that it would be premature to discontinue the use of dexamethasone during adenotonsillectomy.

R. B. Mitchell, MD

Reference

1. Czarnetzki C, Elia N, Lysakowski C, et al. Dexamethasone and risk of nausea and vomiting and postoperative bleeding after tonsillectomy in children: a randomized trial. *JAMA.* 2008;300:2621-2630.

Changes in Heart Rate Variability After Adenotonsillectomy in Children With Obstructive Sleep Apnea
Muzumdar HV, Sin S, Nikova M, et al (Children's Hosp at Montefiore, Bronx, NY; et al)
Chest 139:1050-1059, 2011

Background.—Obstructive sleep apnea syndrome (OSAS) is associated with cardiovascular morbidity and mortality, and increased sympathetic activity is considered to be a causative link in this association. Higher levels of sympathetic activity have been reported in children with OSAS. Sympathetic predominance is indicated on heart rate variability (HRV) analysis by increased heart rate (HR) and a higher ratio of low-frequency to high-frequency band power (LF/HF). Improvement in OSAS after adenotonsillectomy (AT) in children with OSAS could, therefore, be associated with reduced HR and reduced LF/HF.

Methods.—Changes in HR and time and frequency components of HRV were retrospectively analyzed in 2-min epochs free of respiratory events during light, deep, and rapid-eye-movement (REM) sleep in children with OSAS who underwent polysomnography before and after AT.

Results.—Eighteen children with OSAS, aged 4.9 ± 2.4 years (mean ± SD) were studied. After AT, the apnea-hypopnea index decreased from 31.9 ± 24.8 events/h to 4.1 ± 3.7 events/h. The HR decreased after AT in all stages of sleep (99.8 ± 16.9 beats/min to 80.7 ± 12.9 beats/min [light sleep]; 100.2 ± 15.4 beats/min to 80.5 ± 12.4 beats/min [deep sleep)]; and 106.9 ± 16.4 beats/min to 87.0 ± 12.1 beats/min [REM sleep]), as did the LF/HF (1.6 ± 2.7 to 0.6 ± 0.5 [light sleep]; 1.2 ± 1.6 to 0.5 ± 0.6 [deep sleep]; and 3.0 ± 5.4 to 1.4 ± 1.7 [REM sleep]).

Conclusions.—The proportion of sympathetic activity of the autonomic nervous system declines in children with OSAS after AT in association with improvement in sleep-disordered breathing.

▶ Obstructive sleep apnea syndrome (OSAS) in adults is known to be linked to cardiovascular morbidity. The link in children has been studied less extensively. Adenotonsillectomy (AT) is the accepted first-line option in children with adenotonsillar hypertrophy and OSAS and results in a significant improvement in sleep parameters. This study hypothesized that improvement in OSAS after AT would be associated with a reduction in heart rate and the low-frequency to high-frequency band power (LF/HF). The LF/HF ratio represents sympatho-vagal balance, with an increase in the LF/HF indicating a tilt toward the sympathetic component. This study demonstrates that improvement in OSAS following AT in children is associated with changes in autonomic balance, with decreased LF/HF in all stages of sleep and improvement of OSAS, approaching values similar to those of the control group. Together, the decreases in HR and the LF/HF imply a shift in autonomic balance away from the sympathetic component with reductions in OSAS. The changes in HR after AT were significant in obese and nonobese children, but the obese group had more consistent reductions in the LF/HF, suggesting that obese children with OSAS may have greater autonomic imbalance than nonobese children with OSAS. The clinical implications of these findings are unclear.

R. B. Mitchell, MD

Adverse effects of propranolol when used in the treatment of hemangiomas: A case series of 28 infants
de Graaf M, Breur JMPJ, Raphaël MF, et al (Univ Med Ctr Utrecht, The Netherlands)
J Am Acad Dermatol 65:320-327, 2011

Background.—Infantile hemangioma (IH) is a frequently encountered tumor with a potentially complicated course. Recently, propranolol was discovered to be an effective treatment option.

Objective.—To describe the effects and side effects of propranolol treatment in 28 children with (complicated) IH.

Methods.—A protocol for treatment of IH with propranolol was designed and implemented. Propranolol was administered to 28 children (21 girls and 7 boys, mean age at onset of treatment: 8.8 months).

Results.—All 28 patients had a good response. In two patients, systemic corticosteroid therapy was tapered successfully after propranolol was initiated. Propranolol was also an effective treatment for hemangiomas in 4 patients older than 1 year of age. Side effects that needed intervention and/or close monitoring were not dose dependent and included symptomatic hypoglycemia (n = 2; 1 patient also taking prednisone), hypotension (n = 16, of which 1 is symptomatic), and bronchial hyperreactivity (n = 3).

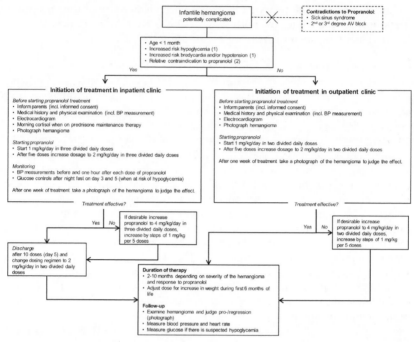

FIGURE 1.—Guidelines for utilization of propranolol in the treatment of (complicated) IH at Wilhelmina's Childrens Hospital. (1) For example, prematurity or dysmaturity and/or simultaneous use of prednisone; (2) relative contraindications to propranolol: impaired cardiac function (when this is secondary to the hemangioma, appropriate treatment is advisable); Sinus bradycardia, hypotension, first-degree atrioventricular block; asthma; and/or bronchial hyperreactivity; diabetes mellitus; chronic renal insufficiency. *AV*, Atrioventricular; *BP*, blood pressure. (Reprinted from the Journal of the American Academy of Dermatology, de Graaf M, Breur JMPJ, Raphaël MF, et al. Adverse effects of propranolol when used in the treatment of hemangiomas: a case series of 28 infants. *J Am Acad Dermatol.* 2011;65:320-327. Copyright 2011, with permission from the American Academy of Dermatology.)

Restless sleep (n = 8), constipation (n = 3) and cold extremities (n = 3) were observed.

Limitations.—Clinical studies are necessary to evaluate the incidence of side effects of propranolol treatment of IH.

Conclusions.—Propranolol appears to be an effective treatment option for IH even in the nonproliferative phase and after the first year of life. Potentially harmful adverse effects include hypoglycemia, bronchospasm, and hypotension (Fig 1).

▶ This report should be read by otolaryngologists who take care of children with infantile hemangiomas (IH). IHs are benign vascular tumors found in up to 10% of white infants. They are characterized by a 3- to 9-month period of rapid growth followed by gradual involution.

Prednisone has been used for treatment of complicated IH, but more recently dramatic results with the use of propranolol have been reported. Propranolol is a nonselective beta-blocker that has been available since 1964 and is widely used in pediatric cardiology. There has been limited experience of propranolol for treatment of IH, and the mechanism of action is poorly understood. This report confirms the impressive results of propranolol as a treatment for IH. It may be a more effective and safer therapeutic drug than systemic corticosteroids. A useful algorithm (Fig 1) is included. Because of potentially harmful side effects, including hypoglycemia, bronchospasm, and hypotension, these patients are preferably treated in a multidisciplinary setting by physicians knowledgeable in the management of IH with propranolol.

R. B. Mitchell, MD

Current Treatment of Parotid Hemangiomas

Weiss I, O TM, Lipari BA, et al (Beth Israel and Roosevelt Hosps, NY; et al)
Laryngoscope 121:1642-1650, 2011

Objectives/Hypothesis.—Parotid hemangiomas are the most common salivary gland tumors in children. Their treatment has posed a challenge because of the lesions' expansive growth, resistance to treatment, and relationship with the facial nerve. Various treatment modalities have been attempted, and promising results have been achieved with surgical resection alone or in conjunction with endovascular sclerotherapy. Recently, bleomycin and oral propranolol have been introduced, and the results thus far are promising. Here we elucidate the treatment options and propose a treatment algorithm for parotid hemangiomas.

Study Design.—Retrospective chart review.

Methods.—We conducted a retrospective chart review of patients from 2004 to 2009 with hemangiomas involving the parotid gland. We included 56 patients and relevant parameters.

Results.—Seventy percent of patients were female. The female-to-male ratio was 2.3 to 1. Thirty-nine percent had unilateral parotid hemangiomas, 12.5% had cutaneous segmental hemangiomas. All 22 patients who underwent systemic steroid therapy responded initially, but 68% of these rebounded after cessation of therapy. Sixteen patients (29%) underwent surgery with excellent results (facial symmetry, restoration of contour, preserved facial nerve function). Seven (44%) patients received sclerotherapy 24 to 48 hours before surgery, and five (8%) received endovascular sclerotherapy alone. Ten patients were treated medically with oral propranolol. Eight of 10 had significant shrinkage of the lesion within the first month of treatment. There were no reported side effects.

Conclusions.—Multiple treatment regimens have been used to successfully treat parotid hemangiomas. Although propranolol is a recent addition, it seems most promising. Further evaluation is warranted (Fig 5).

▶ Hemangiomas are the most common of all childhood tumors. Hemangiomas of the parotid gland are the most common benign salivary gland tumors in children. They occur in up to 10% of all newborn infants and in up to 23% of premature infants. Parotid hemangiomas have posed a surgical challenge because of

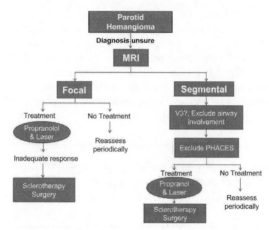

FIGURE 5.—Treatment algorithm. [Color figure can be viewed in the online issue, which is available at wileyonlinelibrary.com.] (Reprinted from Weiss I, O TM, Lipari BA, et al. Current treatment of parotid hemangiomas. *Laryngoscope.* 2011;121:1642-1650, with permission from The American Laryngological, Rhinological and Otological Society, Inc, and John Wiley and Sons (www.interscience.wiley.com).)

their proximity to and frequent involvement of the facial nerve. Several treatment modalities have been implemented. These include conservative management (benign neglect), systemic and intralesional steroids, interferon α-2a (IFN α-2a), vincristine, surgical resection, and, more recently, bleomycin and propranolol. This is a good retrospective review of the different treatment modalities available, and proposes a treatment algorithm for parotid hemangiomas (Fig 5). Treatment of parotid hemangiomas with propranolol, which to date shows few side effects and achieves satisfactory involution, is very promising. They argue that, in the future, this treatment might replace all previous practices. Further investigation is warranted.

R. B. Mitchell, MD

Button battery ingestion: The greek experience and review of the literature
Amanatidou V, Sofidiotou V, Fountas K, et al (Panagiotis and Aglaia Kyriakou Childrens Hosp, Athens, Greece)
Pediatr Emerg Care 27:186-188, 2011

Objectives.—Foreign body ingestion is a common cause of admission in the pediatric emergency room. In the past, button batteries accounted for less than 2% of the foreign bodies ingested by small children, but in the last 2 decades, they show a rapidly increased frequency. The aim of the present study was to evaluate the potential risk after button battery ingestion in relation with the clinical manifestations and to perform a treatment-observation protocol in accordance with the international procedure.

Methods and Results.—In a prospective observational analysis from November 2007 through February 2008, 31 cases of button battery ingestion

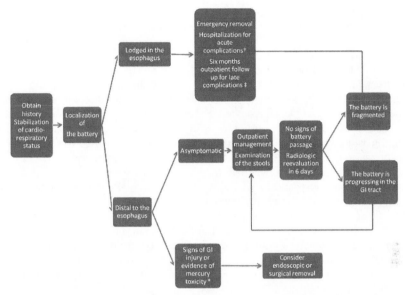

FIGURE 1.—Management of BBI. *GI injury: acute abdomen, vomiting, hematochezia, melena, and fever. Evidence of mercury toxicity: elevated levels and clinical symptoms of mercury poisoning. †Acute complications: esophageal perforation, tracheoesophageal fistula. ‡Delayed complication: esophageal stenosis. (Reprinted from Amanatidou V, Sofidiotou V, Fountas K, et al. Button battery ingestion: the Greek experience and review of the literature. *Pediatr Emerg Care.* 2011;27:186-188.)

were recorded by the Greek Poison Information Center. The interval between the accidental ingestion and first medical contact ranged from 5 minutes to 10 days. After initial evaluation including clinical examination and radiological localization of the foreign body, all cases were treated as outpatients. Reported complications included "black stools" in 9% and diarrhea in 3% of cases. In 1 case, the battery was endoscopically removed.

Conclusions.—The role of primary care physicians in informing the public about the potential danger of button battery digestion is crucial. Pediatricians should educate the parents about this hazard, as part of the routine guidelines for childproofing at home. Once again, prolepsis is the best policy (Fig 1).

▶ This is a good study that summarizes the problems associated with button-battery ingestion. In 80% to 90% of reported cases, the ingested batteries pass through the gastrointestinal (GI) tract without any symptoms, signs, or complications. Most remaining cases have mild GI irritation symptoms, and only a small percentage appear with serious symptoms due to battery's impaction, usually in the esophagus. Major complications or even death appear within a short period. Studies in animal models show mucosal injury as early as 1 hour, progressing to necrosis within 4 hours. In the previous 2 decades, the recorded cases of disk (or button) battery ingestion have shown an increased incidence worldwide, probably in accordance to the increased use of miniature electronic devices. These batteries are small, disk-shaped power units frequently contained in digital watches, hearing aids, cameras, remote controls, toys, and other electronic devices. They contain a variety of heavy metals (mercury, zinc, silver, nickel, lithium) in a strong alkaline electrolyte solution. Among them, mercury batteries are considered to be the most dangerous and are banned in many countries. Current studies indicate that there is a direct correlation between the major complications and the chronic interval from accidental battery ingestion until medical intervention. The diameter of the ingested battery is also strongly related to the risk of esophageal obstruction. Evidence shows that a relatively large-size button battery of more than 15 mm and frequently of 20- to 23-mm diameter is responsible for almost all problems. The most frequent symptom in cases with esophageal impaction is dysphagia; however, approximately one-third of the reported series with serious complications had minimal and nonspecific symptoms with no swallowing difficulties. This may lead to delayed recognition and increase the risk of esophageal perforation. All relevant studies point out that most of these accidents happen in the family environment. Thus, the role of primary care physicians in informing the public of this danger is crucial. Fig 1 summarizes a proposed algorithm that is practical and user-friendly.

R. B. Mitchell, MD

Living With a Craniofacial Condition: Development of the Craniofacial Experiences Questionnaire (CFEQ) for Adolescents and Their Parents

Roberts RM, Shute R (Univ of Adelaide, South Australia, Australia; Flinders Univ, Adelaide, South Australia, Australia)
Cleft Palate Craniofac J 48:727-735, 2011

Objective.—To develop a new instrument (the Craniofacial Experiences Questionnaire, CFEQ) to measure both stressors and positive aspects of living with a craniofacial condition from adolescent and parent perspectives, and to examine its validity and reliability. A secondary aim was to explore experiences reported according to age, gender, and diagnosis.

Design.—Self-report and parent report questionnaires (CFEQ, Youth Self Report [YSR], Child Behavior Checklist [CBCL], Behavioral and Emotional Rating Scale [BERS]) were completed by adolescents with congenital craniofacial conditions and their parents.

Participants.—Fifty adolescents with craniofacial conditions and 55 of their parents.

Results.—Internal reliability of the stressor and positive aspects scales was acceptable (.81 to .92) but was lower for some stressor subscales (.50−.86). Higher stressor scale scores were related to poorer adjustment (CBCL $r = .55$, YSR $r = .37$). There were no consistent differences in the stressful or positive experiences of young people with craniofacial conditions according to gender or age. There were no differences in stressors reported according to diagnosis.

Conclusions.—The CFEQ shows promise as a clinical and research tool for investigating the stressors and positive experiences of young people with craniofacial conditions. Consistent with the literature on chronic pediatric conditions, there were few differences in experiences of young people according to diagnosis. Furthermore, the lack of gender or age differences supports the need for clinicians to comprehensively assess the experiences of young people regardless of demographic variables.

▶ Craniofacial anomalies (CFAs) comprise a diverse group of congenital deformities in the growth of the head and facial bones. The most common is cleft lip and palate. Other CFAs, although rare, as a group represent half the children seen with CFAs. Associated difficulties include problems with feeding, growth, dental development, speech and language, and chronic ear infections. Management frequently involves many investigations, appointments, clinic meetings, orthodontic treatment, and several operations. It is therefore important to be able to measure condition-related stressors to increase both our understanding of the experiences of these young people and the factors related to positive outcomes. The authors argue that available instruments do not target this specific population that would otherwise be neglected. Participants were recruited from families involved in a longitudinal study of adolescents with CFAs in Australia. The Craniofacial Experiences Questionnaire (CFEQ) was constructed based on previous work by the authors. Both a parent version (CFEQ-P) and young person's version (CFEQ) were developed with equivalent items worded appropriately. This study was aimed at looking at the internal validity and reliability of the instrument. Respondents were asked to indicate how often each experience had happened to them (or to their adolescent) in the past year, from "never" (1) to "always" (4). The instrument shows promise as a clinical and research tool for investigating both the stressful and positive experiences of young people with craniofacial conditions. It will be important in the future to test the instrument on a larger patient population to assess the test-retest reliability of the questionnaire. It is likely to become a widely used tool in children with craniofacial anomalies.

R. B. Mitchell, MD

Outcomes

Does Concomitant Mastoidectomy Improve Outcomes for Patients Undergoing Repair of Tympanic Membrane Perforations?

Hall JE, McRackan TR, Labadie RF (Vanderbilt Univ Med Ctr, Nashville, TN)
Laryngoscope 121:1598-1600, 2011

Background.—Tympanoplasty with or without mastoidectomy is a common procedure but failures of perforation closure can occur. Whether mastoidectomy is needed is a controversial topic, with proponents of the combined procedure contending that the surgical opening of the mastoid pneumatic system buffers pressure changes in the middle ear and permits debridement of infected tissue and devitalized bone. Recent studies tend to refute this position. The current literature was searched to determine the best practice.

Methods.—The literature review identified five studies reporting the outcomes of tympanoplasty with or without mastoidectomy to treat non-cholesteatomatous chronic suppurative otitis media (CSOM).

Results.—In 323 patients Balyan et al found no statistically significant differences in terms of graft success, mean residual gap differences, or dry or draining ears. They concluded that mastoidectomy is an avoidable procedure in noncholesteatomatous CSOM. In contrast, McGrew et al studied 320 patients having tympanoplasty alone and 144 having the combined procedure and found no statistically significant differences in perforation repair success or postoperative airbone gap. Mastoidectomy tended to be performed more often in younger patients, those with a higher percentage of ipsilateral pressure equalization tube placement, and those with contralateral otologic disease. Long-term, patients with tympanoplasty alone were more likely to need later otologic procedures than patients with the combined procedure. There were significant trends toward better hearing outcomes and less need for subsequent procedures when the mastoidectomy was performed. In 251 patients Mishiro et al found that mastoidectomy was not helpful, a finding also echoed in Toros et al's study of 46 patients. In 47 pediatric patients having mastoidectomy for noncholesteatomatous CSOM, Rickers et al found that 42% of patients had normal tympanic membranes at a median of 15 years postoperatively, but 40% of patients needed at least one subsequent procedure.

Conclusions.—Tympanoplasty alone may be sufficient to repair simple, uncomplicated tympanic membrane perforation. A large prospective, randomized, multi-institution analysis of mastoidectomy with tympanoplasty is needed to provide sufficient data on the need and indications for mastoidectomy. However, because most surgeons currently combine the procedures, it is unlikely that such a study will be conducted soon.

▶ Controversy currently exists among otologists regarding the appropriate treatment of tympanic membrane perforations (by tympanoplasty alone or with mastoidectomy) resulting from chronic suppurative otitis media without cholesteatoma. Several recent studies investigating tympanoplasty with or without mastoidectomy refute the claim that mastoidectomy improves otologic outcomes following perforation repair. This is a review of the current literature in an effort to elucidate the best practice. The authors review 4 retrospective case-controlled studies with internal controls (level 3 evidence) and 1 retrospective cohort study (level 4 evidence). A large prospective, randomized, multi-institutional analysis of mastoidectomy with tympanoplasty would provide much needed data regarding the necessity of and indications for mastoidectomy in this patient population. As evidenced in the literature, tympanoplasty alone may be sufficient for repair of simple and uncomplicated tympanic membrane perforations. Although these studies included children and adults, the conclusion is particularly important in children, in whom a more conservative plan is often sought.

R. B. Mitchell, MD

A Prospective Study of the Effect of Gastroesophageal Reflux Disease Treatment on Children With Otitis Media

McCoul ED, Goldstein NA, Koliskor B, et al (State Univ of New York—Downstate Med Ctr, Brooklyn)

Arch Otolaryngol Head Neck Surg 137:35-41, 2011

Objectives.—To demonstrate improvements in validated quality-of-life measures for otitis media and gastroesophageal reflux disease (GERD) and an objective score for pediatric reflux obtained by fiberoptic laryngoscopy after treatment with antireflux precautions and therapy in children diagnosed as having either recurrent acute otitis media or otitis media with effusion and GERD.

Design.—Prospective, before-and-after intervention study.

Setting.—Hospital-based pediatric otolaryngology practice.

Participants.—Population-based sample of 47 patients (mean age, 19.5 months).

Intervention.—Standard antireflux therapy for 2 consecutive 12-week periods.

Main Outcome Measures.—Otitis Media 6-Item quality-of-life survey, Infant GERD Questionnaire—Revised, GERD Symptom Questionnaire for Young Children, Pediatric Reflux Finding Score, and speech awareness threshold.

Results.—Follow-up data were available for 37 patients. Mean (SD) change scores for Otitis Media 6-Item quality-of-life survey were 1.6 (1.1) at visit 2 and 1.5 (1.1) at visit 3 ($P<.001$ and $P=.004$, respectively). Change scores were significantly improved for Infant GERD Questionnaire—Revised and GERD Symptom Questionnaire for Young Children at visit 2 and for Infant GERD Questionnaire—Revised at visit 3. Mean (SD) change scores for the Pediatric Reflux Finding Score were 6.4 (4.9) at visit 2 and 8.0 (7.2) at visit 3 ($P<.001$ and $P=.03$, respectively). Hearing loss was significantly improved following therapy, as were laryngeal findings of reflux on fiberoptic laryngoscopy. Otitis media was considered by the examining physician to be clinically improved in 28 of 37 children (76%; 95% confidence interval, 60%-87%) at visit 2 and in 6 of 10 children (60%; 95% confidence interval, 31%-83%) at visit 3. Nine children (19.1%) required myringotomy tube placement.

Conclusions.—Children with otitis media with effusion or recurrent acute otitis media and GERD have improved quality of life following treatment with antireflux therapy. Control of gastroesophageal reflux may play a role in the management of otitis media and avoidance of tympanostomy.

▶ Gastroesophageal reflux disease (GERD) may account for a wide variety of symptoms in children. Equally, otitis media with effusion (OME) and recurrent acute otitis media are commonly seen in children. The objectives of this study were to demonstrate subjective improvement on validated quality-of-life surveys for otitis media and GERD after antireflux therapy, as well as objective improvement on audiometry and fiberoptic laryngoscopy (FOL). Because GERD and

OME are 2 of the most prevalent diseases in young children, a number of investigators have taken preliminary steps to demonstrate a causative link between the diseases. Of particular interest has been the presence of gastric enzymes in the middle ear space. This study reports that validated measures of the disease burden of otitis media and GERD showed significant improvement with antireflux therapy. Hearing loss demonstrated on audiometric testing was significantly improved following therapy, as were laryngeal findings of reflux on FOL, although a validated scale for assessment is lacking. The authors conclude that reduction of gastroesophageal reflux may play a role in the prevention of otitis media. This study lacks a control population and randomization. Nonetheless, it reports encouraging data on an important subject. Additional high-quality clinical trials are warranted.

R. B. Mitchell, MD

Can We Predict a Difficult Intubation in Cleft Lip/Palate Patients?

Arteau-Gauthier I, Leclerc JE, Godbout A (Laval Univ, Quebec, Canada; Centre Hospitalier Universitaire de Québec, Canada)
J Otolaryngol Head Neck Surg 40:413-419, 2011

Objective.—To find predictors of a difficult intubation in infants with an isolated or a syndromic cleft lip/palate.

Study Design.—Retrospective review: single-blind trial.

Settings.—Tertiary care centre.

Methods.—A total of 145 infants born with cleft lip/palate were enrolled. Three clinical and seven lip/palate anatomic parameters were evaluated. The grade of intubation was determined by the anesthesiologist at the time of the labioplasty/staphylorrhaphy surgery at 3 and 10 months, respectively.

Main Outcome Measure.—Intubation grade.

Results.—The relative risk of a difficult intubation in the cleft lip, cleft palate without the Pierre Robin sequence, cleft lip-palate, and cleft palate with Pierre Robin sequence groups was 0, 2.7, 10, and 23%, respectively. The infants born with the Pierre Robin sequence had a statistically significant higher intubation grade. The degree of difficulty was increased in cases with early airway and feeding problems ($p < .0001$). Within the group of cleft palate patients without any lip malformation, a wider cleft was associated with a higher intubation grade with statistical significance ($p = .0323$).

Conclusions.—Infants born with Pierre Robin sequence have a statistically significantly higher risk of difficult intubation. Within this group, of all the studied factors, a clinical history of early airway and feeding problems was the best predictor of a difficult endotracheal intubation. In cleft palate patients without any cleft lip, larger width of the cleft is also a significant predictor.

▶ The otolaryngologist is often called as a backup for patients with a potentially difficult airway, such as cleft lip/palate (CLP) patients. Several techniques have been developed to overcome any difficult situations. However, we felt that it would be useful to find some readily available predictors of a difficult airway intubation that would be easy for an airway team to use. The main objective of this study was to search for criteria predicting a difficult airway and develop safe clinical conduct for better airway control. Four groups of patients were identified: cleft lip, cleft lip + cleft palate, isolated cleft palate, and cleft palate associated with Pierre Robin sequence (PRS). The grade of intubation was written on the anesthesiology report sheet according to the Cormack and Lehane classification 4: grade I, visualization of the entire laryngeal aperture; grade II, visualization limited to the posterior portion of the laryngeal aperture; grade III, visualization limited to the epiglottis or its tip; and grade IV, visualization of the soft palate only. For the purpose of this study, grades I and II were classified as an easy laryngoscopy; intubation and grades III and IV were classified as a difficult one. The study was conducted at a tertiary care, academic university—based medical center. Although this study was retrospective, it was based on data from an established prospective database. The methodology was also straightforward. The risks of a difficult intubation (grades III and IV) for cleft lip, cleft palate without PRS, cleft lip-palate, and cleft palate with PRS were 0%, 2.7%, 10%, and 23%, respectively. The latter (PRS) was the only statistically significant result in the study group. The best predictor of a difficult intubation in the PRS patients was the severity of the respiratory and feeding problems in the first few months of life. Of the anatomic measurements, only a larger width of the cleft at the hard palate level showed a relationship with difficult intubation. Thus, most CLP patients do not pose intubation problems. The minority who do pose them have PRS or a wide cleft palate.

R. B. Mitchell, MD

Adenotonsillectomy improves slow-wave activity in children with obstructive sleep apnoea
Ben-Israel N, Zigel Y, Tal A, et al (Ben-Gurion Univ of the Negev, Beer-Sheva, Israel)
Eur Respir J 37:1144-1150, 2011

The aim of the present study was to estimate slow-wave activity (SWA), a marker of sleep homeostasis, in children with obstructive sleep apnoea (OSA) before and after adenotonsillectomy (AT) compared with untreated OSA children (comparison group).

14 children with OSA (mean ± SD age 6.4 ± 2.5 yrs; apnoea—hypopnoea index (AHI) 10.0 ± 10.3 events·h^{-1}) who underwent AT were consecutively recruited to the study. The comparison group comprised six retrospectively recruited children (age 5.4 ± 2.2 yrs; AHI 9.4 ± 7.6 events·h^{-1}) with OSA that did not undergo treatment. Electroencephalogram (derivation C3/A2) was analysed using spectral and waveform analysis to determine SWA energy and slow-wave slope. The same procedure was repeated 5.4 and 19 months later for the AT and comparison groups, respectively.

AT improved respiration without a change in duration of sleep stages. Following AT, >50% elevation of SWA during the first two sleep cycles (p<0.01) and a more physiological decay of SWA across the night (p<0.0001) were noted. The slow-wave slope increased by >30% following AT (p<0.03). No significant changes were found in SWA in the comparison group.

Sleep homeostasis is considerably impaired in pre-pubescent children with OSA. AT restores more physiological sleep homeostasis in children with OSA. SWA analysis may provide a useful addition to standard sleep-stage analyses in children with OSA.

▶ Adenotonsillectomy (AT) has been shown to improve the apnea-hypopnea index (AHI) in children with obstructive sleep apnea (OSA). However, pediatric OSA is thought to cause substantial neurobehavioral morbidity, at least in part through sleep fragmentation. Previous polysomnography data have revealed no consistent differences following AT. Some studies demonstrated improvement in sleep efficiency, decreased stage 1 sleep, and increased slow-wave sleep (SWS). This study explored SWA in children with OSA before and after AT compared with untreated OSA (comparison group). Spectral analysis of slow-wave activity (SWA), used in this study, is a quantitative measure of SWS dynamics and represents a physiologic marker of homeostatic regulation of sleep. Stronger cortical connections would produce stronger network synchronization and, thus, a higher level of SWA, whereas weaker connections would reduce network synchronization and thereby SWA. Children with untreated OSA exhibit decreased SWA level and slope during the night, indicating reduced sleep homeostasis. AT led to more physiologic sleep homeostasis in children with OSA. The study concludes that SWA analysis may provide a useful addition to standard sleep-stage analyses in children with OSA. This study has a small population and is an attempt to link SWS to outcomes following AT. Ultimately what is needed is a way of predicting neurobehavioral morbidity based on PSG and a way of predicting outcomes following AT.

R. B. Mitchell, MD

Incidence of Revision Adenoidectomy in Children
Grindle CR, Murray RC, Chennupati SK, et al (Connecticut Children's Med Ctr, Hartford; Nemours—Al duPont Hosp for Children, Wilmington, DE; Drexel Univ College of Medicine, Philadelphia, PA)
Laryngoscope 121:2128-2130, 2011

Objective/Hypothesis.—Adenoidectomy is a frequently performed procedure in the pediatric population. Revision rates and indications for a second procedure in children are scarce.

Study Design.—Retrospective cohort study.

Methods.—Patient records at a multistate pediatric healthcare system were searched for all CPT codes that included adenoidectomy in children less than 12 years of age for a 5-year period (2005–2010). A subset of patients was identified for whom the same CPT codes appeared more than once in this 5-year period. The indication, age, gender, adenoid size, and technique of adenoidectomy were recorded.

Results.—A total of 23,612 occurrences of the CPT codes were identified. The subset of patients with multiple CPT codes, indicating revision adenoidectomy, included 304 records (1.3%). Mean age at first procedure was 2.8 years (SD = 1.7 years). Mean age at second procedure was 4.7 years (SD = 1.99 years). Mean interval between procedures was 1.8 years (SD = 1.1 years).

Conclusions.—Revision adenoidectomy occurs at a rate of 1.3%. Reasons for revision include persistence symptoms ranging from adenoiditis to recurrent otitis to obstructive sleep apnea.

▶ This is a good and straightforward approach to looking at the rate of revision adenoidectomies. Otolaryngologists have all seen children who regress after initial adenoidectomy, and studies have suggested that regrowth of adenoid tissue may occur in 19% to 26% of children. The options are watchful waiting versus revision surgery. Some children may require revision adenoidectomy because symptoms have recurred or have never resolved. In this study, there were 23 612 records identified for adenoidectomy or adenotonsillectomy in children younger than 12 years, and a search for second occurrence of CPT code showed 304 records, giving a revision rate of 1.3%. The initial procedure was performed at age 2.8 years, and the reoccurrence of symptoms were noted by 4.7 years. Thus, the authors conclude that regrowth of adenoid tissue with recurrence of symptoms is rare and indications for revision are typically recurrence or persistence of initial presenting symptoms. The rate of revision surgery was present regardless of the method used for adenoidectomies. This retrospective study defines the minimum rate of revision adenoidectomies. The number of children with recurrent adenoid hypertrophy who do not seek revision surgery is likely to be higher and remains unknown. Otolaryngologists should make greater effort to perform more complete adenoidectomies to reduce unnecessary health care costs associated with revision surgery.

R. B. Mitchell, MD

Accuracy of prenatal three-dimensional ultrasound in the diagnosis of cleft hard palate when cleft lip is present
Bäumler M, Faure J-M, Bigorre M, et al (Hôpital Arnaud de Villeneuve, Montpellier, France; et al)
Ultrasound Obstet Gynecol 38:440-444, 2011

Objective.—To investigate the accuracy of prenatal axial three-dimensional (3D) ultrasound in predicting the absence or presence of cleft palate in the presence of cleft lip.

Methods.—Between March 2005 and January 2009, there were 81 cases with a prenatal two-dimensional (2D) ultrasound screening diagnosis of unilateral or bilateral cleft lip at 22–25 weeks of gestation referred to our tertiary care center. Of these, 79 fetuses were included in this prospective study and two were excluded. Axial 3D ultrasound imaging of the fetal palate was performed and the diagnoses were compared with clinical findings at delivery. The frequencies of intact and cleft palate, the degree of association between the prenatal predictions and postnatal findings and the probability of detection of cleft lip and palate were determined.

Results.—Of 79 prenatal predictions, 77 (97%) were correct and the association between the prenatal predictions and postnatal findings was strong. The sensitivity for detection of cleft lip and palate within this high-risk population was 100% and the specificity was 90%. In one of the excluded cases, the palate could not be visualized due to a fetal prone position. There were chromosomal anomalies in 4% of cases and associated structural or growth anomalies in 23%, termination of pregnancy was carried out in 4% and intrauterine fetal demise occurred in 3%.

Conclusion.—Axial 3D ultrasound of the fetal palate has high accuracy in identifying prenatal cleft palate when cleft lip is diagnosed at midtrimester 2D ultrasound screening.

▶ Prenatal ultrasound imaging of the fetal palate has advanced in recent years, and different 2-dimensional (2D) and 3-dimensional (3D) ultrasound techniques have been reported to have different visualization rates of the hard and soft palate. The aim of this study was to calculate the accuracy of an axial 3D ultrasound technique in predicting clefting of the fetal hard palate in high-risk cases, that is, when cleft lip is detected by 2D ultrasound scan at the midtrimester screening, comparing prenatal ultrasound predictions with postnatal clinical findings on examination of the newborn's palate. They use the STARD (Standards for Reporting of Diagnostic Accuracy) recommendations for reporting the accuracy of a diagnostic procedure, a method that minimizes bias. They report axial 3D ultrasound imaging to have good predictive power in terms of sensitivity, specificity, contingency, and phi and that there was a strong association between the prenatal diagnoses and postnatal findings. In only 2 of 79 cases was there an error in prediction. The conclusion is that axial 3D ultrasound scan has an important role when cleft lip is detected on screening in allowing the parents and the prenatal counseling team to obtain accurate information about whether the hard palate is cleft. Another clinical-practice use they recommend would be for the screening of high-risk patients with familial history or environmental risk factors. The study is based on experience in a tertiary referral center, in which the operators are well trained to examine the palate using 3D ultrasound scan. More studies are needed to look at the role of this modality in less-experienced centers.

R. B. Mitchell, MD

Efficacy of Neonatal Release of Ankyloglossia: A Randomized Trial

Buryk M, Bloom D, Shope T (Naval Med Ctr Portsmouth, VA)
Pediatrics 128:280-288, 2011

Background.—Ankyloglossia has been associated with a variety of infant-feeding problems. Frenotomy commonly is performed for relief of ankyloglossia, but there has been a lack of convincing data to support this practice.

Objectives.—Our primary objective was to determine whether frenotomy for infants with ankyloglossia improved maternal nipple pain and ability to breastfeed. A secondary objective was to determine whether frenotomy improved the length of breastfeeding.

Methods.—Over a 12-month period, neonates who had difficulty breastfeeding and significant ankyloglossia were enrolled in this randomized, single-blinded, controlled trial and assigned to either a frenotomy (30 infants) or a sham procedure (28 infants). Breastfeeding was assessed by a preintervention and postintervention nipple-pain scale and the Infant Breastfeeding Assessment Tool. The same tools were used at the 2-week follow-up and regularly scheduled follow-ups over a 1-year period. The infants in the sham group were given a frenotomy before or at the 2-week follow-up if it was desired.

Results.—Both groups demonstrated statistically significantly decreased pain scores after the intervention. The frenotomy group improved significantly more than the sham group ($P<.001$). Breastfeeding scores significantly improved in the frenotomy group ($P=.029$) without a significant change in the control group. All but 1 parent in the sham group elected to have the procedure performed when their infant reached 2 weeks of age, which prevented additional comparisons between the 2 groups.

Conclusions.—We demonstrated immediate improvement in nipple-pain and breastfeeding scores, despite a placebo effect on nipple pain. This should provide convincing evidence for those seeking a frenotomy for infants with signficant ankyloglossia.

▶ Ankyloglossia, or tongue-tie, is an anatomic variation in which the lingual frenulum is unusually thick, tight, or short. Reported incidence of this condition among newborns varies from 1.7% to 4.8%. There is debate about the role or need to perform a frenulectomy in these neonates. This is a well-designed study that is often difficult to conduct in a condition where referral to an otolaryngologist generally preselects children who end up receiving surgical therapy. The authors address the shortcomings of previous studies. This study is a randomized, controlled, blinded design; only infants with breastfeeding problems were enrolled; and it used validated and reliable tools for grading ankyloglossia and measuring pain and maternal report of breastfeeding adequacy. Using this methodology, they detected a significant placebo effect but also an additive statistically significant treatment effect of immediate improvements in nipple pain and maternal report of breastfeeding adequacy. They conclude that when frenulectomy is performed for clinically significant ankyloglossia, there is a clear and immediate improvement in reported maternal nipple pain and infant breastfeeding scores. This should provide compelling evidence for pediatricians, otolaryngologists, oral surgeons, and lactation consultants to seek frenulectomy when indicated.

R. B. Mitchell, MD

6 Rhinology and Skull Base Surgery

Basic and Clinical Research

Empty Nose Syndrome: Limbic System Activation Observed by Functional Magnetic Resonance Imaging
Freund W, Wunderlich AP, Stöcker T, et al (Univ Hosps Ulm, Germany; Med Imaging Physics, Jülich, Germany)
Laryngoscope 121:2019-2025, 2011

Objectives/Hypothesis.—Empty nose syndrome (ENS) patients have a persistent sense of impaired nasal patency despite radical resection of nasal turbinates. The aim of this study was to elucidate differences in cerebral activation during free breathing and after inhalation of a fragrance (lemonene) and a pseudodecongestant (menthol) over a nasofacial mask. Our hypothesis was that menthol would be perceived as beneficial and that cerebral activation would show differences in areas corresponding to emotional suffering and air hunger in ENS patients.

Study Design.—Prospective, controlled intervention with lemonene and menthol during functional magnetic resonance imaging (f-MRI) experiment.

Methods.—Ten right-handed ENS patients were compared to 15 controls using f-MRI and fully automated data analysis with SPM software. Nasal patency was measured with rhinomanometry and rated on a four-point scale.

Results.—Despite similar objective nasal flow, ENS patients rated nasal patency significantly worse than did controls. Menthol was perceived to increase nasal patency. In patients, f-MRI data showed different activation of temporal cortex areas after inhalation of menthol. The comparison of patients and controls showed ENS-specific activation of temporal and cerebellar areas and amygdala during the rating task itself.

Conclusions.—Our experiments showed different cerebral processing of the feeling of nasal patency in ENS patients with prominent activation of areas belonging to the limbic system. The beneficial effect of menthol seems to correspond to activation differences in the temporal pole. These results demonstrate a neuronal substrate for both symptoms and their relief in ENS patients.

▶ This is a controlled study using functional magnetic resonance imaging (fMRI) to evaluate empty nose syndrome (ENS)—a challenging problem that can result from radical resection of the nasal turbinates. In these cases, it is suspected that nasal functioning (including humidifying, warming, and clearing) are deteriorated by a significant reduction of respiratory mucosa, but patients most frequently complain of paradoxical nasal obstruction. As clinicians know too well, the pathophysiology of ENS is poorly understood, and treatment options are often poor. This study used fMRI to elucidate differences in cerebral activation during free breathing and after inhalation of a fragrance (limonene) and a pseudodecongestant (menthol) in 10 ENS and 15 control patients. Interestingly, they found that despite similar objective nasal flow, ENS patients rated nasal patency significantly worse than controls and that Menthol was perceived to increase nasal patency. The fMRI data showed different activation of areas of the brain after inhalation of menthol, and the group suggested that these experiments showed different cerebral processing of the feeling of nasal patency in ENS patients with prominent activation of areas belonging to the limbic system. The authors propose to use the beneficial effects of menthol for the treatment of ENS (by maybe adding it to ointment, for example), which is an intriguing idea. Clearly, further work is needed, but adding menthol to the topical treatment of ENS seems like a low-risk strategy that may help this difficult-to-treat group of patients.

R. Sindwani, MD

Efficacy of using a hydrodebrider and of citric acid/zwitterionic surfactant on a *Staphylococcus aureus* bacterial biofilm in the sheep model of rhinosinusitis
Valentine R, Jervis-Bardy J, Psaltis A, et al (Head and Neck Surgery Univ of Adelaide and Flinders Univ, Australia)
Am J Rhinol Allergy 25:323-326, 2011

Background.—Biofilms in chronic rhinosinusitis (CRS) patients are associated with recalcitrant disease patterns. Citric acid/zwitterionic surfactant (CAZS) has been shown to have significant efficacy at in vitro biofilm eradication. Unique hydrodebrider systems have been shown to have effective antibiofilm efficacy. The aim of this study was to evaluate the efficacy of the CAZS/hydrodebrider treatment on *Staphylococcus aureus* biofilms in the sheep model of CRS.

Methods.—Forty-two sheep frontal sinuses were inoculated with *S. aureus*, followed by 7 days of biofilm growth. Sinuses were randomized to one of nine treatment groups: control, hydrodebrider with saline or CAZS (killed on day 0 or day 7 posttreatment), CAZS, or saline flush (killed on day 0 or day 7 posttreatment). Confocal scanning laser microscopy (CSLM) was used to confirm extent of biofilm reduction. Samples of each sinus were taken, assessing cilia morphology using electron microscopy.

Results.—A mean of 37.22 ± 9.65% of control (no treatment) CSLM images taken showed biofilms. Both CAZS flush and CAZS/hydrodebrider treatments showed initial improvements in biofilms but biofilm regrowth followed treatment, 14.74 ± 9.58% to 18.91 ± 12.14% and 15.60 ± 13.92% to 24.70 ± 3.66%, respectively ($p > 0.05$). Saline/hydrodebrider treatments showed a nonsignificant improvement in biofilm treatment, which was maintained, 18.34 ± 11.85% to 12.04 ± 10.28% ($p > 0.05$). Cilial morphology grade was significantly worse in the CAZS treatment groups ($p > 0.05$).

Conclusion.—CAZS solution (with and without a hydrodebrider system) can significantly adversely affect cilia morphology. The hydrodebrider system, when combined with saline, may be a useful treatment adjunct for mucosal biofilms.

▶ The presence of bacterial biofilms in recalcitrant chronic rhinosinusitis (CRS) patients has been well documented and has been shown to contribute to adverse effects on postoperative outcomes. This study is one of several initiatives to actually use our understanding of the presence of biofilms in CRS and try to explore methods of disrupting them. Effective biofilm removal has been hypothesized to include 2 main components: a chemical surfactant that interacts with the calcium—ion bridges of the biofilm and disrupts the extracellular polymeric substance (EPS) structure and a device that allows a shear force to be delivered to the mucosal surface. Recently, an agent that combines citric acid and zwitterionic surfactant (CAZS) has been developed. Citric acid combines with the calcium—ion bridges to disrupt the chemical binding of the EPS chains, and the zwitterionic surfactant dissolves the disconnected chains.[1] The physical debridement component was provided by the new Hydrodebrider irrigation system from Medtronic (Jacksonville, FL). The authors tested the effectiveness of this treatment in sheep frontal sinuses inoculated with *Staphylococcus aureus* biofilm. Both CAZS flush and CAZS/hydrodebrider treatments showed initial improvements in biofilms, but regrowth followed treatment. Saline/hydrodebrider treatments showed a nonsignificant improvement in biofilm treatment, which was maintained. The authors concluded that CAZS solution showed ciliary toxicity and suggested that the microdebrider (with saline) may show promise in this application. It was interesting that all treatments evaluated in this study showed a biofilm clearance effect, albeit for only a while. Several topically deliverable techniques have been investigated for the treatment of bacterial biofilms in CRS, including baby shampoo, antibiotic and antifungal therapies, and even Manuka honey. With the improved understanding of the molecular and chemical mechanism of biofilm formation and sustenance, we can hopefully continue to trial targeted treatment strategies for recalcitrant CRS. More work on the role of the microdebrider, possibly too simplistic a solution, is required.

R. Sindwani, MD

Reference

1. Desrosiers M, Myntti M, James G. Methods for removing bacterial biofilms: In vitro study using clinical chronic rhinosinusitis specimens. *Am J Rhinol.* 2007; 21:527-532.

Mepolizumab, a humanized anti–IL-5 mAb, as a treatment option for severe nasal polyposis

Gevaert P, Van Bruaene N, Cattaert T, et al (Ghent Univ, Belgium; Univ of Liège, Belgium; et al)

J Allergy Clin Immunol 128:989-995, 2011

Background.—Approximately 85% of nasal polyps (NPs) in white subjects are characterized by prominent eosinophilia. IL-5 is the key driver of eosinophilic differentiation and survival.

Objective.—We sought to investigate the therapeutic potential of inhibiting IL-5 with a humanized mAb as treatment for severe nasal polyposis.

Methods.—Thirty patients with severe nasal polyposis (grade 3 or 4 or recurrent after surgery) refractory to corticosteroid therapy were randomized in a double-blind fashion to receive either 2 single intravenous injections (28 days apart) of 750 mg of mepolizumab (n = 20) or placebo (n = 10). Change from baseline in NP score was assessed monthly until 1 month after the last dose (week 8). Computed tomographic scans were also performed at week 8.

Results.—Twelve of 20 patients receiving mepolizumab had a significantly improved NP score and computed tomographic scan score compared with 1 of 10 patients receiving placebo at week 8 versus baseline.

Conclusion.—Mepolizumab achieved a statistically significant reduction in NP size for at least 1 month after dosing in 12 of 20 patients. IL-5 inhibition is a potential novel therapeutic approach in patients with severe eosinophilic nasal polyposis.

▶ This double-blind, placebo-controlled study evaluated the effectiveness of mepolizumab, a humanized anti–interleukin (IL)-5 mAb, as a treatment option for severe nasal polyposis (NP). The premise for the trial was that chronic rhinositis (CRS) with NP (CRSwNP) is characterized by a dominant TH2 eosinophilic inflammation with high levels of IL-5 and IgE,[1-3] whereas CRS without NP (CRSsNP) shows more of a TH1 milieu. The authors hypothesized that blocking IL-5 should have a positive effect, because this cytokine seems to play a key role in the chemotaxis, activation, and survival of eosinophils.[4,5] In this study, 30 patients with severe refractory nasal polyposis were randomly assigned to receive either 2 single intravenous doses 1 month apart of mepolizumab (n = 20) or placebo (n = 10). Outcomes included NP scores assessed monthly, computed tomography (CT) scores, and symptomatic improvement. The study found on objective outcomes (CT and NP scores) there was a significant positive effect over placebo in the treatment group, but there was no associated significant improvement in symptoms. The authors suggested this could be a power issue, which certainly is one possibility. Although tempered by these modest objective improvements and lack of significant subjective changes, the results of this study are encouraging and deserve further consideration. On a theoretical level, interfering with IL-5 does make sense, although it appears that the interplay between cytokines, polyp formation/progression, and symptom manifestation are more complicated than expected. This is an exciting area of study.

R. Sindwani, MD

References

1. Hamilos DL, Leung DY, Wood R, et al. Evidence for distinct cytokine expression in allergic versus nonallergic chronic sinusitis. *J Allergy Clin Immunol.* 1995;96: 537-544.
2. Bachert C, Gevaert P, Holtappels G, et al. Total and specific IgE in nasal polyps is related to local eosinophilic inflammation. *J Allergy Clin Immunol.* 2001;107: 607-614.
3. Riechelmann H, Deutschle T, Rozsasi A, Keck T, Polzehl D, Bürner H. Nasal biomarker profiles in acute and chronic rhinosinusitis. *Clin Exp Allergy.* 2005; 35:1186-1191.
4. Sanderson CJ. Interleukin-5, eosinophils, and disease. *Blood.* 1992;79:3101-3109.
5. Gevaert P, Bachert C, Holtappels G, et al. Enhanced soluble interleukin-5 receptor alpha expression in nasal polyposis. *Allergy.* 2003;58:371-379.

Evidence for Distinct Histologic Profile of Nasal Polyps With and Without Eosinophilia

Payne SC, Early SB, Huyett P, et al (Univ of Virginia Health System, Charlottesville; Carter Ctr for Immunology Res, Charlottesville, VA; et al)
Laryngoscope 121:2262-2267, 2011

Objective/Hypothesis.—To evaluate the histology, RNA, and protein signatures of nasal polyps (NPs) in order to demonstrate specific subtypes of disease and differentiate "idiopathic" NPs based on tissue eosinophilia.

Study Design.—Prospective laboratory-based study.

Methods.—NP tissue was obtained from patients referred to the University of Virginia Health System for sinus surgery. Histology analyses included hematoxylin-eosin, Gomori's trichrome, toluidine blue, and chloroacetate staining. RNA and protein were extracted from tissue and cytokine transcript or protein concentrations determined.

Results.—Idiopathic NPs can be divided into distinct subsets characterized by absence (NE) and presence (E) of prominent eosinophilia. The validity of this distinction is supported by the demonstration that NE polyps are further distinguished by glandular hypertrophy, dense collagen deposition, and mononuclear cellular infiltrate. In contrast, E-NP display edema, rare glandularity, and minimal collagen deposition except within the basement membrane. Total mast cell numbers were reduced in E-NP, whereas connective tissue mast cells were increased in NE-NP. Consistent with the distinctive pattern of increased fibrosis, NE-NP displayed increased transforming growth factor-β and vascular endothelial growth factor transcripts. Similarly, NE-NPs had higher concentrations of transforming growth factor-β, fibroblast growth factor-β, and platelet-derived growth factor protein.

Conclusions.—Idiopathic NPs can be distinguished by NE and E and are supported by the observations that these display distinct histologic, gene, and protein expression patterns. The findings suggest that as unique diseases, idiopathic NPs will require distinct therapeutic interventions.

▶ This laboratory study on nasal polyp tissue sought to evaluate the histology, RNA, and protein signatures of nasal polyps (NPs). The authors provide evidence that there are specific subtypes of NPs and differentiate idiopathic NPs (polyps not associated with allergic fungal sinusitis, aspirin salicylic acid intolerance, or cystic fibrosis) based on the presence or absence of tissue eosinophilia. This study demonstrates other elements that support that these 2 phenotypes are significantly different. For example, when compared with noneosinophilic idiopathic NPs, eosinophilic NPs show glandular hypertrophy, dense collagen deposition, and mononuclear cellular infiltrate. Other differences, including histologic gender and protein expression, are also highlighted. Based on these unique differentiating factors, the authors strongly argue that idiopathic NPs should be subcategorized as with or without eosinophilia and that these are in fact 2 distinct disease entities that may benefit from distinct therapeutic interventions. Further work is necessary, but these results are intriguing and may have significant implications for delivering tailored therapies to polyps patients. Certainly, there is a marked swell in the thinking that chronic rhinosinusitis is not just 1 condition but a group of heterogeneous disorders, and work such as this is assisting in trying to further stratify it.

R. Sindwani, MD

Immunohistochemical Characterization of Human Olfactory Tissue

Holbrook EH, Wu E, Curry WT, et al (Harvard Med School, Boston, MA; The Tufts Univ School of Medicine, Boston, MA; Massachusetts General Hosp, Boston)
Laryngoscope 121:1687-1701, 2011

Objectives/Hypothesis.—The pathophysiology underlying human olfactory disorders is poorly understood because biopsying the olfactory epithelium (OE) can be unrepresentative and extensive immunohistochemical analysis is lacking. Autopsy tissue enriches our grasp of normal and abnormal olfactory immunohistology and guides the sampling of the OE by biopsy. Furthermore, a comparison of the molecular phenotype of olfactory epithelial cells between rodents and humans will improve our ability to correlate human histopathology with olfactory dysfunction.

Study Design.—An immunohistochemical analysis of human olfactory tissue using a comprehensive battery of proven antibodies.

Methods.—Human olfactory mucosa obtained from 21 autopsy specimens was analyzed with immunohistochemistry. The position and extent of olfactory mucosa was assayed by staining whole mounts (WMs) with neuronal markers. Sections of the OE were analyzed with an extensive group of antibodies directed against cytoskeletal proteins and transcription factors, as were surgical specimens from an esthesioneuroblastoma.

Results.—Neuron-rich epithelium is always found inferior to the cribriform plate, even at advanced age, despite the interruptions in the neuroepithelial sheet caused by patchy respiratory metaplasia. The pattern of immunostaining with our antibody panel identifies two distinct types of basal cell progenitors in human OE similar to rodents. The panel also clarifies the complex composition of esthesioneuroblastoma.

Conclusions.—The extent of human olfactory mucosa at autopsy can easily be delineated as a function of age and neurologic disease. The similarities in human versus rodent OE will enable us to translate knowledge from experimental animals to humans and will extend our understanding of human olfactory pathophysiology (Fig 1).

▶ Although strides have been made in the recent past in olfaction basic science research, there is still a great deal to be learned in this area. A major issue to date

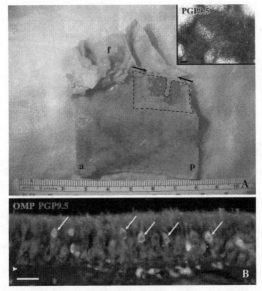

FIGURE 1.—Autopsy specimens provide tissue for both a comprehensive perspective of the extent of neuronal staining and a detailed characterization of olfactory mucosa. (A) Whole-mount staining of the left septum taken from a 75-year-old male with Alzheimer's. The edges of the whole mount stripped from the underlying bone are delineated by dashed lines. The thin rectangular defect extending from the superior boarder corresponds to the region removed from the whole-mount for histology. The pattern of PGP9.5 staining of the mucosal WM is represented in red and is superimposed on a photograph taken of the septum after removal of the mucosa. The inset is a higher power magnification of the actual PGP9.5 staining at the surface of the WM. Notice the circular patches of nonneuronal epithelium at the edges of the olfactory boarder and within the olfactory region seen in the whole-mount representation and inset. Arrows indicate anterior and posterior extent of the cribriform plate, f = frontal sinus; a = anterior; p = posterior; scale bar = 50 μ. (B) Section of epithelium from specimen shown in (A) fluorescently double labeled with OMP and PGP9.5 antibodies. PGP9.5 labels mature and immature ONs and OMP labels only the mature neurons. In this specimen the double labeled mature neurons (arrows) are relatively few compared to the abundant PGP9.5(+)/OMP(−) immature neurons. Arrowhead = basement membrane; scale bar = 25 μ. For interpretation of the references to color in this figure legend, the reader is referred to web version of this article. (Reprinted from Holbrook EH, Wu E, Curry WT, et al. Immunohistochemical characterization of human olfactory tissue. *Laryngoscope.* 2011;121:1687-1701, with permission from The American Laryngological, Rhinological and Otological Society, Inc, and John Wiley and Sons (www.interscience.wiley.com).)

has been the small biopsy samples that have been analyzed. This study attempts to lay the ground work for in-depth study of the olfactory organ by examining entire block specimens from autopsy specimens. A structural and immunohisto-chemical analysis of human olfactory tissue from 21 autopsy specimens was conducted. The position and extent of olfactory mucosa was assayed by stain-ing whole mounts with neuronal markers (Fig 1). Neuron-rich epithelium is always found inferior to the cribriform plate, even at advanced age, despite the interruptions in the neuroepithelial sheet caused by patchy respiratory meta-plasia. This study shows that human olfactory mucosa is very similar to rodents with respect to constituent cells and molecular phenotypes. The similarities identified will improve confidence in future investigations evaluating patho-physiology of olfactory disorders using murine models.

R. Sindwani, MD

Histological features of the nasal mucosa in hematopoietic stem cell transplantation
Ortiz É, Sakano E, Meirelles LR, et al (UNICAMP Campinas, Sao Paulo, Brazil)
Am J Rhinol Allergy 25:e191-e195, 2011

Background.—Immunosuppression is the leading cause of recurrent sinus infections after hematopoietic stem cell transplant (HSCT), with increased incidence of sinusitis in patients with chronic graft versus host disease (GVHD). Histological descriptions of the oral mucosa, lung ciliary epithe-lium, and intestinal mucosa related to HSCT have been described. However, few have described the nasal mucosa. We, therefore, sought to elucidate the histological and ultrastructural features of the nasal mucosa in patients after HSCT to better understand the pathophysiology of the immune response.

Methods.—Uncinate processes from 24 HSCT patients and 12 immuno-competent patients were subjected to histological analyses via light and transmission electron microscopy (TEM).

Results.—TEM revealed aberrant cilia structure, altered mitochondria quantity, microvilli, and cytoplasm vacuolization. All HSCT patients with rhinosinusitis had significant loss or absence of cilia ($p = 0.018$). Apoptotic bodies were increased and Goblet cells decreased in nasal epithelium from patients with chronic GVHD ($p = 0.04$).

Conclusion.—This tissue destruction likely enhances pathogen penetra-tion resulting in recurrent infection (Fig 1).

▶ It is thought that immunosuppression is the main cause of the increased inci-dence of recurrent or chronic sinusitis in patients undergoing hematopoietic stem cell transplant (HSCT). However, other factors could also include pro-longed antibiotic administration, immunosuppressants, radiotherapy, chemo-therapy, diabetes, prolonged hospitalization, and, notably, graft versus host disease (GVHD). This study examined the histologic and morphologic features of nasal mucosa in patients with HSCT and explored changes seen in patients with GVHD. Electron microscopic examination demonstrated aberrant cilia

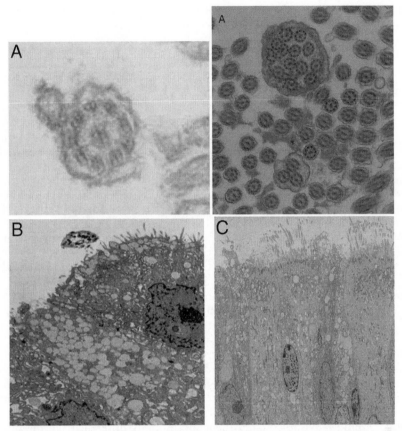

FIGURE 1.—(A, A) Transmission electron microscopy (16,700–6000×): structural abnormalities in the epithelium of the hematopoietic stem cell transplant (HSCT) patients. (B) Nasal epithelium without cilia in the HSCT patients. (C) Cytoplasm vacuolization of the ciliated cell in the HSCT patient. (Courtesy of Ortiz É, Sakano E, Meirelles LR, et al. Histological features of the nasal mucosa in hematopoietic stem cell transplantation. *Am J Rhinol Allergy.* 2011;25:e191-e195, with permission from OceanSide Publications, Inc.)

structure, altered mitochondria quantity, microvilli, and cytoplasm vacuolization (Fig 1). All HSCT patients with sinusitis had significant loss or absence of cilia, and apoptotic bodies were increased and goblet cells decreased in nasal epithelium in patients with chronic GVHD. The histological alterations demonstrated in this study are significant, and the authors propose that the tissue destruction identified is the key reason for the increased susceptibility of these patients to sinus infection. Ciliary motility and the structural integrity of the epithelium of course serves as an important mechanical barrier to infection. The authors also point out that viral or bacterial infections do not seem to be the main source of tissue damage in patients with GVHD associated with HSCT, but rather the destruction is from the GVHD itself. This tissue injury likely facilitates bacterial and viral penetration, resulting in recurrence or exacerbation of the infection.

R. Sindwani, MD

General

Revisiting Human Nose Anatomy: Phylogenic and Ontogenic Perspectives
Jankowski R (Université Henri Poincaré, Nancy, France)
Laryngoscope 121:2461-2467, 2011

This review suggests revisiting nose anatomy by considering the ethmoidal labyrinths as part of the olfactory nose and not as paranasal sinuses.

Phylogenetically, the olfactory and respiratory organs of the most primitive vertebrates are separated. Exaptation, a mechanism of evolution, may explain the fusion of the olfactory and respiratory organs in dipnoi. The respiratory and olfactory noses remain anatomically separated by the transverse lamina in most mammals, whose olfactory labyrinth is a blind recess housing the ethmoturbinates. In humans, the partitioning between the olfactory cleft and the ethmoid labyrinth seems to be a consequence of ethmoid bone remodeling induced by the acquisition of an upright posture. The ethmoid bone is derived from the cartilaginous nasal capsule of primitive vertebrates and considered to be a highly conserved region among the bony elements of the skull base. It appears to be involved only in housing and protecting the olfactory function.

During the early stages of human fetal development, rupture of the oronasal membrane leads to the integration of the primary olfactory sac in the future respiratory organ. The cartilaginous nasal capsule appears in the tissue under the brain and around the olfactory channels. Its early fetal development is classically regarded as the beginning of paranasal sinus formation. From phylogenic and ontogenic perspectives, it may be regarded as the development of the olfactory labyrinth as modified by the remodeling process of the human face and skull base. The endochondral bony origin of the ethmoid labyrinths makes them substantially different from the other paranasal sinuses.

▶ This is a very unique and fascinating article that explores the evolutionary origins and changes associated with sinonasal anatomy. It specifically examines the ethmoid bone from phylogenetic and ontogenic perspectives. The work revisits the anatomy of the human nose from the stance that the ethmoidal labyrinths are part of the olfactory nose and not of the paranasal sinuses as generally held. Through detailed comparative anatomy, the author makes the case that phylogenetically, the olfactory and respiratory organs of the most primitive vertebrates are separated. He argues that through exaptation (a mechanism of evolution) the olfactory and respiratory organs eventually fused. The respiratory and olfactory noses remain anatomically separated in most mammals, and in humans, the partitioning between the olfactory cleft and the ethmoid labyrinth seems to be a consequence of ethmoid bone remodeling induced by the acquisition of an upright posture. This article is very well written and an interesting read.

R. Sindwani, MD

Exostoses of the Paranasal Sinuses

Ramakrishnan JB, Pirron JA, Perepletchikov A, et al (Univ of Pittsburgh, PA; Starmedica Lomas Verdas Hosp, Mexico City, Mexico)
Laryngoscope 120:2532-2534, 2010

While bony exostoses of the external auditory canal have long been recognized as a complication of cold-water swimming, bony exostoses of the paranasal sinuses have not been previously reported. We present an unusual case of multiple exostoses of the paranasal sinuses, which began coincident with nasal irrigation with cold gentamicin solution. The patient had had prior endoscopic sinus surgery. Topical antibiotic gentamicin irrigation lessened recurrence of bacterial sinus episodes. He admitted to using the irrigation directly from the refrigerator daily for two years. A biopsy was consistent with exostosis. Patients should be counseled to avoid irrigating their paranasal sinuses with cold irrigants (Figs 1 and 3).

▶ This is a very unique case report. It is the first report in the literature demonstrating multiple small exostoses of the paranasal sinuses caused by cold nasal irrigations in a patient with chronic rhinosinusitis after sinus surgery. After surgery, the patient used cold gentamicin irrigations (directly from the refrigerator) and over time developed multiple, enlarging cystic-appearing lesions in his sinuses that were asymptomatic (Fig 1). These were biopsied and consistent with lamellar bone, akin to what is seen with external auditory canal exostosis (Fig 3). He was advised to continue his daily practice of gentamicin irrigations.

Exostoses occur more commonly in the external auditory canal (EAC) and can occur over a wide age range (usually between 10 and 50 years of age). Exostoses of the ear (also known as "surfer's ear") are thought to be a reactive process from repeated stimulation by cold water because it occurs predominantly in patients

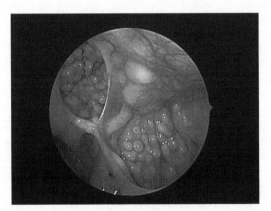

FIGURE 1.—Left-sided nasal endoscopy demonstrates numerous small cystic-appearing masses that were regularly scattered throughout the postsurgical maxillary and ethmoid sinus cavity. [Color figure can be viewed in the online issue, which is available at wileyonlinelibrary.com.] (Reprinted from Ramakrishnan JB, Pirron JA, Perepletchikov A, et al. Exostoses of the paranasal sinuses. *Laryngoscope.* 2010;120:2532-2534, with permission from The American Laryngological, Rhinological and Otological Society, Inc, and John Wiley and Sons, www.interscience.wiley.com.)

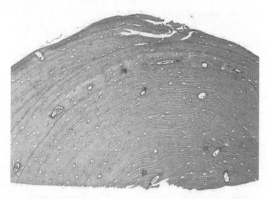

FIGURE 3.—Low-power histopathologic section of the biopsy of the sinus lesion. [Color figure can be viewed in the online issue, which is available at wileyonlinelibrary.com.] (Reprinted from Ramakrishnan JB, Pirron JA, Perepletchikov A, et al. Exostoses of the paranasal sinuses. *Laryngoscope.* 2010;120:2532-2534, with permission from The American Laryngological, Rhinological and Otological Society, Inc, and John Wiley and Sons, www.interscience.wiley.com.)

exposed to repeated and prolonged cold-water exposure, such as lifeguards, kayakers, and cold-water surfers. Interestingly, studies have shown that the more years of cold-water surfing one does, the greater the risk of developing EAC exostoses of any kind (12% per year). The authors recommend that patients avoid cold irrigation of their nose and sinuses. Amazingly, we have also seen a few patients with this clinical picture, and our biopsies also showed bony changes consistent with (bilateral, multiple) sinus exostoses. The following are a few things to highlight about this unique condition: (1) these lesions are benign but can grow; (2) they appear to occur in postoperative, open sinus cavities (ethmoid and maxillary in this case report, presumably because the cold solution can then directly strike the sinus walls); (3) treatment is to stop cold irrigations and provide surveillance; and (4) the possibility of Gardner syndrome should be explored. As the authors review, Gardner syndrome is an autosomal dominant disease characterized by multiple polyps in the colon and extracolonic tumors, such as osteomas of the skull, thyroid cancer, epidermoid cysts, fibromas, and sebaceous cysts. The long-term sequelae or clinical implications (if any) of multiple exostoses of the paranasal sinuses is unknown.

R. Sindwani, MD

The natural history of epistaxis in patients with hereditary hemorrhagic telangiectasia in the Norwegian population: A cross-sectional study
Dheyauldeen S, Abdelnoor M, Bachmann-Harildstad G (Oslo University Hospital/Rikshospitalet, Norway; Oslo Univ Hosp, Ulleval, Norway; Oslo Univ, Nordbyhagen, Norway)
Am J Rhinol Allergy 25:214-218, 2011

Background.—Epistaxis is usually the first and most common symptom in hereditary hemorrhagic telangiectasia (HHT), which is known also as

Rendu-Osler-Weber syndrome. The severity of HHT-associated epistaxis is highly variable and can affect the patient's quality of life. In the literature, the natural history of epistaxis in HHT patients has been described in a few countries but not from the Norwegian population.

Objective.—This work focused on the natural history of epistaxis in the Norwegian population in a cross-sectional study.

Material and Methods.—Ninety-eight patients with three or four Curaçao criteria were included. The severity of epistaxis was graded depending on epistaxis intensity, frequency, and the amount of blood transfusion during a period of 4 weeks. The epistaxis grades were studied in association with age, gender, gene mutation, age of onset, and whether the patient had or had not been treated for epistaxis during the last 2 years.

Results.—Most of the HHT patients (90%) complained of mild-to-moderate epistaxis. Seventy-seven percent of the patients started epistaxis by or before the age of 20 years. The progression of HHT-associated epistaxis with age could not be proved statistically in this study. There was no statistically significant difference in the grades of epistaxis between HHT1 and HHT2 type, neither between female and male patients. Most of the patients started epistaxis by or before the age of 20 years. There was a significant difference in the grade of epistaxis between non-*ENG*, non-*ALK1* carrier patients, and *ENG* or *ALK1* carrier patients.

Conclusion.—Compared with other populations, the grading of epistaxis in Norwegian patients with HHT gave generally similar results. A multi-center epidemiological study is required to get a larger study population. A common internationally accepted grading or classification system for epistaxis in HHT is highly recommended.

▶ Most of the studies in the literature focus on the benefit and risk of the various treatment modalities of epistaxis associated with hereditary hemorrhagic telangiectasia. This cross-sectional study describes the natural history of epistaxis in the Norwegian population by focusing on the grade of epistaxis in relation to other factors such as sex, age, gene mutation type, and age of epistaxis onset. Ninety-eight patients were studied. Epistaxis severity was examined from a variety of angles including intensity, frequency, and the amount of blood transfusions. Interesting findings included that the majority of patients felt their epistaxis was mild to moderate in severity and that almost 80% started having problems with nosebleeds by age 20. Many clinicians likely suspect that epistaxis gets worse with increasing age, but this was not established statistically by the study. In fact, no major associations were found between epistaxis severity and the other parameters looked at which underscores that this is a highly variable symptom.

R. Sindwani, MD

Sinonasal Malignancies in Children: A 10-Year, Single-Institutional Review

Zevallos JP, Jain KS, Roberts D, et al (Univ of Texas M.D. Anderson Cancer Ctr, Houston; State Univ of New York, Syracuse)
Laryngoscope 121:2001-2003, 2011

Objectives.—Sinonasal malignancies in children are rare, histologically diverse tumors that present diagnostic and management challenges. The purpose of this study is to review the experience of a single cancer center in the management of pediatric sinonasal malignancies.

Study Design.—Retrospective review.

Methods.—Retrospective chart review.

Results.—Forty-four patients were identified. The median age was 12 years (range: 2–17), 54% were female, and the maxillary sinus was the most common primary site. Facial swelling and pain were the most common presenting complaints. Thirty-four patients (76%) in this series had paranasal sinus sarcomas, three patients had esthesioneuroblastomas, and eight patients had carcinomas. The 5-year overall survival, disease-specific survival, and recurrence rate for the entire group was 71%, 81%, and 43%, respectively.

Conclusions.—Pediatric sinonasal malignancies are rare, locally aggressive tumors associated with nonspecific signs and symptoms. Multimodality treatment can result in 5-year overall and disease-specific survival rates of over 70%. A multidisciplinary team approach is essential to optimize outcomes and limit the morbidity of treatment (Table 2).

▶ Sinonasal malignancies in children are rare and challenging to manage. This single cancer center experience with pediatric sinonasal malignancies over a 10-year period reports the outcomes of 44 children (ages 2–17) with sinonasal cancers. The maxillary sinus was the most common primary site, with facial swelling and pain representing the most common complaints. It is noteworthy that 50% of patients had no sinonasal symptoms at all. Among those with sinonasal complaints, obstruction and epistaxis were the most common. As shown in Table 2, sinus sarcomas, carcinomas, and esthesioneuroblastoma were the histologies most encountered. This article highlights the rarity and nonspecific presentation of sinonasal malignancies in kids. A recent review of SEER data by Shapiro et al[1] also underscored the rarity of these lesions in kids, with only 63 cases identified over a 17-year period. This has precluded the development of

TABLE 2.—Histologic Characteristics

Histology	Number (%)
Sarcoma	34
Squamous cell carcinoma	4
Esthesioneuroblastoma	3
Adenoid cystic carcinoma	1
Adenocarcinoma	1
Carcinoma ex-pleomorphic	1

well-established treatment protocols, and critical studies examining treatment modalities are lacking. The risks of surgical resection in the sinonasal region and skull base, as well as long-term effects of radiation therapy in this region, are important considerations when treating children. Although an open surgical approach was used in most cases in this series, evolving endoscopic approaches to the sinonasal region and skull base show promise in limiting surgical morbidity in adults and may play an expanding role in pediatrics as well. Data are lacking and further studies are needed to assess the adaptability of endoscopic approaches to pediatric sinonasal malignancies. A multidisciplinary team approach that includes otolaryngology, neurosurgery, medical and radiation oncologists, and pediatricians is critical to maximize outcomes.

R. Sindwani, MD

Reference

1. Shapiro NL, Bhattacharyya N. Staging and survival for sinus cancer in the pediatric population. *Int J Pediatr Otorhinolaryngol.* 2009;73:1568-1571.

Do Biofilms Contribute to the Initiation and Recalcitrance of Chronic Rhinosinusitis?

Foreman A, Jervis-Bardy J, Wormald P-J (Univ of Adelaide and Flinders Univ, Australia)
Laryngoscope 121:1085-1091, 2011

Chronic rhinosinusitis is a common disease whose underlying aetiopathogenesis has not been completely understood. Amongst a range of other potential environmental triggers in this disease, a role has recently been proposed for bacterial biofilms. Adopting the biofilm paradigm to explain the initiation and maintenance of this disease may help to clarify previous inconsistencies in this disease that have resulted in the role of bacteria being questioned. Of particular interest is the association of bacterial biofilms with recalcitrant disease states. Over the last five years, research has progressed rapidly since biofilms were first identified on the surface of diseased sinonasal mucosa. Their presence there has now been associated with more severe disease that is often recalcitrant to current management paradigms. Technological advances are allowing accurate characterization of the bacterial and fungal species within these biofilms, which would appear to be an important step in improving our understanding of how these bacterial communities might interact with the host to cause disease. This is an unanswered, yet highly important, question in this field of research that will undoubtedly be an area of investigation in the near future. As the body of evidence suggesting biofilms may be involved in this disease grows, research interest has switched to the development of antibiofilm therapies. Given the unique properties of bacteria existing in this form, biofilm eradication strategies will need to incorporate novel medical therapies into established surgical practices as we attempt to improve the outcomes of our most difficult patients.

▶ The role of biofilms in chronic rhinosinusitis (CRS) remains an intriguing and hot area of research in the field of rhinology. This contemporary review thoroughly explores the available evidence on the role of biofilms in the initiation and recalcitrance of CRS. The authors examine the growing body of knowledge of biofilms, which has expanded from the initial studies back in 2004 that demonstrated these entities on the mucosa of patients with CRS to more recent investigations that have associated their presence with more severe disease. The authors conclude that in aggregate, the literature suggests that biofilms may play a role in CRS initiation and maintenance. However, they do caution that a number of unanswered questions remain that complicate the story. For example, a definitive link between biofilms and the host is required to prove they are intimately involved in the pathogenesis (let alone as the sole case) of CRS, and even if biofilms do play a significant role, we have much to learn about how to interfere or eradicate them to improve the disease process and ameliorate patient symptoms. Further inquiry will undoubtedly follow in the years to come. This review is an excellent summary of the current level of understanding of the role of biofilms in CRS.

R. Sindwani, MD

Regional and Specialty Variations in the Treatment of Chronic Rhinosinusitis
Lee LN, Bhattacharyya N (Massachusetts Eye and Ear Infirmary, Boston; Brigham and Women's Hosp, MA)
Laryngoscope 121:1092-1097, 2011

Objectives/Hypothesis.—To identify regional and specialty differences in the medical treatment of chronic rhinosinusitis (CRS).

Study Design.—Cross-sectional analysis of a national database.

Methods.—Ambulatory visits for CRS were extracted from the National Ambulatory Medical Care Survey (NAMCS) for years 2005 to 2006. Medication utilization associated with CRS (antibiotics, antihistamines, nasal steroids, and oral steroids) was tabulated for medication class and individual drug. Statistical analyses were conducted to determine variations in medication class and specific drug utilization by U.S. geographic region and physician specialty, specifically primary care physicians (PCP) versus otolaryngologists (ORL).

Results.—Among an estimated 36.2 ± 0.3 million visits for CRS (mean age, 36.8 ± 1.4 years; $60.1 \pm 1.9\%$ female), the ratio of PCP to ORL visits was 10:1. The percent of clinician visits with prescriptions for antibiotics ($47.3 \pm 3.0\%$ of overall visits), nasal steroids ($10.8 \pm 1.4\%$) and oral steroids ($2.8 \pm 0.7\%$) did not vary significantly by geographic region ($P = .79, .66,$ and .34, respectively). Antihistamines were prescribed significantly more often in the South ($15.3 \pm 3.4\%$ of visits vs. $11.3 \pm 1.8\%$

nationally, $P = .04$). PCPs were significantly more likely to prescribe antibiotics compared to ORLs (53.3 ± 2.9% vs. 27.4 ± 4.2%, respectively,
$P < .001$) and less likely to prescribe both nasal steroids (9.7 ± 1.5% vs.
17.5 ± 2.8%, $P = .01$) and oral steroids (2.3 ± 0.7% vs. 6.6 ± 2.0%,
$P = .01$). Significant differences existed for specific drugs prescribed according to specialty.

Conclusions.—There are significant variations in the outpatient medical
treatment of CRS according to geography and specialty. This study highlights the need for evidence-based medical treatment protocols for CRS.

▶ In this era of health care reform and cost containment, variations in health
care practice patterns are being scrutinized. There is growing concern over
the wide variation in physician use of different diagnostic tests and treatments
for the same diagnosis, as these varying management approaches often differ
greatly in cost as well as effectiveness. This study used a Centers for Medicare
and Medicaid Services database to explore regional and specialty differences in
the medical treatment of chronic rhinosinusitis (CRS) between 2005 and 2006.
Differences in practice patterns between primary care physicians (PCPs) and
otolaryngologists (ORLs) were analyzed. Among an estimated 36 million visits
for CRS, the ratio of PCP to ORL visits was 10:1. The percentage of clinician
visits with prescriptions for most medications (except antihistamines) did not
vary much geographically, but PCPs were significantly more likely to prescribe
antibiotics than ORLs. The study concluded that the medical treatment of CRS
varies significantly across geographic regions and across physician specialties.
The authors suggested that an evidence-based treatment protocol is needed so
that patients can receive consistent treatment for CRS regardless of their
geographic region or specialty of their physician. The results of this study
further emphasize the need for evidence-based practice, as well as further
high level of evidence in rhinology to minimize waste of valuable health care
resources. In line with a key tenet of quality and health care delivery, minimizing
variations in medical practice is being emphasized as a method to improve
delivery of quality care and to reduce costs.

R. Sindwani, MD

**Microbiology of Acute and Chronic Maxillary Sinusitis in Smokers and
Nonsmokers**
Brook I, Hausfeld JN (Georgetown Univ School of Medicine, Washington, DC)
Ann Otol Rhinol Laryngol 120:707-712, 2011

Objectives.—We evaluated the microbiology of sinus aspirates of smokers
and nonsmokers with acute and chronic maxillary sinusitis.

Methods.—Cultures were obtained from 458 patients, 244 (87 smokers
and 157 nonsmokers) of whom had acute maxillary sinusitis and 214 (84
smokers and 130 nonsmokers) of whom had chronic maxillary sinusitis,
between 2001 and 2007.

Results.—A greater number of *Staphylococcus aureus*, methicillin-resistant *S aureus* (MRSA), and beta-lactamase—producing bacteria (BLPB) were found in the 87 smokers with acute sinusitis than in the nonsmokers with acute sinusitis ($p < 0.005$, $p < 0.025$, and $p < 0.05$, respectively). A greater number of these organisms were found in the 84 smokers with chronic sinusitis than in the nonsmokers ($p < 0.01$, $p < 0.025$, and $p < 0.001$, respectively). Eighty-five BLPB isolates were recovered from 73 patients (30%) with acute sinusitis. These included *Moraxella catarrhalis*, *S aureus*, *Haemophilus influenzae*, *Prevotella* spp, and *Fusobacterium* spp; 40 BLPB isolates were found in smokers, and 45 in nonsmokers ($p < 0.05$). One hundred twenty-five BLPB isolates were recovered from 91 patients (43%) with chronic sinusitis, including *M catarrhalis*, *Bacteroides fragilis* group, *S aureus*, *H influenzae*, *Prevotella* spp, and *Fusobacterium* spp; 69 BLPB isolates were found in smokers, and 56 in nonsmokers ($p < 0.001$). Antimicrobial therapy had been administered in the past month to 130 patients (28%; 60 smokers and 70 nonsmokers; $p < 0.025$). Both MRSA and BLPB were isolated more often from these individuals ($p < 0.025$). However, the higher isolation rates of MRSA and BLPB in smokers were independent of previous antimicrobial therapy.

Conclusions.—These data illustrate a greater frequency of isolation of *S aureus*, MRSA, and BLPB in patients with acute and chronic sinusitis who smoke.

▶ In case we needed yet another reason to quit smoking, this article demonstrates a greater number of *Staphylococcus aureus*, methicillin-resistant *S aureus*, and beta-lactamase—producing bacteria (BLPB) in smokers with acute and chronic sinusitis when compared with nonsmokers. One of the more interesting parts of the discussion is a review of some of the microbiology-related effects of smoking. For example, smoking is associated with enhanced epithelial binding of bacteria to epithelium of smokers and lower numbers of inhibiting organisms, and tobacco smoke also inhibits antimicrobial function of leukocytes and T and B cells. Smokers are at increased risk of respiratory tract infections, exposing them to more antibiotics than nonsmokers, which translates to increased resistance rates (as shown in this study).

R. Sindwani, MD

Paranasal sinus computed tomography anatomy: a surgeon's perspective
Ramakrishnan Y, Zammit-Maempel I, Jones NS, et al (Freeman Hosp, Newcastle, UK)
J Laryngol Otol 125:1141-1147, 2011

Computed tomography scans serve as a critical 'roadmap' for functional endoscopic sinus surgery. A systematic evaluation of such scans, and an awareness of any anatomical variants that may modify one's surgical approach, allow one to pre-empt complications. This article describes, from a novice's perspective, two methods of evaluating paranasal sinus computed tomography scans: a quick assessment technique; and a stepwise, operative approach covering radiological features relevant to pre- and peri-operative management.

▶ This article provides an excellent review of computed tomography (CT) sinus anatomy and presents a stepwise checklist approach to basic endoscopic sinus surgery. It highlights key features of a CT scan that should be reviewed prior to every case, including skull base anatomy and asymmetry and location of the anterior ethmoid artery to name a few (Fig 2 in the original article). The take-away messages from this article include: (1) always correlate the patient's symptoms with the radiologic and clinical findings from surgery; (2) evaluate CT scans in all 3 planes; and (3) identify key anatomic variations that should modify one's operative approach to avoid complications.

R. Sindwani, MD

Sphenoid sinus fungus ball: Our experience

Pagella F, Pusateri A, Matti E, et al (Univ of Pavia, Italy; et al)
Am J Rhinol Allergy 25:276-280, 2011

Background.—Fungal rhinosinusitis is a common disease of the paranasal sinuses. The fungus ball (FB) is defined as an extramucosal mycotic proliferation that fills one or more paranasal sinuses. Sphenoid sinus is an uncommon localization of this disease, as reported in the literature. This study describes our experience in the diagnosis and treatment of sphenoid sinus FB (SSFB), with a particular focus on the surgical approach to the sphenoid sinus.

Methods.—We retrospectively analyzed the clinical records of patients affected by FB of the sphenoid sinus, who underwent endoscopic sinus surgery (ESS) in our institutions between 1995 and 2009. We described the surgical technique, the methods of mycological and histopathological evaluation, as well as the perioperative and postoperative management.

Results.—From 1995 to 2009, 226 patients affected by sinonasal FB underwent ESS in our institutions. A sphenoid localization was found in 56 patients (24.78%; mean age, 62 years). Cephalea was the most common symptom, and 14.3% of patients complained of ocular symptoms. We performed a direct paraseptal sphenoidotomy in 31 patients (55.4%) and a transethmoidal sphenoidotomy in 25 patients (44.6%). Histology unveiled fungal hyphae with absent mucosal invasion in all cases. Cultural results revealed positivity for mycotic colonization in 26 cases (46.4%, most commonly Aspergillus fumigatus). Follow-up ranged from 12 to 181 months with a mean of 70.7 months.

Conclusion.—The description of our experience in the diagnosis and treatment of SSFB underlines the importance of a precise diagnostic pathway in case of sphenoidal disease. Nowadays, in our opinion, the

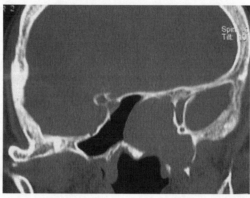

FIGURE 1.—Computed tomography (CT) study of a left sphenoid sinus fungus ball (SSFB; coronal view). (Courtesy of Pagella F, Pusateri A, Matti E, et al. Sphenoid sinus fungus ball: our experience. *Am J Rhinol Allergy.* 2011;25:276-280, OceanSide Publications, Inc.)

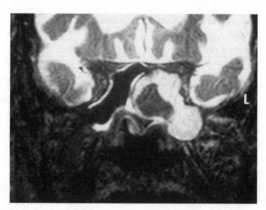

FIGURE 2.—Magnetic resonance imaging (MRI) study of a left sphenoid sinus fungus ball (SSFB; T2-weighted sequence, coronal view). (Courtesy of Pagella F, Pusateri A, Matti E, et al. Sphenoid sinus fungus ball: our experience. *Am J Rhinol Allergy.* 2011;25:276-280, OceanSide Publications, Inc.)

paraseptal direct sphenoidotomy represents the less invasive, fastest and most anatomically conservative approach to the sphenoid sinus in case of SSFB (Figs 1-3).

▶ This article represents a large experience with the diagnosis and management of sphenoid sinus fungal balls (SSFB), which is an uncommon location. The authors review the presentation and management of these lesions, including surgical route used to access the sphenoid sinus. Between 1995 and 2009, 226 patients with sinonasal FB were encountered, with 56 of these representing SS lesions (24.78%; mean age, 62 years). As far as presenting symptoms, headache was the most common, but 14% of patients also had ocular symptoms, most of which resolved with surgical intervention. One case of blindness was also

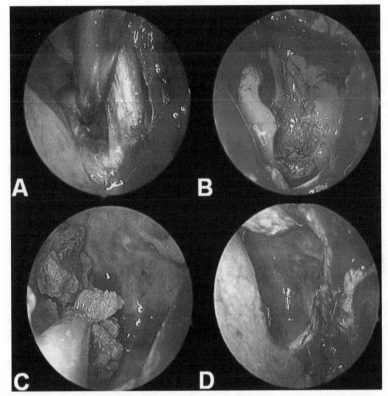

FIGURE 3.—Surgical steps of a paraspetal direct sphenoidotomy for a sphenoid sinus fungus ball (SSFB). (*A*) The left sphenoidal ostium is enlarged with microdebrider after a partial resection of the middle turbinate; (*B*) the left sphenoid sinus appears filled of a clay-like dense material; (*C*) the fungal debris is removed; (*D*) the left sphenoid sinus at the end of the procedure. (Courtesy of Pagella F, Pusateri A, Matti E, et al. Sphenoid sinus fungus ball: our experience. *Am J Rhinol Allergy.* 2011;25:276-280, Ocean-Side Publications, Inc.)

seen, which did not resolve with surgery. The authors highlight the complex anatomy around the SS and underscore why sphenoid pathology should be considered in patients with persistent headache or visual symptoms. Computed tomography and characteristic magnetic resonance imaging findings are also described (Figs 1 and 2). Surgically, most cases used the direct paraseptal (transnasal) approach to the sphenoid sinus passing between the middle and superior turbinates and the septum, as opposed to the transethmoidal route. Unfortunately, the authors did not provide details as to the rationale for which route was selected in any given procedure and why. They did comment that "the paraseptal direct sphenoidotomy represents the less invasive, fastest and most anatomically conservative approach to the sphenoid," which I completely agree with. Sometimes resecting a small portion of the middle turbinate can provide increased exposure, which can be helpful in cases in which the fungal ball is more adherent or when the lateral recess of a well-pneumatized sphenoid sinus needs to be accessed. As long as the ethmoid sinuses are not involved in disease, the transseptal route is the best, least invasive approach.

R. Sindwani, MD

Paranasal sinus mucoceles with ophthalmologic manifestations: A 17-year review of 96 cases
Kim Y-S, Kim K, Lee J-G, et al (Yonsei Univ College of Medicine, Seoul, Korea)
Am J Rhinol Allergy 25:272-275, 2011

Background.—The purpose of this study was to assess the characteristics of paranasal sinus mucoceles with ophthalmologic manifestations with a focus on optic neuropathy.

Methods.—From January 1993 to May 2010, 96 consecutive patients diagnosed with paranasal sinus mucoceles with ophthalmologic manifestations were investigated. Clinical and therapeutic factors and demographics were reviewed from medical records. Statistical associations between clinical and therapeutic factors and visual outcomes after surgery were also analyzed.

Results.—A total of 352 patients were diagnosed with paranasal sinus mucoceles and underwent surgical treatment. Ninety-six of them presented with ophthalmologic symptoms, and periorbital swelling and pain were the most common symptoms (36.4%) in those patients. Among the 96 patients with ophthalmologic manifestations, 18 (18.8%) were diagnosed with optic neuropathy based on the deterioration of their visual acuity and unilateral relative afferent papillary defect. Ten of these 18 patients showed improvements in their vision after surgical intervention. The statistical analysis of the association between clinical and therapeutic factors and visual outcomes showed that the presence of infection was the only significant factor ($p = 0.023$).

Conclusion.—Paranasal sinus mucoceles present various ophthalmologic manifestations. Among them, optic neuropathy may be one of the most devastating conditions. In treating optic neuropathy caused by mucoceles, the presence of infection was the only factor that had any influence on postoperative visual outcomes. Therefore, we conclude that not only surgical drainage and ventilation of the sinus are necessary, but infection control is also a vital factor in treating mucoceles with optic neuropathy (Table 5).

▶ This is one of the largest series in the literature on sinus mucoceles with ophthalmologic manifestations, with a focus on optic neuropathy. Periorbital swelling and pain were the most common symptoms, and 18 (18.8%) of 96 patients were diagnosed with optic neuropathy. Of the 18 patients, 10 showed improvements in their vision after surgical intervention. The majority of cases with optic neuropathy (15/18 [83%]) involved the ethmoid sinus, and not the sphenoid sinus as might be suspected (Table 5). The study examined multiple clinical factors involved in poor vision outcomes, but it is interesting that only the presence of infection was a significant association, leading the authors to

TABLE 5.—Clinical Features of Patients With Optic Neuropathy Caused by Paranasal Sinus Mucoceles

Case No.	Origins	Presence of Infection	Symptom Duration (Days)	Lamina Papyracea Dehiscence	Steroid Pulse Treatment	Preoperative Vision	Postoperative Vision	Follow-up (mo)
1	E (L)	Y	14	N	N	20/32	20/32	21
2	E (L)	N	7	N	N	20/40	20/40	10
3	E (L)	N	2	N	N	20/30	20/25*	8
4#	E (L)	N	18	N	N	20/60	20/60	3
5§	E (L)	N	2	Y	Y	LP(+)	HM*	22
6	E (R)	N	10	N	N	20/40	20/25*	3
7	E (R)	Y	11	Y	Y	LP(−)	LP(−)	12
8	E (R)	N	30	N	N	20/40	20/30*	13
9	E, F (R)	N	5	N	N	20/50	20/30*	11
10	E, S (L)	N	17	N	Y	20/30	20/20*	9
11	E, S (R)	N	7	N	N	LP(−)	LP(−)	5
12#	E, S (B)	N	21	N	N	20/1200	20/25*	3
13	F (L)	N	21	N	N	20/200	20/60*	10
14	S (R)	N	10	N	N	20/25	20/20*	7
15	S (R)	Y	3	N	Y	LP(−)	LP(−)	24
16	S (R)	Y	2	N	Y	LP(−)	LP(−)	9
17	S (R)	N	3	N	N	LP(−)	LP(−)	7
18	Clinoid (R)	N	15	N	N	LP(+)	20/200*	25

No. = number of patients; E = ethmoid sinus; F = frontal sinus; S = sphenoid sinus; R = right; L = left; LP = light perception; HM = hand motion detection.
*Improvement of one or more Snellen lines in vision.
#Patients with visual field defect.
§Patients with abnormal appearance of optic disc.

encourage appropriate infection control in addition to surgery so as to maximize outcomes. The article does a nice job of exploring some interesting points such as the mechanisms at play in vision loss, which may not be simple compression. Another proposed mechanism, for example, causing optic neuropathy, is the spread of infection through congenital bony dehiscence and bony perforation of the vessels between the sinuses and orbits. The authors assert that the key mechanism of irreversible nerve injury is postinflammatory insults and not solely compression-induced ischemia. This concept may also tie in with the finding that the presence of infection (ie, mucopyocele) is a poor prognosticator for vision outcomes.

R. Sindwani, MD

A new approach to the treatment of nasal bone fracture: The clinical usefulness of closed reduction using a C-arm
Han DSY, Han YS, Park JH (Kosin Univ Gaspel Hosp, Seo-gu, Busan, Republic of Korea)
J Plast Reconstr Aesthet Surg 64:937-943, 2011

Closed reduction is commonly conducted for the treatment of a nasal bone fracture unless a concurrent fracture or a severe nasal septum fracture is observed. As the reduction, however, is not conducted through the direct gross observation of the fracture site, it is difficult to obtain a good result from it. Accordingly, a supplementary process is required.

Closed reduction with a C-arm was conducted within the period from March 2009 to January 2010 on 50 patients with nasal bone fractures, to treat these fractures or to evaluate the postoperative conditions of such. The usefulness of the C-arm was evaluated by comparing the afore-mentioned closed reduction with a C-arm with the closed reduction without a C-arm that was conducted on 64 patients with nasal bone fractures within the period from January 2008 to February 2009.

The complication morbidity and re-operation rate were significantly lower in the patient group with closed reduction with a C-arm, and the radiologic examination also showed a significant difference.

If closed reduction is conducted on patients with nasal bone fractures using a C-arm, an accurate result can be obtained by observing the fractured bone indirectly with continuous imaging during the operation, and the operation result can be immediately assessed in the operating room, thereby reducing the frequencies of complications and re-operation (Fig 5, Table 1).

▶ Nasal bone fractures are the most common form of injury resulting from facial trauma. They are typically managed using a closed technique, which has the disadvantage of not allowing direct observation, especially in the setting of

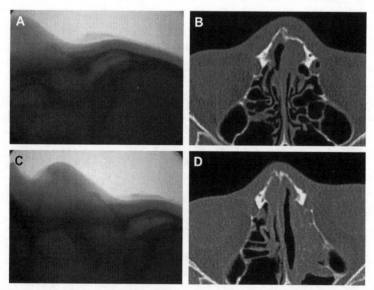

FIGURE 5.—A and B: The dorsum fracture of the nasal bone was found in a 15-year old patient on 9th day after injury in a preoperative nasal lateral view and CT via a C-arm. C and D: The fracture was almost completely reduced after closed reduction with a C-arm. (Reprinted from Journal of Plastic, Reconstructive & Aesthetic Surgery, Han DSY, Han YS, Park JH. A new approach to the treatment of nasal bone fracture: the clinical usefulness of closed reduction using a C-arm. *J Plast Reconstr Aesthet Surg.* 2011; 64:937-943. Copyright 2011, with permission from British Association of Plastic, Reconstructive and Aesthetic Surgeons.)

TABLE 1.—Postoperative Results and Complications

	Conventional Closed Reduction	Closed Reduction with C-Arm
No. of Patients	64	50
Postoperative complications (%)	21 (32.8)	4 (8)
Nasal deformity (%)	12 (18.8)	2 (4)
Dysfunction of nasal cavity (%)	9 (14.1)	2 (4)
Secondary operation (%)	4 (6.3)	0 (0)
Aver. sore of specialist[a]	2.9	4.0

[a]A significant difference was found as t-value was -13.394 and p-value was 0.000.

traumatic swelling where the bony fragments are located, before or after reduction. This, of course, greatly affects the outcome of the procedure. This study explores the benefits of augmenting this procedure by using a C-arm (Fig 5). The usefulness of the C-arm was evaluated by comparing the outcomes in 50 patients whose nasal bone fractures were reduced using this technology with the outcomes in a group of 64 patients whose fractures were reduced without the use of the C-arm. As shown in Table 1, the morbidity and reoperation rates were significantly lower when the C-arm was used. The advantages of using the C-arm seem intuitive: better diagnosis of nasal bone fractures and immediate confirmation of adequate, or rather ideal, reduction and fragment alignment prior to the conclusion of the procedure. It is surprising that this technique has not caught on, and I suspect that over time surgeons will appreciate the use of this technique and invest the extra time taken to ensure that their fracture reductions are ideal.

R. Sindwani, MD

Lack of efficacy of long-term, low-dose azithromycin in chronic rhinosinusitis: a randomized controlled trial

Videler WJ, Badia L, Harvey RJ, et al (Academic Med Centre, Amsterdam, the Netherlands; Nose & Ear Hosp, London, UK; et al)
Allergy 66:1457-1468, 2011

Background.—In persistent chronic rhinosinusitis (CRS), conventional treatment is often insufficient. Long-term, low-dose administration of macrolides has been suggested as a treatment option. The MACS (Macrolides in chronic rhinosinusitis) study is a randomized placebo-controlled trial evaluating the efficacy of azithromycin (AZM) in CRS.

Methods.—We describe a group of patients with recalcitrant CRS with and without nasal polyps unresponsive to optimal medical and (in 92% also) surgical treatment. Patients were treated with AZM or placebo. AZM was given for 3 days at 500 mg during the first week, followed by 500 mg per week for the next 11 weeks. Patients were monitored until 3 months post-therapy. The assessments included Sino-Nasal Outcome Test-22 (SNOT-22), a Patient Response Rating Scale, Visual Analogue

Scale (VAS), Short Form-36 (SF-36), rigid nasal endoscopy, peak nasal inspiratory flow (PNIF), Sniffin' Sticks smell tests and endoscopically guided middle meatus cultures.

Results.—Sixty patients with a median age of 49 years were included. Fifty per cent had asthma and 58% had undergone revision sinus surgery. In the SNOT-22, Patient Response Rating Scale, VAS scores and SF-36, no significant difference between the AZM and the placebo groups was demonstrated. Nasal endoscopic findings, PNIF results, smell tests and microbiology showed no relevant significant differences between the groups either.

Conclusion.—At the investigated dose of AZM over 3 months, no significant benefit was found over placebo. Possible reasons could be disease severity in the investigated group, under-dosage of AZM and under-powering of the study. Therefore, more research is urgently required (Fig 1).

▶ Besides antibacterial properties, macrolides have been shown to possess immunomodulatory properties similar to those of corticosteroids. In animal studies, macrolides have increased mucociliary transport, reduced goblet cell secretion, accelerated apoptosis of neutrophils, reduced expression of cell surface adhesion molecules, and decreased levels of cytokines implicated in

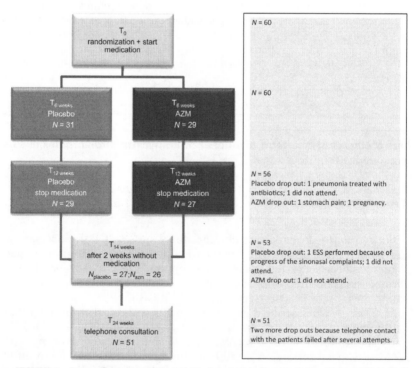

FIGURE 1.—Patient flow chart of the MACS clinical trial. (Reprinted from Videler WJ, Badia L, Harvey RJ, et al. Lack of efficacy of long-term, low-dose azithromycin in chronic rhinosinusitis: a randomized controlled trial. *Allergy.* 2011;66:1457-1468, with permission from John Wiley and Sons (www.interscience.wiley.com).)

chronic rhinosinusitis (CRS). So considering the use of these drugs in refractory CRS makes sense. This study built on a growing interest in the use of low-dose macrolides in CRS to look at the effectiveness of low-dose azithromycin (AZM) for CRS with and without polyps. The Macrolides in Chronic Rhinosinusitis Study (MACS) was well performed and used sound methodology (Fig 1). Patients were treated with placebo or AZM (for 3 days at 500 mg during the first week, followed by 500 mg per week for the next 11 weeks) and followed for 3 months. Evaluations with a variety of reliable outcome tools showed no significant difference between the AZM and placebo. The MACS trial is only the second randomized, placebo-controlled trial on macrolides in the treatment for CRS and, like the first, it did not demonstrate any significant benefits. Further study using other members of the macrolide family, other dosage schemes, and different treatment periods need to be explored before the use of this therapy in CRS is advocated.

R. Sindwani, MD

Adjuvant therapy with flutamide for presurgical volume reduction in juvenile nasopharyngeal angiofibroma

Thakar A, Gupta G, Bhalla AS, et al (All India Inst of Med Sciences, New Delhi)
Head Neck 33:1747-1753, 2011

Background.—Although 2 studies totaling 11 cases have indicated some benefit of anti-androgen treatment with flutamide on juvenile nasopharyngeal angiofibroma (JNA), it is not part of contemporary practice.

Methods.—Our approach was through a prospective, single-arm, before-and-after study, in which 20 patients with advanced JNA (Radkowski stage IIB—IIIB) were administered flutamide (per oral: $10 \text{ mg kg}^{-1} \text{ day}^{-1} \times$ 6 weeks) prior to surgical excision. Pretherapy and posttherapy tumor volume measurements were established by MRI. Periodic assessments were recorded of liver, kidney functions, testosterone levels, and secondary sexual characteristics.

Results.—Prepubertal and postpubertal cases responded differently ($p < .05$). Prepubertal cases had inconsistent and minimal responses; 13/ 15 postpubertal cases demonstrated measurable volume reduction (mean, 16.5%; maximum, 40%). Two cases with optic nerve compression had visual improvement. Volume reduction correlated with serum testosterone level ($r = .53; p < .05$). No significant toxicity was noted, with the exception of transient breast tenderness.

Conclusions.—Prepubertal and postpubertal patients differ in their response to flutamide. In postpubertal patients, 6 weeks preoperative use is safe and leads to partial tumor regression. Tumor regression from adjacent vital structures may facilitate surgical excision and limit morbidity (Fig 1, Table 2).

▶ The exclusivity of juvenile nasopharyngeal angiofibroma (JNA) to male adolescents has long pointed to a hormonal connection, and prior work has

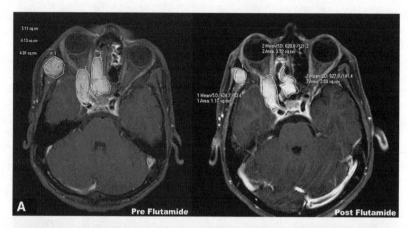

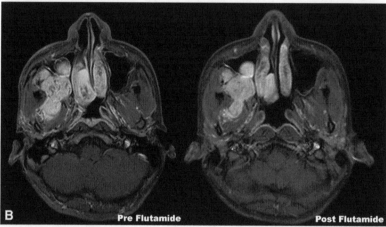

FIGURE 1.—(A) Pre- and postflutamide axial MR images (stage IIIB juvenile nasopharyngeal angiofibroma [JNA], scans at level of internal carotid artery). Postflutamide tumor regression is noted in the ethmoids, temporal fossa, superior orbital fissure, and middle cranial fossa. (B) Pre- and postflutamide axial MR images (stage IIC JNA, scans at level of fossa of Rosenmuller). Postflutamide tumor regression is noted in the posterior nose and the infratemporal fossa. (Reprinted from Thakar A, Gupta G, Bhalla AS, et al. Adjuvant therapy with flutamide for presurgical volume reduction in juvenile nasopharyngeal angiofibroma. *Head Neck.* 2011;33:1747-1753, with permission from John Wiley and Sons.)

noted increased tumor growth with testosterone and a regression with estrogen. The concept of trying to treat or at least reduce the volume of JNAs with antitestosterone agents is not new, but because of the side effects (including feminization) these hormonal therapies were largely abandoned. Flutamide is an orally active nonsteroidal androgen antagonist with a favorable side effect profile that has been used in children for other conditions. This study looks at the outcomes of 20 patients with advanced JNA who were administered flutamide daily for 6 weeks for volume reduction prior to surgical excision. Pretherapy and posttherapy volume measurements were calculated using MRI (Fig 1). The study found that although reduction was inconsistent and minimal in

TABLE 2.—Pretreatment and Posttreatment Tumor Volumes and Percentage Reduction in Tumor Volume

Serial No.	Age, y	Tumor Stage	Volume, cm^3 Pretherapy	Volume, cm^3 Posttherapy	% Volume Reduction
1	20	IIIA	70.2	65.3	7%
2	11	IIC	90.8	85.8	6%
3	14	IIC	101.8	65.9	35%
4	12	IIIB*	32.7	28.9	12%
5	15	IIIB	146.8	97.4	34%
6	14	IIIA	60.4	57.0	6%
7	16	IIIA	135.8	127.5	6%
8	19	IIC	68.2	57.8	15%
9	25	IIIB	63.8	55.1	14%
10	12	IIIB	103.0	111.4	−8%
11	12	IIIA	190.2	242.9	−28%
12	14	IIIB*	232.7	191.5	18%
13	15	IIIA	63.8	64.8	−2%
14	15	IIIB	64.7	48.7	25%
15	19	IIIB	57.3	55.1	4%
16	18	IIC	130.5	97.0	25%
17	17	IIIA	61.9	37.0	40%
18	15	IIIB	114.8	98.3	14%
19	21	IIIB	54.7	50.8	7%
20	10	IIB*	13.4	12.4	7%

*Cases 4, 12, and 20 were recurrent tumors. Staging as depicted is based on the tumor extent following recurrence.

prepubescent male patients, those treated demonstrated significant volume reduction (mean, 16.5%; maximum, 40%; Table 2). No significant toxicity was noted. The authors recommended the use of this agent in postpubescent male patients preoperatively and suggested that tumor regression from adjacent vital structures may facilitate surgical excision. This is the largest and most well-analyzed study on the use of this agent for volume reduction in JNA. Other studies contained much smaller numbers, and although they both showed volume reduction with flutamide (29% and 7%, respectively), they arrived at conflicting recommendations. The impressive results of this large study call into question the lack of enthusiasm in the literature for this agent and put forward conservative and well-thought-out considerations for its use, including reducing tumor volumes preoperatively for advanced lesions and possibly exploring applications for residual disease intracranially as well. With time and the benefit of further scientific discourse, this novel concept may find a role; however, this will likely be limited to advanced disease only because contemporary surgical techniques for modest-to-large lesions are effective with minimal morbidity, and accepting any potential risks of hormonal therapy just to "facilitate" surgery is not necessary.

R. Sindwani, MD

Postoperative Care for Samter's Triad Patients Undergoing Endoscopic Sinus Surgery: A Double-Blinded, Randomized Controlled Trial

Rotenberg BW, Zhang I, Arra I, et al (The Univ of Western Ontario, London, Ontario, Canada)
Laryngoscope 121:2702-2705, 2011

Objectives/Hypothesis.—Evidence is lacking to guide the postoperative management of Samter's triad patients with chronic rhinosinusitis with polyposis (CRSwP) undergoing endoscopic sinus surgery (ESS). The purpose of this study was to compare three different standardized medication regimens prescribed to these patients after ESS.

Study Design.—Three-arm, randomized, double-blinded, controlled trial.

Methods.—Patients with Samter's triad undergoing ESS were postoperatively randomized into three medication regimens, those being saline irrigation alone (control group A), saline irrigation plus separate budesonide nasal spray (group B), and saline irrigation mixed with budesonide nasal spray (group C). Outcome measures were Sino-Nasal Outcome Test scores, Lund-Mackay computed tomography scores, and Lund-Kennedy endoscopic scores taken at preoperative baseline, and then at 6 months and 1 year postoperatively. Side effect profiles were also measured (adrenocorticotropic hormone blood level ranges and intraocular pressure at the same interval points). Analysis of variance and χ^2 analyses were conducted using a Bonferroni correction method and routine descriptive statistics. Inter- and intragroup comparisons were made.

Results.—Sixty subjects were recruited. All groups were equivalent at baseline in all outcomes. All intragroup analyses showed statistically and clinically significant improvement in disease status as compared to baseline ($P < .0167$), with a sustained but lessened improvement at 1 year. However, no statistically or clinically significant differences were observed between groups at any time point ($P > .05$). There was no treatment effect noted.

Conclusions.—In this study, nasal steroids did not confer any additional benefit over saline alone as post-ESS care for the Samter's triad CRSwP patient population.

▶ Samter triad (or AERD) patients generally are considered to have especially recalcitrant nasal polyps and can be challenging to treat. This very well designed and thoughtfully conducted study compared 3 different medication regimens prescribed to Samter patients following endoscopic sinus surgery (ESS). The 3 arms in this randomized, double-blinded, controlled trial were postoperative saline irrigation alone (control group, A), saline irrigation plus separate twice-daily budesonide nasal spray (group B), and saline irrigation mixed with budesonide (group C). Sixty study patients were evaluated using SNOT scores, Lund-Mackay computed tomography scores, and Lund-Kennedy endoscopic scores taken at preoperative baseline and then at 6 months and 1 year postoperatively. Although all patients improved from baseline, there was no difference found between any of the groups at either time point during the study. There was no treatment effect noted. The authors concluded that nasal steroids did not confer any additional benefit over saline alone as post-ESS care for the Samter triad patients, which was supported by their findings. Although well designed, this study has some major limitations. First, the compliance of patients was not monitored or ensured, and second, the patients were only formally evaluated twice in the year after surgery. The findings of this study are surprising, as many clinicians have migrated to the use of more concentrated topical steroid delivery through irrigations, which makes sense in this group of challenging patients. Further investigation into the use and efficacy of this practice is needed.

R. Sindwani, MD

Outcomes

Olfactory Outcomes After Endoscopic Transsphenoidal Pituitary Surgery
Rotenberg BW, Saunders S, Duggal N (Univ of Western Ontario, London, Canada)
Laryngoscope 121:1611-1613, 2011

Background.—Olfaction has been demonstrated to have a great impact on patients' lives. Transsphenoidal endoscopic pituitary surgery is associated with potentially significant damage to olfactory tissues, but to date this issue has been only poorly documented in the literature.

Study Design.—Prospective cohort study comparing olfactory outcomes pre- and postpituitary surgery.

Method.—Patients were administered the University of Pennsylvania Smell Identification Test (UPSIT) preoperatively and again at 6 months postoperatively. The endoscopic transsphenoidal pituitary surgery was carried out using a full middle turbinate preservation protocol. A Hadad-Bassagasteguy (HB) vascularized septal flap was raised in each case. Secondary outcomes included Lund-Kennedy endoscopy scores (LKES) and patient self-report of olfactory disturbance. The results were analysed using a paired *t*-tests.

Results.—Seventeen patients met inclusion criteria for the study. Mean preoperative UPSIT value was 37.2 (normosmia), and mean postoperative UPSIT value was 30.8 (moderate hyposmia) ($P < .001$). All patients were fully healed with normal LKES scores by 6 months. All patients complained of their olfactory dysfunction.

Conclusions.—This study is the first to describe postoperative olfactory perturbations suffered by patients undergoing endoscopic transsphenoidal pituitary surgery. We hypothesize that olfactory impairment results from use of the HB flap. We recommend that the possibility of permanent olfactory changes be added to routine patient counseling and consent for this procedure, and that HB flaps be raised judiciously during trannssphenoidal endoscopic procedures.

▶ For reasons including quality of life and concerns over safety, permanent loss in olfaction is considered a major problem for patients. There has been growing interest in olfactory outcomes following transsphenoidal pituitary surgery.

This well-designed and thoughtful prospective study uses the University of Pennsylvania Smell Identification Test (UPSIT) to examine the issue of olfactory loss in patients 6 months following thyroid stimulating hormone (TSH). Importantly, the authors describe their technique of bilateral middle turbinate preservation, endoscopic TSH using a Hadad-Bassagasteguy (HB) septal flap for reconstruction. They admit to resecting the inferior portion of the superior turbinate and inferior posterior ethmoids in some cases. Patients were administered the UPSIT preoperatively and again at 6 months postoperation. In this study of 17 patients, the mean preoperative UPSIT value of 37.2 (normosmia) and mean postoperative UPSIT value of 30.8 (moderate hyposmia) were significantly different ($P < .001$). Despite being well healed at 6 months, all patients complained of smell disturbance postoperatively. The authors blamed the reduction in smell on the HB flap and suspect that this technique for repair compromised olfactory fibers in the superior septum/nasal cavity and advised the possibility of permanent olfactory changes be added to routine patient counseling and consent and that HB flaps be raised judiciously. In the article, the authors discuss important issues, including whether the routine use of an HB flap is "overkill" for routine TSH, given that this area heals very well and the risk of CSF leak during this type of surgery is fairly small. There are of course other techniques of repair available if this situation is encountered during the course of surgery. I wonder, as the authors must also be wondering, whether the use of the HB flap routinely, especially in light of these findings, should be reconsidered. Another possibility here is that it is not simply the use of a vascularized septal flap that is to blame but the geometry or possibly the precise technique being used in this case to harvest or inset the tissues. For example, could the use of cautery during harvest (even though at low settings) be implicated here? This study raises some very important questions, and further investigations looking at different techniques and using control groups, would be worthwhile.

R. Sindwani, MD

Complications in Endoscopic Sinus Surgery for Chronic Rhinosinusitis: A 25-Year Experience
Stankiewicz JA, Lal D, Connor M, et al (Loyola Univ Med Ctr, Maywood, IL; Mayo Clinic Hosp, Phoenix, AZ; San Antonio Military Med Ctr, TX)
Laryngoscope 121:2684-2701, 2011

Objectives/Hypothesis.—The aim of this study was to review complications occurring as a result of endoscopic sinus surgery by one surgeon in an academic practice during a 25-year period.

Study Design.—Retrospective clinical study.

Methods.—A register of complications was tabulated during a period of 25 years for endoscopic sinus surgery performed for chronic rhinosinusitis in 3,402 patients (6,148 sides). All complications were reviewed as a whole and were not divided into major or minor categories.

Results.—A total of 105 patients were found to have complicated endoscopic sinus surgery, for an overall patient complication rate of 0.031, or 0.017 per operated side. The most common complications were hemorrhage (n = 41), orbital complications (n = 29), and CSF leak (n = 19). The following factors were noted to have increased risk for complications: age, revision surgery, nasal polyps, anatomic variation, extensive disease, overall health, medications, and underlying factors. Certain types of instrumentation such as powered instrumentation placed patients at greater risk. The use of image guidance or surgical experience did not eliminate complications from occurring.

Conclusions.—Complications of endoscopic sinus surgery still occur 25 years after the initial introduction of the surgery in 1985. Many complications can be managed without a bad outcome. The key to prevention is knowledge of anatomy, preparation, anticipation, and experience. Even then, complications can occur in the most experienced hands. Patients most at risk for complications include those with revision surgery, extensive disease, skull base anatomic or radiologic variations or dehiscences related to disease or previous surgery, and the use of powered instrumentation (Figs 8 and 12, Table 1).

▶ This sobering article reports the complications occurring as a result of endoscopic sinus surgery (ESS) by a senior rhinologist in an academic practice during a 25-year career. The article discusses major complications that were encountered, their management, and techniques for avoidance in a manner that it serves generally as an excellent overall review for ESS complications. In reviewing some of the grave complications presented, the reader should bear in mind that these patients were seen in a tertiary-level rhinology practice and that many of the earlier procedures were performed when ESS was initially

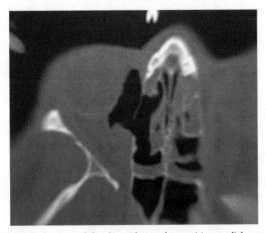

FIGURE 8.—Microdebrider injury left orbit with complete excision medial rectus. (Reprinted from Stankiewicz JA, Lal D, Connor M, et al. Complications in endoscopic sinus surgery for chronic rhinosinusitis: a 25-year experience. *Laryngoscope.* 2011;121:2684-2701, with permission from The American Laryngological, Rhinological and Otological Society, Inc, and John Wiley and Sons (www.interscience.wiley.com).)

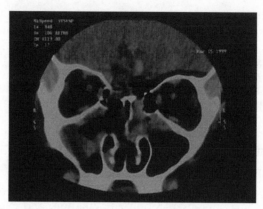

FIGURE 12.—Postoperative coronal computerized axial tomography scan showing low-lying skull base and skull base injury. [Color figure can be viewed in the online issue, which is available at wileyonlinelibrary. com.]. (Reprinted from Stankiewicz JA, Lal D, Connor M, et al. Complications in endoscopic sinus surgery for chronic rhinosinusitis: a 25-year experience. *Laryngoscope.* 2011;121:2684-2701, with permission from The American Laryngological, Rhinological and Otological Society, Inc, and John Wiley and Sons (www.interscience.wiley.com).)

TABLE 1.—Complications in 3,402 Endoscopic Sinus Patients from 1985 to 2010

	Complications	Patients
1	Hemorrhage	41
	Intraoperative	4
	Postoperative	37
2	CSF leak	19
3	Orbital hematoma	20
4	Orbital subcutaneous emphysema	4
5	Meningitis	2
6	DVT pulmonary embolism	4
7	Facial numbness	4
8	Toxic shock	2
9	Blindness	4
	Permanent	2
	Temporary	2
10	Cardiac shock	1
11	Brain injury/death	1
12	Check hematoma	1
13	Postoperative chest pain	1
14	Diplopia	1
	Total	105

CSF = cerebrospinal fluid; DVT = deep vein thrombosis.

taking form (circa 1985), and it wasn't until much later that surgical navigation and other contemporary instrumentation became available. This registry spans 25 years and includes 3402 patients (6148 sides) who underwent ESS for chronic rhinosinusitis. A total of 105 complications are presented for an overall complication rate of 0.031, or 0.017 per operated side. Complications are shown in Table 1, with the most common being hemorrhage (n = 41), orbital complications (n = 29), and cerebrospinal fluid leak (n = 19). Factors noted to have increased risk for complications were age, revision surgery (62% in this study), nasal polyps, anatomic variation, extensive disease, overall health, medications, and use of powered instrumentation. The presentation and management of orbital complications is particularly insightful and worthwhile to review. The authors stress that quick action to recognize complications intra- or postoperatively often allows for immediate treatment limiting morbidity or mortality. Even in experienced hands, however, complications can and do occur. Dr Stankiewicz should be congratulated for the candor and honesty with which he has presented his experience, which serves as an excellent learning tool for novice and experienced surgeons alike.

R. Sindwani, MD

Contemporary Management of Sinonasal Cancer

Robbins KT, Ferlito A, Silver CE, et al (Southern Illinois Univ School of Medicine, Springfield; Univ of Udine, Italy; Albert Einstein College of Medicine, Bronx, NY; et al)

Head Neck 33:1352-1365, 2011

Background.—Sinonasal cancer is a relatively uncommon entity encountered by head and neck oncologists, rhinologists, and skull base surgeons. Recent innovations in surgical and nonsurgical therapeutic modalities raise the question of whether there has been any measurable improvement for treatment outcomes.

Methods.—A retrospective review of data from recent studies that focus on surgery, radiation, and chemotherapy, or combinations thereof, was conducted.

Results.—Surgery continues to be the preferred treatment and provides the best results, albeit with an inherent bias based on patient selection. For advanced disease (T4 lesions), the survival rate remains only modest. Complications of treatment, including both surgical and radiation therapy, have been reduced.

Conclusions.—There is a need to improve the efficacy of treatment for this disease. Recommendations for the future direction of therapeutic investigations are outlined.

▶ Even when the histologically and biologically diverse tumors of the sinonasal tract are combined, sinonasal cancers are quite rare and represent only 3% of head and neck malignancies. In addition to the confounding issues of rarity and wide biological diversity, the complex anatomy of the region, which makes surgical resection or aggressive radiotherapy feasible, is another complicating feature in the management of these tumors. As has been stated at many a journal club across the country, these factors have made it very difficult to conduct meaningful trials designed to improve upon traditional treatment strategies or even to compare the results of some studies. Current management continues to hold surgical resection as the mainstay, which is then often followed by radiotherapy. Surgical approaches have evolved of late to include less minimally invasive techniques including fully endoscopic approaches to tumor resection. Studies comparing traditional open approaches to endoscopic techniques are difficult to interpret for a variety of reasons—most notably, selection bias. However, the authors underscore that despite the refinements in surgical techniques, there is no convincing evidence that disease control outcomes have improved and remain quite modest. The article highlights that applying nonsurgical treatment modalities, including radiation and chemotherapy as alternatives or adjuncts, is feasible for some tumors and potentially could improve treatment outcomes as these modalities continue to evolve. This contemporary review of the management of sinonasal cancers highlights some of the challenges in interpreting the literature on this topic and also sheds some light on potential avenues for future improvements in the management of these patients, as seen through the eyes of a very reputable group of coauthors. It is an excellent review of the topic (and its associated controversies) and is a must read.

R. Sindwani, MD

Association between severity of asthma and degree of chronic rhinosinusitis

Lin DC, Chandra RK, Tan BK, et al (Northwestern Univ Feinberg School of Medicine, Chicago, IL)
Am J Rhinol Allergy 25:205-208, 2011

Background.—There is a clinical association between asthma and chronic rhinosinusitis (CRS). This study was designed to determine whether severity of coexistent asthma affects the clinical presentation of CRS.

Methods.—Cross-sectional analysis was performed of prospectively collected data in 187 patients with CRS who were evaluated in a large, tertiary academic nasal and sinus center. Patients were stratified into three groups based on asthma status using National Institutes of Health criteria: (1) nonasthmatic, (2) intermittent/mild asthma, (3) or moderate/severe asthma.

Results.—Mean Lund-Mackay scores were 9.7, 11.6, and 15.6, respectively. ANOVA testing with post-hoc Tukey analysis revealed that Lund-MacKay scores were significantly greater in group 3 than either group 1 ($p < 0.05$) or group 2 ($p < 0.01$). The prevalence of allergic sensitization was 72.4, 82.8, and 100% in groups 1, 2, and 3, respectively ($p = 0.03$). The prevalence of nasal polyposis was 31.4% in group 1, 48.3% in group 2, and 94.4% in group 3 ($p < 0.0001$). No differences were observed regarding demographic factors or the incidence of the triad of aspirin sensitivity, asthma, and nasal polyposis among those with different severities of asthma.

Conclusion.—Increasing severity of asthma is associated with advancing radiological severity of CRS and a greater prevalence of allergic sensitization and nasal polyposis. This large adult series shows that asthma severity may have a significant correlation with the presentation of CRS. This study adds to the growing support for the unified airway theory.

▶ This study explores whether the severity of coexistent asthma affects the clinical presentation of chronic rhinosinusitis (CRS) and lends support to the unified airway hypothesis. One hundred eighty-seven CRS patients were stratified into 3 groups based on asthma status using National Institutes of Health criteria and computed tomography (CT) scores; atopy and presence of polyps were compared. Not surprisingly, increasing severity of asthma was associated with advancing radiologic severity of CRS, greater allergies, and nasal polyposis. Although the association linking upper airway disease and lower airway disease is becoming more and more compelling, the exact mechanism responsible for this connection is unclear. The article comments on some of the putative mechanisms in the literature, including aspiration of inflamed sinus secretions into the lower airways, excessive drying of the lower airways by mouth breathing as a consequence of nasal obstruction, production of bacterial toxins that induce partial B-blockade, and production in the infected sinus of cytokines and bronchoconstrictive mediators.[1] More recent evidence suggests that a systemic inflammatory process, possibly mediated by eosinophils, may be central to the unified airway.[2] More information on the mechanistic underpinnings connecting the upper and lower airways are expected in the future.

R. Sindwani, MD

References

1. Marney SR Jr. Pathophysiology of reactive airway disease and sinusitis. *Ann Otol Rhinol Laryngol.* 1996;105:98-100.
2. Joe SA, Thakkar K. Chronic rhinosinusitis and asthma. *Otolaryngol Clin North Am.* 2008;41:297-309.

Evidence-based applications of mitomycin C in the nose

Karkos PD, Leong SC, Sastry A, et al (Univ Hosp Aintree, Bristol, UK; Southmead Hosp, Bristol, UK; et al)
Am J Otolaryngol 32:422-425, 2011

Background.—Mitomycin C (MMC) is an antimitotic drug that may, when applied topically, prevent postoperative stenosis. Its use remains controversial. This review aims to provide otolaryngologists with an update of the evidence on the applications of this agent in the nose and sinuses.

Methods.—A systematic review was performed. Inclusion criteria were as follows: English literature, original articles, reviews, and case series. Exclusion criteria were as follows: animal and in vitro studies, nonendoscopic and nonsinonasal applications of MMC, and external lacrimal surgery. Studies that used other ways of dilating stenoses in conjunction with MMC were excluded.

Results.—Out of 48 studies published, 9 fulfilled our inclusion criteria, totaling 322 patients. Eighty-five percent were primary and 15% were

TABLE 2.—Type of Sinonasal Operation, Follow-up in Months, and Outcome Measures Used

Reference	Type of Operation	No. of Patients	Duration of TOP (min)	FUp	Outcome Measures
Kim et al [8]*	ESS	38	5	3 (min)	Ex, CT
Dolmetch et al [9]	DCR	71	5	12.3 (mean)	Ex, dye test, SR
Konstantinidis et al [10]*	ESS	30	5	7.2 (mean)	Ex CT, AN, SR
Nemet et al [11]	DCR	5	5	15.4 (mean)	Ex, dye test, SR
Amonoo-Kuofi et al [12]	ESS	28	5	19 (mean)	Ex
Kim et al [13]*	ESS	20	5	13.3 (mean)	Ex, MCST, AN
Gupta and Motwani [14]*	ESS	30	4	3 (max)	Ex, SR
Chan et al [15]*	ESS	45	4	1-6 (range)	Ex, AN
Chung et al [16]*	ESS	55	4	4.1 (mean)	Ex

Editor's Note: Please refer to original journal article for full references.

*References with asterisk are double-blind, randomized, controlled trials. TOP indicates topical application; FUp, follow-up (mean, minimum, maximum, or range); Ex, outpatient endoscopic examination; CT, computerized tomography sinuses; SR, subjective symptom resolution; MCST, mucociliary clearance saccharin test; AN, anatomical measurement of ostia.

revision cases. Follow-up ranged from 1 to 42 months. Main outcome measures used were endoscopic examination, anatomical measurements, radiological scoring systems, dye tests, and subjective symptom resolution. Main overall outcomes from studies where extrapolation of data was feasible were (1) patency rate, which ranged from 63% to 94.4% (mean, 81.3%); (2) adhesions: 5.1% (MMC) vs 15.05 (control); and (3) stenosis: 14.05% (MMC) vs 32.6% (control).

Conclusions.—There appears to be a favorable short-term effect of MMC, but no robust evidence regarding long-term prevention of restenosis. Larger homogenous and multicenter randomized trials are needed to assess the long-term effects of MMC in sinonasal surgery (Table 2).

▶ The use of mitomycin C (MMC) to decrease stenosis and adhesions after endoscopic sinus surgery remains controversial, and the evidence in the literature is conflicting. This systematic review included 6 double-blinded randomized controlled trials and 3 nonrandomized studies.

In 5 of the 6 randomized trials, there appeared to be a favorable effect of MMC on maintaining patency and reducing adhesion formation (Table 2). One randomized study showed that 1-time intraoperative topical MMC was not effective. None of the studies found any adverse effects or systemic toxicity when MMC was applied in a maximum concentration of 0.6 mg/mL and a maximum dose of 1.5 mL. The authors concluded that there appears to be a favorable short-term effect of MMC, but no robust evidence regarding its long-term prevention of restenosis, and noted the need for larger studies with a longer follow-up. Although this analysis suggests that there appears to be a favorable short-term effect of MMC, several confounding factors make these findings difficult to interpret, including the concentration of MMC used, the method of application, the duration and timing of application, and its use in primary or revision surgery. Further inquiry is required.

R. Sindwani, MD

Health State Utility Values in Patients Undergoing Endoscopic Sinus Surgery

Soler ZM, Wittenberg E, Schlosser RJ, et al (Med Univ of South Carolina, Charleston; Brandeis Univ, Waltham, MA; et al)
Laryngoscope 121:2672-2678, 2011

Objectives/Hypothesis.—The primary study goal was to measure health state utility values in patients with chronic rhinosinusitis (CRS) before and after undergoing endoscopic sinus surgery (ESS). A secondary goal was to assess the meaning of these values by comparing them with other chronic disease processes and currently available medical or surgical treatments.

Study Design.—Prospective, observational cohort study.

Methods.—Adults with CRS were enrolled after electing ESS and were observed for a 5-year period. Baseline demographic and medical comorbidities were recorded for each patient, as well as findings from computed tomography (CT), endoscopy, olfaction, and disease-specific quality of life scores. Utility values were derived using the Short-Form 6D (SF-6D) at baseline and again after surgery.

Results.—The mean SF-6D utility value for the baseline health state of all patients with CRS (n = 232) was 0.65 (95% confidence interval [CI]: 0.63-0.66). Baseline utility values correlated with disease-specific quality

Utility Scores for Various Health States

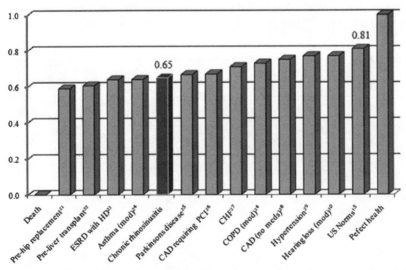

FIGURE 2.—Utility scores for various health states. ESRD = end-stage renal disease; HD = hemodialysis; mod = moderate; CAD = coronary artery disease; PCI = percutaneous coronary intervention; CHF = congestive heart failure; COPD = chronic obstructive pulmonary disease; meds = medications; US = United States. (Reprinted from Soler ZM, Wittenberg E, Schlosser RJ, et al. Health state utility values in patients undergoing endoscopic sinus surgery. *Laryngoscope.* 2011;121:2672-2678, with permission from The American Laryngological, Rhinological and Otological Society, Inc, and John Wiley and Sons (www.interscience.wiley.com).)

of life as measured by the Rhinosinusitis Disability Index ($r = -0.660$; $P < .001$), but not baseline CT, endoscopy, or olfactory scores. Follow-up utility values (≥ 6 months) after ESS improved by 0.087 (95% CI: 0.06-0.12; $P < .001$) in patients with no history of sinus surgery and 0.062 (95% CI: 0.04-0.09; $P < .001$) in those undergoing a revision procedure.

Conclusions.—Patients with CRS who failed medical therapy and elected to undergo ESS reported health state utility values that were significantly lower than the US population norm. Utility values showed improvement after ESS, which was statistically and clinically significant. These results provide the initial data necessary for formal cost-effectiveness analyses incorporating ESS (Figs 2 and 3).

▶ It is well known that chronic rhinosinusitis (CRS) significantly affects patients and that endoscopic sinus surgery (ESS) improves quality of life (QOL) in affected individuals. Prior studies have demonstrated sustained improvements in QOL after ESS, providing justification for surgical treatment in refractory patients. This study takes a unique look at the impact of surgery on CRS using health state utility values. The article explains that health state values, or "utilities" are a measure of preference-based health-related QOL (HRQOL) often used by health economists. Utility values represent an individual's valuation or preference for being in a particular health state from 0 (death) to 1 (perfect health). Utility values are also useful for economic evaluations of medical interventions. In this

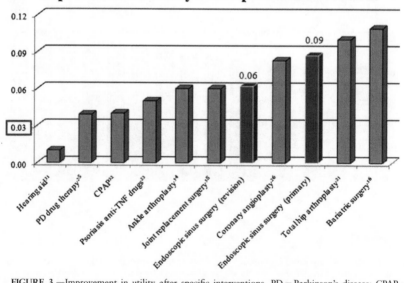

FIGURE 3.—Improvement in utility after specific interventions. PD = Parkinson's disease; CPAP = continuous positive airway pressure; TNF = tumor necrosis factor alpha. (Reprinted from Soler ZM, Wittenberg E, Schlosser RJ, et al. Health state utility values in patients undergoing endoscopic sinus surgery. *Laryngoscope.* 2011;121:2672-2678, with permission from The American Laryngological, Rhinological and Otological Society, Inc, and John Wiley and Sons (www.interscience.wiley.com).)

study, adults with CRS were followed for 5 years after sinus surgery with utility values derived using the Short-Form 6D (SF-6D) at baseline and again after surgery. An interesting finding was that the baseline (preop) utility values for CRS were poor and correlated only with the Rhinosinusitis Disability Index scores and notably not with CT, olfaction, or endoscopy. The utility decline for presurgical CRS patients was comparable to that for many other chronic diseases, which was noteworthy (Fig 1). There was significant improvement in values postoperatively, and patients who underwent ESS reported health state utility values that were significantly lower than the US population norm. The analysis demonstrated that the level of impact that ESS had on CRS was similar to what other established interventions have on other chronic disease states (Fig 2). This type of in-depth analysis continues to add to the evidence available showing the positive impact of ESS on patients with CRS and will no doubt foster meaningful studies on the cost-effectiveness of this intervention.

R. Sindwani, MD

Silent sinus syndrome: dynamic changes in the position of the orbital floor after restoration of normal sinus pressure
Sivasubramaniam R, Sacks R, Thornton M (The Canberra Hosp, Australian Capital Territory, New South Wales, Australia; Concord General Hosp, New South Wales, Australia; St Vincent's Univ Hosp, Dublin, Ireland)
J Laryngol Otol 125:1239-1243, 2011

Background.—Silent sinus syndrome is characterised by spontaneous enophthalmos and hypoglobus, in association with chronic atelectasis of the maxillary sinus, and in the absence of signs or symptoms of intrinsic sinonasal inflammatory disease. Traditionally, correction of the enophthalmos involved reconstruction of the orbital floor, which was performed simultaneously with sinus surgery. Recently, there has been increasing evidence to support the performance of uncinectomy and antrostomy alone, then orbital floor reconstruction as a second-stage procedure if needed.

Methods.—We performed a retrospective review of 23 cases of chronic maxillary atelectasis managed in our unit with endoscopic uncinectomy and antrostomy alone. All patients were operated upon by the same surgeon.

Results.—Twenty-two of the 23 patients had either complete or partial resolution. One patient had ongoing enophthalmos, and was considered for an orbital floor reconstruction as a second-stage procedure.

Conclusion.—Our case series demonstrates that dynamic changes in orbital floor position can occur after sinus re-ventilation. These findings support the approach of delaying orbital floor reconstruction in cases of silent sinus syndrome treated with sinus re-ventilation, as such reconstruction may prove unnecessary over time (Fig 1).

▶ This is a large series that examines what happens to the orbital floor in silent sinus syndrome over time if endoscopic sinus surgery alone is performed and the sinus simply reventilated. Traditionally, correction of the enophthalmos involved

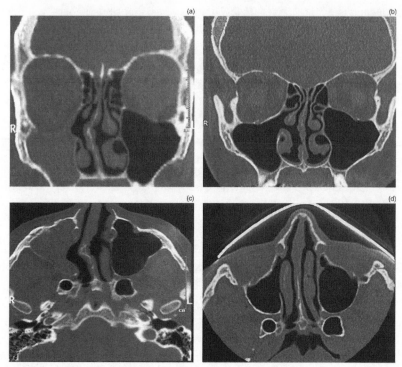

FIGURE 1.—(a) Coronal and (b) following uncinectomy and middle meatal antrostomy, parts (c) axial computed tomography views of a hypoplastic right maxillary antrum in a patient with silent sinus syndrome and (d) show corresponding views indicating remodelling of the orbital floor and orbital medial wall, 10 years post-surgery. (Reprinted from Sivasubramaniam R, Sacks R, Thornton M. Silent sinus syndrome: dynamic changes in the position of the orbital floor after restoration of normal sinus pressure. *J Laryngol Otol.* 2011;125:1239-1243, with permission of Cambridge University Press.)

reconstruction of the orbital floor, which has been advocated by some authors at the same setting of the initial sinus surgery. The authors report their experience of 23 cases of silent sinus syndrome in which only endoscopic uncinectomy and antrostomy alone were performed. Only 1 patient of 23 in this study had ongoing enophthalmos postoperatively and was then considered for an orbital floor reconstruction as a second-stage procedure. As far as the results presented, only the following was reported with respect to direct evidence that there was any movement or return to a more normal position of the orbital floor postoperatively: 14 of 18 patients with enophthalmos (78%) had complete resolution, whereas 3 (17%) had partial resolution (ie, no aesthetic concerns). Fig 1 shows comparative preoperative and postoperative images demonstrating changes in orbital floor position (actually, only the coronals in panels a and b demonstrate this in a meaningful way; panels b and c are at different cuts and more difficult to interpret with regard to floor position to my review). The article went on to report that these changes became evident around 18 months postoperatively, beginning at 6 months postoperatively but provided no further data. The authors concluded that dynamic changes in orbital floor position can occur after sinus ventilation and that their findings support the approach of delaying orbital floor reconstruction, as such reconstruction may prove unnecessary over time. Although I agree with the approach and also recommend staged orbital floor reconstruction only after sinus surgery for silent sinus syndrome, I must admit that the data presented in this article is essentially qualitative and would be far more convincing if actual measurements of floor changes radiographically (or otherwise) were provided (or done). The assertion that "dynamic changes in orbital floor position can occur" by the authors, even if true, is frankly left as a leap of faith given the way the results of this study are presented. Although the data provided in the article were not very thorough with regard to how the "return to normal" of the orbital floor transpired (again, unfortunately no measurements or data-driven time course were provided), the results of the study are of interest and at least suggest that dynamic changes in orbital floor position may occur after sinus reventilation.

R. Sindwani, MD

Surgical Technique

The Frontal Intersinus Septum Takedown Procedure: Revisiting a Technique for Surgically Refractory Unilateral Frontal Sinus Disease
Reh DD, Melvin T-AN, Bolger WE, et al (Johns Hopkins School of Medicine, Baltimore, MD; Mayo Clinic Florida, Jacksonville)
Laryngoscope 121:1805-1809, 2011

Objectives/Hypothesis.—Unilateral frontal sinus obstruction presents a surgical challenge when outflow tract osteoneogenesis or dense scarring is present. Frontal sinus obliteration is often employed as a last resort, but this procedure has potential long-term complications. In some cases, endoscopic modified Lothrop or unilateral drillout procedures may be effective options; however, restenosis rates are often high. Here we report our experience using frontal intersinus septum takedown (FISST) to address unilateral obstruction while preserving the opposite frontal outflow tract.

Study Design.—A retrospective review was performed of 12 patients with unilateral frontal sinus opacification due to irreversible frontal recess obstruction who underwent FISST. Surgical outcomes were assessed based on symptoms and computed tomography (CT) resolution of frontal sinus disease.

Results.—All 12 patients undergoing FISST had significant improvement in their symptoms. Ten postoperative CT scans were available for review, all showing continued patency of the interfrontal connection, and nine out of 10 with resolution of radiographic frontal sinus disease. Eleven of the procedures were performed via trephination, and one was achieved endoscopically.

Conclusions.—In patients with one obstructed frontal sinus and a functional contralateral sinus, removal of the intersinus septum allows for adequate sinus drainage and significant clinical improvement. The success of FISST may be surprising given knowledge of mucociliary clearance

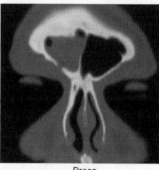 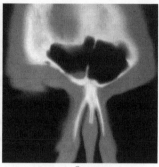

Preop   Postop

FIGURE 2.—A 47-year-old male with history of frontal sinusitis and multiple prior endoscopic surgeries, including trephination. The right frontal recess had significant bony obstruction. The left frontal sinus was healthy. To avoid a frontal sinus obliteration, the patient opted for FISST procedure with right frontal sinus trephination. The patient remains symptom-free for 4.5 years. (Reprinted from Reh DD, Melvin T-AN, Bolger WE, et al. The frontal intersinus septum takedown procedure: revisiting a technique for surgically refractory unilateral frontal sinus disease. *Laryngoscope.* 2011;121:1805-1809, with permission from The American Laryngological, Rhinological and Otological Society, Inc, and John Wiley and Sons (www.interscience.wiley.com).)

patterns, but may be effective because of the naturally dependent position of the frontal sinus ostium (Fig 2).

▶ Unilateral chronic frontal sinusitis presents a surgical challenge when the frontal outflow tract is inaccessible because of osteoneogenesis, dense scarring, trauma, or a decompressed orbit. Options for treatment of this scenario would generally consist of an osteoplastic flap (OPF) obliteration or an endoscopic-modified lothrop procedure (EMLP). This article describes the management of refractory unilateral chronic frontal sinusitis using a technique that resects the interfrontal sinus septum and opens the diseased sinus into the contralateral normal side. The authors describe the indications and technique of the frontal intersinus septum takedown (FISST) to address unilateral obstruction while preserving the opposite frontal outflow tract in 12 patients. Outcomes including symptoms and computed tomography showed that the large majority did well. Eleven of the procedures were performed via trephination, and 1 was achieved endoscopically. The authors concluded that the FISST procedure is a safe and effective option in the unique setting presented, and may avoid the need for OPF or EMLP, which carry more morbidity and are more technically demanding to perform. They also admit that the success of this technique may be surprising given knowledge of mucociliary clearance patterns, but hypothesized that it worked because of the naturally dependent position of the frontal sinus ostium, which seems reasonable. A pre requisite for attempting this technique, of course, is that there is a healthy contra-lateral frontal sinus with a patent frontal recess. It should also be noted that the concept of removing the intersinus septum via an external approach (trephination) to treat unilateral disease is not new—having been described previously in 2 studies.[1,2] In 11 of 12 of the cases presented, a trephine was used to access the frontal sinus interior, although the current study described the use of endoscopes through the trephine for septal take-down. Only in 1 case was the intersinus septum removed through a strictly endoscopic technique—the truly novel concept/technique described in this report. In either case, care should be taken to remove the inferior portion of the intersinus septum to the frontal floor to maximize the effects of gravity on clearance.

R. Sindwani, MD

References

1. Pope TH Jr, Thompson WR Jr. Treatment of chronic unilateral frontal sinusitis by removal of the interfrontal septum. *South Med J*. 1976;69:755-756.
2. Goode RL, Strelzow V, Fee WE Jr. Frontal sinus septectomy for chronic unilateral sinusitis. *Otolaryngol Head Neck Surg*. 1980;88:18-21.

Study of the Nasoseptal Flap for Endoscopic Anterior Cranial Base Reconstruction

Pinheiro-Neto CD, Ramos HF, Peris-Celda M, et al (Univ of Pittsburgh Med Ctr, PA; et al)
Laryngoscope 121:2514-2520, 2011

Objectives/Hypothesis.—Measure the dimensions of the nasoseptal (NS) flap and the anterior skull base (ASB) defect. Verify whether the flap is sufficient to cover the defect. Study the anatomy of the septal artery (SA).

Study Design.—Anatomical and radiological study.

Methods.—After endoscopic craniofacial resection, sufficiency of the flap to cover the ASB defect was assessed. The SA was dissected. The number of branches in the pedicle and the distance between the artery and the sphenoid ostium were noted. Radiologic study analyzing CT scans of 30 patients for comparison among measurements of the NS flap and the ASB defect was performed.

Results.—In all cases the flap was sufficient to cover the ASB. Two branches of the SA were found in the pedicle in 71.4%. The distance between the SA and the sphenoid ostium was 9.3 mm. The reconstruction area of the flap (17.12 cm^2) was larger than the defect area (8.64 cm^2) ($P < .001$). The difference between the superior length of the flap and the anterior-posterior distance of the defect was ≤5 mm in 26.7%. Comparison between the anterior flap width and the anterior defect width revealed that in 33% the difference was ≤5 mm.

Conclusions.—The dimensions of NS flap are sufficient to cover completely the ASB defect. The anterior edge of the defect presents increased risk for failure in coverage. Additional width adding the nasal floor mucosa to the flap is important to decrease the risk of gap in the anterior orbit-orbit defect. It is more common to find two branches of the SA in the pedicle (Figs 1 and 2).

▶ This cadaver and radiographic study evaluates the dimensions of the nasoseptal flap and evaluates the ability of the flap to cover the entirety of the

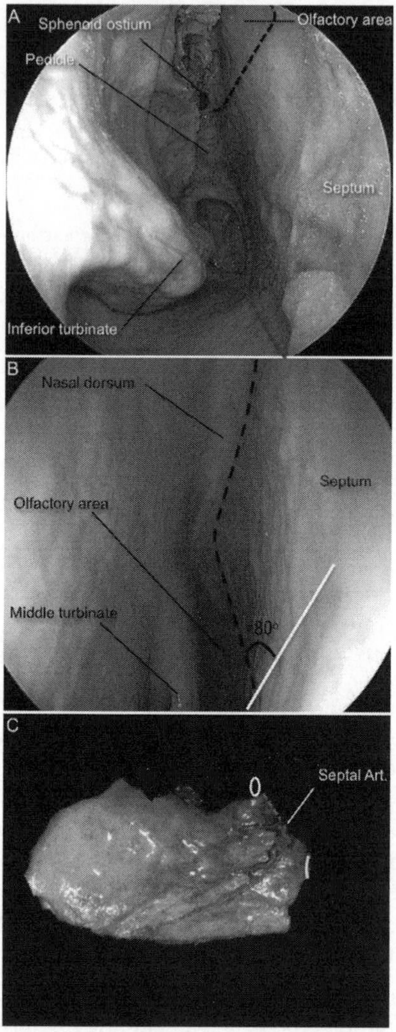

FIGURE 1.—(A) Image obtained from a dissection with a 0-degree endoscope of a right nasal cavity. Inferior dashed line shows the inferior incision for the nasoseptal flap. Notice the contour in the posterior border of the vomer and the incision prolonged anteriorly between the septum and the nasal floor. Superior dashed line shows the superior cut. Observe the preservation of part of the superior septal mucosa, which contains the olfactory neuroepithelium. (B) Image from a dissection with a 0-degree endoscope looking at nasal dorsum in the right side. Dashed line shows that the superior incision turns toward the nasal dorsum in an angle of approximately 80 degrees at the level of the middle turbinate attachment. (C) Image from the subperichondrial/subperiosteal surface of the flap. Notice two branches of the septal artery below the sphenoid ostium. Circle represents the sphenoid ostium. Dashed line shows the distance from the sphenoid ostium to the septal artery. Continuous line corresponds to the arch of the choana. Art = artery. [Color figure can be viewed in the online issue, which is available at wileyonlinelibrary.com.] (Reprinted from Pinheiro-Neto CD, Ramos HF, Peris-Celda M, et al. Study of the nasoseptal flap for endoscopic anterior cranial base reconstruction. *Laryngoscope.* 2011;121:2514-2520, with permission from The American Laryngological, Rhinological and Otological Society, Inc, and John Wiley and Sons (www.interscience.wiley.com).)

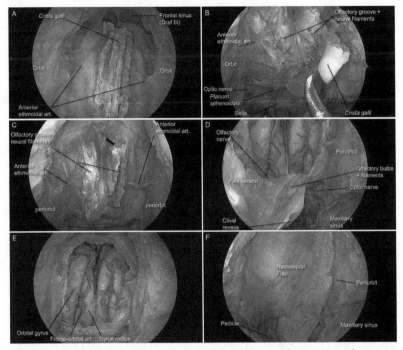

FIGURE 2.—(A) Image obtained from a dissection with a 45-degree endoscope. Notice the exposure of the entire anterior cranial base after bilateral sphenoethmoidectomy, bilateral maxillary antrostomy, superior septectomy, and Draf III frontal sinusotomy. (B) Image obtained from a dissection with a 0-degree endoscope showing the resection of the crista galli from the underlying dura mater. (C) Image from a 0-degree endoscope. After the crista galli was removed, observe the dural depression from the crista (arrow). Notice the exposure of the dura of the anterior cranial base. The anterior limit of the bony resection of the skull base is the anterior border of the crista galli and the posterior limit is the anterior border of the planum sphenoidale (continuous line). The lateral limits are the orbits. (D) Image from a 0-degree endoscope of a dissection of a cadaver injected with colored silicone. Notice the transection of the falx cerebri and exposure of the olfactory bulbs and nerves. (E) Image from a 45-degree endoscope of a dissection of a cadaver injected with colored silicone. See the final aspect of the anterior cranial base defect. Notice that the dural incisions have the same limits of the bony resection. (F) Image from a 0-degree endoscope after the flap is placed to cover the anterior cranial base defect. Observe the flap covering completely the defect with no over traction in the pedicle, which is positioned toward the right orbit. Art = artery. [Color figure can be viewed in the online issue, which is available at wileyonlinelibrary.com.] (Reprinted from Pinheiro-Neto CD, Ramos HF, Peris-Celda M, et al. Study of the nasoseptal flap for endoscopic anterior cranial base reconstruction. *Laryngoscope.* 2011;121:2514-2520, with permission from The American Laryngological, Rhinological and Otological Society, Inc, and John Wiley and Sons (www. interscience.wiley.com).)

anterior skull base. Fig 1 shows the fashioning of the flap, which is based on the septal branch of the small pulmonary arteries, which courses across the inferior face of the sphenoid sinus, and Fig 2 shows how it can be used to completely cover a maximal skull base defect created by a craniofacial defect created by a resection performed endoscopically. This well-done analysis provides measurements and dimensions for the flap and shows that the nasoseptal flap is sufficient to cover this entire region. The authors do comment that the anterior region of the skull base is of course where the reach of the flap becomes most exaggerated because of geometry and the region where risk of failure is greatest. I agree that this flap should be considered the work horse pedicled flap for endoscopic reconstruction of larger skull base defects. It is readily available and easy to harvest and it can be fashioned in varying sizes to fit the situation. A noteworthy point is that the flap can be enlarged by extending the inferior margin during harvest down to the nasal cavity floor—if a larger size is desired, such as in the scenario being discussed (ie, total anterior skull base defect).

R. Sindwani, MD

Endoscopic Maxillary Antrostomy: Not Just a Simple Procedure
Kennedy DW, Adappa ND (Hosp of the Univ of Pennsylvania, Philadelphia)
Laryngoscope 121:2142-2145, 2011

The endoscopic middle meatal maxillary antrostomy is one of the most commonly performed endoscopic procedures. Despite this, at our tertiary institution, we commonly see failed antrostomies requiring revision surgery. Accordingly, we describe in a stepwise fashion strategies helpful in creating a patent and naturally function maxillary antrostomy (Figs 1 and 2).

▶ This "How I Do It" article by Drs Kennedy and Adappa is an excellent review of the nuances and important considerations in performing an endoscopic maxillary antrostomy correctly. It is a must read. The authors make the notable point that although often considered the easiest portion of the operation, this is far from the truth. Because of the lack of specificity of available landmarks, performing a proper and effective antrostomy can be more challenging than is sometimes appreciated. This is important, of course, because failure to perform a careful antrostomy is a frequent cause of technical failure in endoscopic sinus surgery. This easy-to-read and well-written article touches on critical topics, including the importance of identifying and including the natural ostium in the antrostomy to avoid recirculation, current recommendations of (and reasoning behind) removing the uncinate process for established chrnoic rhinosinusitis, and the ideal shape of a completed antrostomy (pear-shaped). Controversies such as the ideal size of the antrostomy, which the authors admit is currently unclear, are also explored. The step-by-step description of the technique and the use of landmarks such as the maxillary line are an excellent review for even the seasoned otolaryngologist.

R. Sindwani, MD

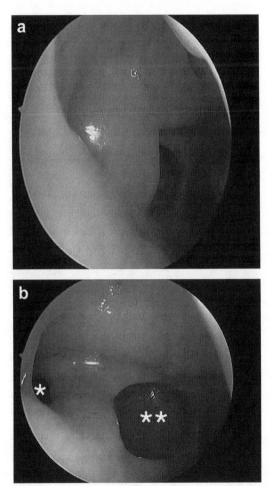

FIGURE 1.—(a) A right maxillary antrostomy made posterior to natural ostium. This results in muco-ciliary recirculation with mucopurulence exiting the anterior natural ostium and subsequently reintrodu-ces through the posterior surgical ostium due to natural ciliary flow. (b) After suctioning of right maxillary antrostomy. (*) Denotes natural ostium, (**) denotes surgical ostium posteriorly. Mucociliary recircula-tion occurs if tissue is left between two ostiums, or scar band formation occurs. The surgical ostium must include the natural ostium to avoid this complication. [Color figure can be viewed in the online issue, which is available at wileyonlinelibrary.com.] (Reprinted from Kennedy DW, Adappa ND, Endo-scopic maxillary antrostomy: not just a simple procedure. *Laryngoscope*. 2011;121:2142-2145, with permission from The American Laryngological, Rhinological and Otological Society, Inc, and John Wiley and Sons (www.interscience.wiley.com).)

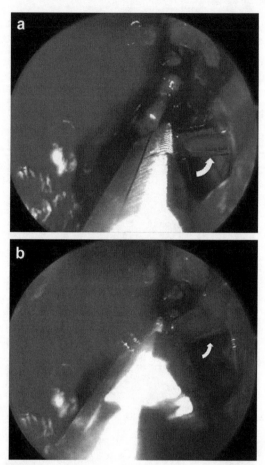

FIGURE 2.—(a) With the backbiter open, gentle rotation of the tip is extremely helpful in removing any residual uncinate process superiorly, in the region of the natural ostium. (b) With complete rotation, the tissue obstructing the natural ostium is then brought into the nasal cavity and can be removed with the backbiter or the microdebrider. [Color figure can be viewed in the online issue, which is available at wileyonlinelibrary. com.] (Reprinted from Kennedy DW, Adappa ND, Endoscopic maxillary antrostomy: not just a simple procedure. *Laryngoscope.* 2011;121:2142-2145, with permission from The American Laryngological, Rhinological and Otological Society, Inc, and John Wiley and Sons (www.interscience.wiley.com).)

Endoscopic devascularisation of sphenopalatine bundle in intractable posterior epistaxis: technique, efficacy and safety

Eladl HM, Elmorsy SM, Khafagy YW (Mansoura Univ, Egypt)
J Laryngol Otol 125:1136-1140, 2011

Objective.—To evaluate endoscopic cauterisation of the sphenopalatine neurovascular bundle, as treatment for intractable posterior epistaxis, with regard to efficacy, safety and post-operative sequelae.

Patients and Methods.—A prospective study reviewed 42 patients with severe posterior epistaxis who were treated with endoscopic cauterisation of the sphenopalatine neurovascular bundle, over a 17-month period.

Results.—Hypertension and hepatic disease were present as predisposing factors in 66.7 and 35.7 per cent of patients, respectively. Branching of the sphenopalatine artery at its foramen was present in more than 85 per cent of patients. The success rate was 100 per cent, with no recurrent epistaxis in the follow-up period. Severe nasal dryness was present in only four patients (9.5 per cent); hypoaesthesia was found in the nasal mucosa of eight patients, without any patient complaints.

Conclusion.—Endoscopic sphenopalatine neurovascular bundle cauterisation is an effective treatment for refractory posterior epistaxis. In this study, neurovascular bundle cauterisation did not cause any neurological deficits or major complications.

▶ Transnasal endoscopic sphenopalatine artery ligation (TESPAL) has become a commonly performed and well-established procedure for the management of posterior epistaxis refractory to conservative therapy. The posterior superior nasal branches of the maxillary nerve course with the sphenopalatine artery through the sphenopalatine foramen. Although neurologic deficit from injury to these structures has not been described, this risk of injury is considered a potential complication when performing SPA ligation.[1] In fact, one of the reported advantages of dissection and clipping the artery (as opposed to simply cauterizing it) is that the nerve branches in the vicinity are preserved. This study tests the validity of this concept by performing cauterization of the distal branches of the SPA without purposely dissecting out the neurovascular bundle in 42 patients. The success rate for epistaxis control was 100% with no cases of rebleeding over the 17-month follow-up period. Although there were a few cases of minor issues that may be nerve injury related (nasal dryness in 4 patients and objective hypoaesthesia in 8 patients without any subjective complaints), the authors concluded that cauterization of the SPA neurovascular bundle did not cause any neurologic deficits or major complications. I think this is a reasonable conclusion based on the data presented. However, it should be noted that while the authors did not formally dissect out the SP neurovascular bundle, they did isolate the SPA trunk and made a point of avoiding excessive cauterization in the area. These 2 factors likely minimized injury and protected some of the posterior superior nasal branches of the maxillary nerve and led to the favorable outcomes observed.

R. Sindwani, MD

Reference

1. Bolger WE, Borgie RC, Melder P. The role of the crista ethmoidalis in endoscopic sphenopalatine artery ligation. *Am J Rhinol.* 1999;13:81-86.

Hot water irrigation as treatment for intractable posterior epistaxis in an out-patient setting

Novoa E, Schlegel-Wagner C (Kantonsspital Luzern, Lucerne, Switzerland)
J Laryngol Otol 126:58-60, 2012

The management of intractable posterior epistaxis is challenging for any physician. Nasal packing, often combined with use of an endonasal balloon system, is painful for the patient, and torturous to maintain for two to three days. If conservative treatment fails, the most commonly used treatment options are currently invasive procedures such as endoscopic coagulation of bleeding arteries, external ligation and, rarely, embolisation. This paper describes a simple, non-invasive technique of treating posterior epistaxis with hot water irrigation. Technical information is presented, and the benefits of the method are discussed (Fig 1).

▶ Managing posterior epistaxis is a challenge for the otolaryngologist and a miserable experience (at best) for the patient because the first line of treatment includes posterior packing. Bleeding refractory to posterior packing can be dealt with using embolization or endoscopic ligation of the sphenopalatine

(a)

(b)

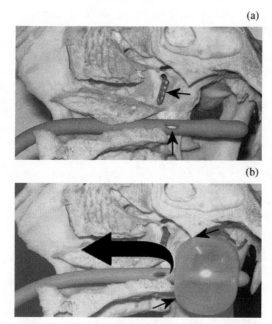

FIGURE 1.—(a) Correct placement of the modified balloon catheter along the inferior meatus, with the orifice of the catheter (arrow) placed underneath the sphenopalatine foramen (second arrow). (b) The large arrow indicates the direction of water flow through the nose during continuous irrigation, while the small arrows show the correct placement of the inflated balloon, anchored within the choana. (Reprinted from Novoa E, Schlegel-Wagner C. Hot water irrigation as treatment for intractable posterior epistaxis in an out-patient setting. *J Laryngol Otol.* 2012;126:58-60, with permission of Cambridge University Press.)

artery. The author describes a simple alternative to all of this: hot water irrigation using a modified balloon catheter system. Stangerup et al[1] have demonstrated that hot water irrigation, using temperatures of up to 50°C, produces vasodilation and edema of the nasal mucosa without the risk for necrosis. The concept behind hot water irrigation to control bleeding is that this mucosal edema leads to local compression of the bleeding vessels, while at the same time triggering and possibly accelerating the clotting cascade. Using a modified irrigation technique (Fig 1), this group reports being able to stop bleeding permanently in up to 82% of cases of intractable posterior epistaxis, with minimal morbidity and discomfort. Further studies of the application of this technique and the experience from patients' perspectives are needed.

R. Sindwani, MD

Reference

1. Stangerup SE, Dommerby H, Lau T. Hot-water irrigation as a treatment of posterior epistaxis. *Rhinology.* 1996;34:18-20.

Endoscopic Transvestibular Paramandibular Exploration of the Infratemporal Fossa and Parapharyngeal Space: A Minimally Invasive Approach to the Middle Cranial Base
Chan JYK, Li RJ, Lim M, et al (Johns Hopkins Med Institutions, Baltimore, MD)
Laryngoscope 121:2075-2080, 2011

Objectives/Hypothesis.—To describe a novel transvestibular endoscopic approach for the exposure, exploration, and resection of lesions in the infratemporal fossa (ITF) and parapharyngeal space (PPS).

Study Design.—Surgical technique and clinical feasibilty of a novel approach to the middle cranial base.

Methods.—The transvestibular endoscopic approach was applied to four patients with lesions involving the ITF and PPS. Through a vertical oral mucosal incision along the ascending ramus of the mandible, an optical corridor to the ITF and PPS was created and maintained with the aid of a Hardy speculum. The contents of the ITF and PPS were explored with the aid of a 0-degree 4-mm rigid endoscope.

Results.—Four patients underwent exploration of their right-sided ITF and PPS. The approach provided exposure and access from the middle cranial base at the level of the foramen ovale to the mid-PPS. Branches of the trigeminal nerve in the ITF were safely explored and preserved. Exposure and visualization of the internal maxillary artery and branches were achieved. Of the four patients, two underwent resection of a primary and a recurrent pleomorphic adenoma, one had chronic pain relief from a large synovial chondromatosis, and one had debulking of a recurrent mucoepidermoid carcinoma. The only complications were self-limiting hypoesthesia of the lip in one patient and transient dysphagia in another patient.

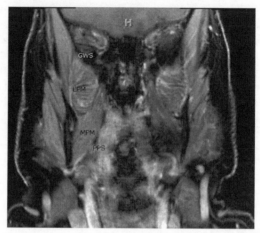

FIGURE 1.—High-resolution coronal T1-weighted magnetic resonance imaging of brain and skull base with gadolinium enhancement demonstrating the infratemporal fossa. The greater wing of the sphenoid (GWS) comprises the skull base in this image. The right lateral pterygoid muscle (LPM) and medial pterygoid muscle (MPM) are shown inserting into the mandible at the condyle and angle, respectively. The parapharyngeal space (PPS) is located medial and inferior to the MPM. The pterygopalatine fossa is located medial to the infratemporal fossa and the two spaces are connected by the pterygomaxillary fissure. (Reprinted from Chan JYK, Li RJ, Lim M, et al. Endoscopic transvestibular paramandibular exploration of the infratemporal fossa and parapharyngeal space: a minimally invasive approach to the middle cranial base. *Laryngoscope*. 2011;121:2075-2080, with permission from The American Laryngological, Rhinological and Otological Society, Inc, and John Wiley and Sons (www.interscience.wiley.com).)

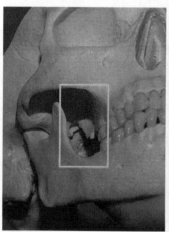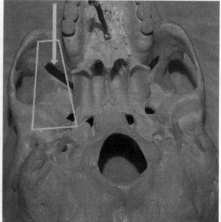

FIGURE 2.—The figure on the left demonstrates the trajectory of the transvestibular approach that is bounded laterally by the ramus of the mandible. In the figure on the right, the infratemporal fossa is identified by the trapezium; seen also are the pterygoid plates medially and the foramen ovale posterior to the arrow. [Color figure can be viewed in the online issue, which is available at wileyonlinelibrary.com.] (Reprinted from Chan JYK, Li RJ, Lim M, et al. Endoscopic transvestibular paramandibular exploration of the infratemporal fossa and parapharyngeal space: a minimally invasive approach to the middle cranial base. *Laryngoscope*. 2011;121:2075-2080, with permission from The American Laryngological, Rhinological and Otological Society, Inc, and John Wiley and Sons (www.interscience.wiley.com).)

Conclusions.—The transvestibular endoscopic approach to the ITF and PPS offers direct and minimally invasive access to select lesions within this region. Further use of this approach will allow us to determine its potential and limitations (Figs 1 and 2).

▶ This article describes a novel approach to the parapharyngeal space (PPS) and infratemporal fossa (ITF) using a "keyhole" technique through the mouth ("transvestibular") in which a hardy speculum and endoscope are used for visualization. The surgical technique and feasibility are described in 4 patients with lesions successfully managed with minimal morbidity. Through a vertical oral mucosal incision along the ascending ramus of the mandible, an optical corridor to the ITF and PPS is created and maintained with a speculum while an endoscope is used for visualization (Figs 1 and 2). For selected lesions, this approach may offer the clear advantage of a shorter, less morbid surgery with quicker recovery compared with traditional lateral and anterior approaches. The endoscopic transvestibular approach described takes advantage of a natural bony window and corridor to the ITF and PPS. The authors espouse the advantages of the light cone offered by the endoscope, which they felt improved visualization and facilitated the technique considerably. They also point out that access to PPS below the level of the mandibular angle is limited with this technique, and for lesions extending below this area, the technique described can be combined with a transcervical approach. This technique is yet another example of surgeons' ongoing efforts to perform minimally invasive surgery through "keyhole" techniques, which are facilitated by the endoscope.

R. Sindwani, MD

A balloon dilatation technique for the treatment of intramaxillary lesions using a Foley catheter in chronic maxillary sinusitis

Park CH, Kim HS, Lee JH, et al (Hallym Univ, Chuncheon, Kangwon, South Korea; et al)

Am J Otolaryngol 32:304-307, 2011

Background.—In chronic maxillary sinusitis, pathologic mucosas of the anterior and lateral walls of the maxillary sinus are difficult to remove. Trocar insertion to the canine fossa is the most commonly used procedure. In the present work, we report a method involving a balloon dilatation technique for treatment of intramaxillary lesions using a Foley catheter in chronic maxillary sinusitis and the outcomes of this approach.

Methods.—Records of 34 patients with intramaxillary sinus lesions who underwent endoscopic sinus surgery were analyzed. After widening the natural ostium, a 10F Foley catheter was inserted through the widening ostium into the maxillary sinus. The intramaxillary lesion was removed by repeated balloon inflation and deflation of the Foley catheter. The patients were followed-up for at least 6 months after the surgery.

Results.—There were no significant intraoperative or postoperative complications. We found that the postoperative symptoms and resolution

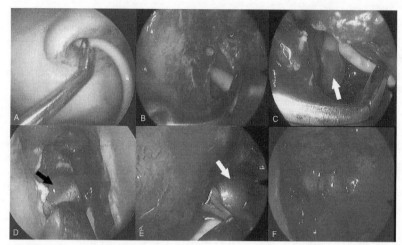

FIGURE 2.—Intraoperative findings. (A) Using upward forceps, Foley catheter was inserted into nasal cavity in the direction toward maxillary sinus. (B) A 10F Foley catheter was inserted through the natural ostium into the maxillary sinus. (C–E) The end of catheter was positioned on edematous mucosas of the anterolateral wall of the maxillary sinus. For balloon inflation, about 10 to 20 cm^3 of normal saline was injected into the Foley catheter. By balloon inflation, the pathologic mucosa was ruptured and the discharge drained away through the natural ostium. (F) After inflating the balloon, most edematous mucosas ruptured and squeezed in the maxillary sinus, finally. White arrow indicates balloon; black arrow, the ruptured pathologic mucosa. (Reprinted from American Journal of Otolaryngology, Park CH, Kim HS, Lee JH, et al. A balloon dilatation technique for the treatment of intramaxillary lesions using a Foley catheter in chronic maxillary sinusitis. *Am J Otolaryngol*. 2011;32:304-307. Copyright 2011 with permission from Elsevier.)

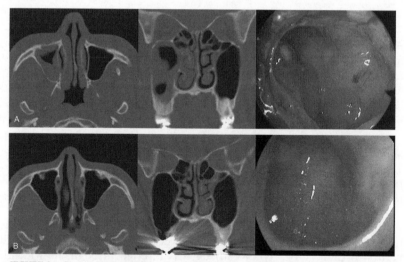

FIGURE 3.—Computer tomographic and endoscopic findings. (A) Preoperative CT shows the mucosal thickness in the right maxillary sinus, and intraoperative endoscopic findings shows the edematous pathologic mucosa in the maxillary sinus. (B) Six months after surgery, the right maxillary sinusitis was resolved completely at postoperative CT. Pathologic mucosa was not seen in the maxillary sinus. (Reprinted from American Journal of Otolaryngology, Park CH, Kim HS, Lee JH, et al. A balloon dilatation technique for the treatment of intramaxillary lesions using a Foley catheter in chronic maxillary sinusitis. *Am J Otolaryngol*. 2011;32:304-307. Copyright 2011 with permission from Elsevier.)

of the lesions in comparison to classic functional endoscopic sinus surgery were not different in authors' experiences.

Conclusion.—The balloon dilatation technique using a Foley catheter is a minimally invasive and effective technique that is not associated with major complications in cases of intramaxillary lesions (Figs 2 and 3).

▶ This article demonstrates creative thinking and shows that rhinology is still looking for the ideal technique of using balloons in the sinuses. The authors describe a creative but "off the wall" technique of treating chronic maxillary sinusitis. A regular 10-F Foley catheter is used to "squish" and rupture intrasinus lesions (ie, sinus retention cysts) and edematous mucosa by repeated inflation and deflation of the catheter (with strategic repositioning) in 34 chronic rhinosinusitis patients (Figs 1 and 2). Although there were no controls, the authors felt the results obtained were comparable with traditional surgical techniques, and no complications were encountered. The authors espoused advantages of this easy-to-perform technique, including the cheap cost of the Foley, the fact that it spares mucosa, and its less invasive nature (compared with a canine fossa approach).

Although I do not think this technique will catch on (sinus retention cysts can readily be removed with angled instruments, and some may not even need to be removed), I do applaud the authors for their creativity and cost-conscious approach to instrument selection.

R. Sindwani, MD

Antegrade transsphenoidal vidian neurectomy: Short-term surgical outcome analysis
Su W-F, Liu S-C, Chiu F-S, et al (Tri-Service General Hosp, Taipei, Taiwan; et al)
Am J Rhinol Allergy 25:e217-e220, 2011

Background.—Vidian neurectomy was an option for treating allergic rhinitis in the past but outcomes varied. A modified transsphenoidal approach is proposed to simplify endoscopic vidian neurectomy. The postoperative evaluation of rhinorrhea, sneezing, and recurrence was investigated.

Methods.—A total of 317 patients with refractory allergic rhinitis underwent 414 transsphenoidal vidian neurectomies from September 2006 to December 2010. A rigid nasal endoscope was used through a transsphenoidal approach to reach the vidian canal inside the sphenoid sinus (type I) or through its anterior opening into the pterygopalatine fossa (type II) and to cut or cauterize the vidian nerve. The surgical outcomes were analyzed for patients with at least 6 months of follow-up.

Results.—Our approach was successful in 90.3% of the 414 vidian neurectomies. Vidian neurectomy was successful via the type I approach in 27 sides and type II approach in 347 sides. The short-term surgical outcomes of 163 patients who underwent a total of 236 vidian neurectomies with at least 6 months of follow-up were analyzed. Immediate, complete cessation of sneezing and rhinorrhea occurred uniformly. Three recurrences were detected during the 1—2 years of follow-up. The symptom of dry eye was reported for 172 surgical sides, but only 6 had persistent symptoms for >6 months.

Conclusion.—The transsphenoidal approach in a vidian neurectomy is a simple method that removes the need for sphenopalatine artery ligation and causes less surgical morbidity. However, the possibility of recurrence of this condition in the long term needs further investigation.

▶ This is a very eye-catching article for several reasons: its large numbers, its innovative and noteworthy technique, and the indications for which it was performed. The study describes an approach to vidian neurectomy by accessing the nerve within the sphenoid sinus rather than accessing it in the pterygopalatine fossa as typically done. The authors describe 2 anatomic scenarios. The type I transsphenoidal approach (intrasphenoidal, Fig 1 in the original article) is used if the prominence over the vidian canal in the floor of the sphenoid sinus can be unroofed directly in the sinus cavity. The type II transsphenoidal (Fig 2 in the original article) approach is used if the prominence over the vidian canal is not obvious in the sphenoid floor and is situated more laterally, in which case the vidian nerve is approached by taking down more of the sphenoid face and skin perfusion pressure. The authors describe their large experience with these techniques in 317 patients (414 procedures) with refractory allergic rhinitis. Yes—refractory allergic rhinitis, where *refractory* was defined as poor response to nasal steroid spray after a 3-month trial (WOW). The patients seemed to do well with improvement in allergic symptoms and minimal morbidity, at least for the short 6-month follow-up period. The authors concluded that the transsphenoidal approach is a simple method for performing a vidian neurectomy because it removes the need for sphenopalatine artery ligation, is more straightforward, and has less attendant morbidity. This does appear true—especially for the type I procedure, which was encountered in only 27 (of only the anatomic scenario in 27 [vs 347]) sides. Clearly, the success and applicability of this technique is entirely based on anatomy, and the authors point out that the type I technique is much easier and simpler and takes less operating room time. The techniques described are innovative and worth noting. However, it should be underscored that vidian neurectomy is generally used for refractory vasomotor rhinitis (VMR), and not allergic rhinitis (AR). Even in VMR, the use of the procedure has been dramatically reduced with the advent of anticholinergic sprays that have been shown to be highly effective for this condition. The indications used for this procedure in this study, AR refractory to 3 months of a nasal steroid spray, are very stringent (to say the least). The application of this procedure (however performed) for the indication described in this article is extremely controversial and not currently advocated.

R. Sindwani, MD

Coblation-assisted endonasal endoscopic resection of juvenile nasopharyngeal angiofibroma

Ye L, Zhou X, Li J, et al (Zhongnan Hosp of Wuhan Univ, Hubei, People's Republic of China)
J Laryngol Otol 125:940-944, 2011

Objective.—Juvenile nasopharyngeal angiofibroma may be successfully resected using endoscopic techniques. However, the use of coblation technology for such resection has not been described. This study aimed to document cases of Fisch class I juvenile nasopharyngeal angiofibroma with limited nasopharyngeal and nasal cavity extension, which were completely resected using an endoscopic coblation technique.

Methods.—We retrospectively studied 23 patients with juvenile nasopharyngeal angiofibroma who underwent resection with either traditional endoscopic instruments ($n = 12$) or coblation ($n = 11$). Intra-operative blood loss and overall operative time were recorded.

Results.—The mean tumour resection time for coblation and traditional endoscopic instruments was 87 and 136 minutes, respectively ($t = 9.962$, $p < 0.001$). Mean intra-operative blood loss was 121 and 420 ml, respectively ($t = 28.944$, $p < 0.001$), a significant difference. Both techniques achieved complete tumour resection with minimal damage to adjacent tissues, and no recurrence in any patient.

Conclusion.—Coblation successfully achieves transnasal endoscopic resection of juvenile nasopharyngeal angiofibroma (Fisch class I), with good surgical margins and minimal blood loss (Figs 2 and 5).

▶ Juvenile nasopharyngeal angiofibroma (JNA) is an uncommon, highly vascular, nonencapsulated tumor that typically occurs in adolescent boys and is associated with significant bleeding during surgical resection. The goal of surgery is complete resection of the tumor, which is usually attempted after selective embolization. This study describes the use of coblation for 11 cases of JNA resection and compares outcomes with those of conventional techniques (12 cases). The authors report that the mean resection time for coblation was significantly shorter than with traditional instrumentation (87 vs 136 minutes, respectively), and there was also significantly less associated blood loss (121 vs 420 mL). There were no complications in either group. Although the tumors included in this study were admittedly small (all Fisch stage 1, Fig 2), the improved outcomes of less bleeding and reduced operating room time achieved with coblation were nonetheless impressive. Coblation involves passing a bipolar, radiofrequency electric current through a medium of normal saline, resulting in the production of a plasma field of highly ionized particles (Fig 5). These ions are able to break down intercellular bonds, resulting in tissue melting at a temperature of approximately 70°C, which results in much less energy transmission than would occur with the use of conventional electrocautery.[1,2] I consider the coblator an excellent tool for resection of any vascularized soft tissue from the sinonasal cavity. The fact that the energy can be delivered in a bipolar fashion also provides a margin of safety to sensitive intracranial and orbital structures in proximity. Another

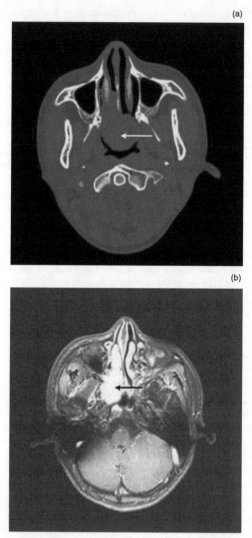

FIGURE 2.—Pre-operative axial (a) computed tomography and (b) magnetic resonance imaging scans showed a soft tissue mass (arrow) in the nasopharynx and nasal cavity. (Reprinted from Ye L, Zhou X, Li J, et al. Coblation-assisted endonasal endoscopic resection of juvenile nasopharyngeal angiofibroma. *J Laryngol Otol.* 2011;125:940-944, with permission of Cambridge University Press.)

significant advantage of this technology not highlighted in the article, is that the coblation wand is malleable and thus permits the surgeon to more easily address any awkward geometry encountered during surgery. I suspect the application of this technology in rhinologic surgery (especially tumor surgery of the skull base) will proliferate in the future.

R. Sindwani, MD

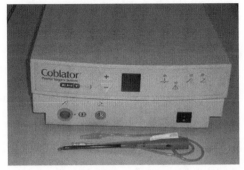

FIGURE 5.—The coblation system. A hook is used to resect the tumour. (Reprinted from Ye L, Zhou X, Li J, et al. Coblation-assisted endonasal endoscopic resection of juvenile nasopharyngeal angiofibroma. *J Laryngol Otol.* 2011;125:940-944, with permission of Cambridge University Press.)

References

1. Noordzij JP, Affleck BD. Coblation versus unipolar electrocautery tonsillectomy: a prospective, randomized, single-blind study in adult patients. *Laryngoscope.* 2006;116:1303-1309.
2. Parsons SP, Cordes SR, Comer B. Comparison of posttonsillectomy pain using the ultrasonic scalpel, coblator, and electrocautery. *Otolaryngol Head Neck Surg.* 2006;134:106-113.

7 Thyroid and Parathyroid

Basic and Clinical Research

Central Lymph Node Metastasis of Unilateral Papillary Thyroid Carcinoma: Patterns and Factors Predictive of Nodal Metastasis, Morbidity, and Recurrence
Roh J-L, Kim J-M, Park CI (Univ of Ulsan College of Medicine, Seoul, Republic of Korea; Chungnam Natl Univ College of Medicine, Daejeon, Republic of Korea)
Ann Surg Oncol 18:2245-2250, 2011

Background.—Although subclinical cervical lymph node (LN) metastases in papillary thyroid carcinoma (PTC) are common, the efficacy of prophylactic central LN dissection (CLND) is unclear. Few prospective studies have assessed the relationships between complete pathologic information regarding tumors and metastatic nodes in the central compartment. We therefore investigated the pattern and predictive indicators of central LN metastasis, morbidity, and recurrence in patients who underwent total thyroidectomy and prophylactic CLND for unilateral PTC and clinically node-negative neck (cN0) disease.

Methods.—This prospective study involved 184 patients with previously untreated unilateral PTC and cN0 who underwent total thyroidectomy and bilateral CLND. Nodal samples were divided into the prelaryngeal/pretracheal and ipsilateral and contralateral paratracheal regions, with each assessed for clinicopathologic predictors of central metastases. Postoperative morbidity and recurrence were assessed.

Results.—Rates of metastasis to ipsilateral and contralateral central compartments were 42.9 and 9.8%, respectively. Multivariate analysis showed that tumor size >1 cm and extrathyroidal extension were independent predictors of ipsilateral metastasis, and ipsilateral metastases independently predicted contralateral metastases ($P < 0.05$ each). Permanent hypoparathyroidism and incidental recurrent nerve paralysis were found in 1.6 and 0% of patients, respectively. After a mean follow-up of 46 months, none of these patients had recurrence in the central compartment.

Conclusions.—Subclinical metastases are highly prevalent in the ipsilateral central neck of patients with PTC >1 cm. Contralateral central metastases, although uncommon, are associated with ipsilateral central metastases. These findings may guide the necessity and extent of prophylactic bilateral or unilateral CLND.

▶ It is generally accepted that in papillary thyroid carcinoma, cervical lymph node metastases do not affect overall survival. However, presence of cervical lymph node metastases is associated with increased incidence of locoregional recurrence, justifying intraoperative removal of clinically or radiographically positive cervical lymph nodes in both lateral and central compartments. On the other hand, the issue of prophylactic cervical lymphadenectomy in clinically and radiographically negative cases remains subject to significant controversy. This holds particularly true for the prophylactic central compartment lymphadenectomy, which is associated with increased risk for recurrent laryngeal nerve injury and permanent hypoparathyroidism. The high incidence of central compartment micrometastases in clinically negative cases (50%-60%) is often used by proponents of prophylactic neck dissection to justify their approach, whereas detractors cite increased incidence of complications without proven benefit of survival or even change in the course of the disease to justify their objection. To make things even more confusing, the American Thyroid Association recently came out with a recommendation to consider lymph node dissection (basically leaving the decision to the individual surgeon) in all patients undergoing thyroidectomy for papillary thyroid carcinoma, regardless of whether the nodes are enlarged. Not unexpectedly, the results of this selected study showed that tumor diameter of greater than 1 cm as well as presence of extrathyroidal tumor extension served as independent predictors for occult central compartment cervical lymph node metastases. Naturally, they cautiously recommend prophylactic central compartment neck dissection in these patients.

At this point, I would like to emphasize that many highly respected thyroid surgeons, based on their experience, their data, and their overall philosophy, recommend observation for clinically and radiographically negative central compartment and surgery only for clinically or radiographically positive nodes. In my practice, in addition to the foregoing outlined philosophy, I use risk stratification to guide my surgical approach: prophylactic central compartment lymphadenectomy in high-risk patients and no lymphadenectomy in patients with low-risk scores.

M. Gapany, MD

An Analysis of Factors Predicting Lateral Cervical Nodal Metastases in Papillary Carcinoma of the Thyroid
Hunt JP, Buchmann LO, Wang L, et al (Univ of Utah Health Sciences Ctr, Salt Lake City)
Arch Otolaryngol Head Neck Surg 137:1141-1145, 2011

Objective.—To analyze the possible correlation between the location of the primary tumor within the thyroid gland and the patterns of central vs lateral compartment lymph node metastasis.

Design.—Retrospective analysis of papillary thyroid carcinoma (PTC) treated in an academic university setting from July 1, 2004, through August 31, 2010.

Setting.—Head and neck oncology clinic.

Patients.—Those receiving surgical therapy for PTC at the University of Utah.

Main Outcome Measures.—Tumor characteristics of patients with central vs lateral nodal metastatic disease in PTC.

Results.—Two hundred one patients with PTC met inclusion criteria. There were 136 females (67.7%), and the mean age was 44.8 years. Histologic subtypes included 68 follicular variants of PTC, 111 conventional variants of PTC, and 22 patients with both follicular and conventional PTC variants. Metastatic nodal disease was confirmed histologically in 81 patients (40.3%): 42 with central nodal disease only (20.9%), 10 with lateral disease only (5.0%), and 29 with both central and lateral nodal disease (14.4%). Positive lateral compartment nodal metastasis correlated with distant metastases ($P < .01$), extrathyroid extension ($P < .05$), histologic subtype (conventional PTC greater than follicular variant PTC) ($P < .05$), and tumor location within the thyroid lobe ($P < .01$). Tumors involving the superior aspect of the thyroid lobe were more likely to be associated with metastasis to the lateral cervical lymph nodes ($P < .01$), and 76.9% of patients with lateral cervical lymph node disease had involvement of the superior aspect of the lobe. Thyroid microcarcinomas were not associated with lateral cervical compartments in this study.

Conclusions.—The intrathyroidal location of PTC predicts the pattern of nodal spread. Therefore, patients with PTC involving the superior aspect of the lobe should undergo specific imaging evaluation of the lateral neck compartments to determine the need for lateral compartment neck dissection (Tables 2 and 3).

▶ It is commonly agreed that presence of cervical lymph node metastases in well-differentiated thyroid cancer is associated with significant risk for regional

TABLE 2.—Risk Factors for Lateral Compartment Lymphatic Spread[a]

| Variable | Lateral Compartment Lymph Nodes | | P Value |
	Absent (n = 162)	Present (n = 39)	
Age, mean, y	46	37	.03
Male sex	45 (28)	17 (44)	.06
Histologic feature			.02
Conventional variant papillary thyroid carcinoma	83 (51)	28 (72)	
Follicular variant papillary thyroid carcinoma	62 (38)	6 (15)	
Both variants	17 (10)	5 (13)	
Multifocal tumor	79 (49)	23 (59)	.25
Tumor size, cm	1.5	1.5	.20
Extrathyroid extension	30 (19)	14 (36)	.02
Distant metastasis	1 (1)	4 (10)	<.01
Tumor location, superior pole	61 (38)	30 (77)	<.01

[a]Data are given as number (percentage) unless otherwise indicated.

TABLE 3.—Risk Factors for Central Compartment Lymphatic Spread[a]

Variable	Central Compartment Lymph Nodes		P Value
	Absent (n = 126)	Present (n = 75)	
Age, mean, y	46	37	<.01
Male sex	34 (27)	28 (37)	.12
Histologic feature			<.01
Conventional variant papillary thyroid carcinoma	51 (40)	60 (80)	
Follicular variant papillary thyroid carcinoma	60 (48)	8 (11)	
Both variants	15 (12)	7 (9)	
Multifocal tumor	65 (52)	37 (49)	.76
Tumor size, cm	1.2	2.0	<.01
Extrathyroid extension	17 (13)	27 (36)	<.01
Distant metastasis	0	5 (7)	.02
Tumor location, inferior pole	67 (53)	56 (75)	<.01

[a]Data are given as number (percentage) unless otherwise indicated.

and local recurrence. This is an interesting study that attempts to identify preoperative risks for cervical lymph node involvement in well-differentiated thyroid carcinoma. The findings are summarized in Tables 2 and 3 of the article. The authors have made an interesting observation, linking the location of the tumor in the superior aspect of the thyroid lobe with increased risk of lateral compartment lymph node metastases. In their study, patients who presented with the tumor in the superior aspect of the thyroid lobe were 4.5 times more likely to have lateral compartment cervical lymph node metastases. As expected, other prognostic factors, such as presence of extra-thyroidal tumor extension as well as tumor size were associated with lateral or central compartment lymph node metastases. This study underscores the importance of preoperative ultrasound localization of the primary tumor in the thyroid gland. A thorough search for presence of lateral cervical lymph node metastases should be undertaken in patients with superior thyroid pole tumors.

M. Gapany, MD

Clinical and Molecular Features of Papillary Thyroid Cancer in Adolescents and Young Adults
Vriens MR, Moses W, Weng J, et al (Univ of California at San Francisco; et al)
Cancer 117:259-267, 2011

Background.—Age disparities in thyroid cancer incidence and outcome among adolescents and young adults (AYAs) with thyroid cancer are under reported. In this study, the authors compared the molecular and clinical features of papillary thyroid cancer (PTC) in AYAs with the same features among patients in other age groups.

Methods.—One thousand eleven patients underwent initial treatment for PTC at the University of California at San Francisco. Patients were subdivided into 2 age groups: ages 15 to 39 years (the AYA group) and aged ≥40 years. Demographic, clinical, and survival data in the cohort also were compared with data from the National Cancer Instsitute's Surveillance, Epidemiology, and End Results (SEER) Program. In a subset of the study cohort, the primary tumors were analyzed by genome-wide expression analyses, genotyping for common somatic mutations, and pathway-specific gene expression arrays between the age groups.

Results.—The percentage of women and the lymph node metastasis rate were significantly higher in the AYA group. In the AYA group, the rate of distant metastasis was lower. Disease-free survival and median overall survival were significantly higher in the AYA group. The better survival in AYA patients also was apparent in the national SEER data. An unsupervised cluster analysis of gene expression data revealed no distinct clustering by age in 96 PTC samples. The frequency and type of somatic mutations in the primary tumors did not differ significantly between age groups (the AYA group vs the group aged ≥40 years). Six genes (extracellular matrix protein 1 [*ECM1*], v-erb-2 erythroblastic leukemia viral oncogene homolog 2 [*ERBB2*], urinary plasminogen activator [*UPA*], 6-phosphofructo-2-kinase/fructose-2,6-biphosphatase 2 [*PFKFB2*], meis homeobox 2 [*MEIS2*], and carbonic anhydrase II [*CA2*]) had significant differential expression between age groups.

Conclusions.—The extent of disease at presentation and the survival of patients with PTC differed between AYAs and older patients. The current results indicated that these differences may be caused by several candidate genes and that these genes are expressed differentially and may play an important role in tumor cell biology. However, no distinct gene expression profiles exist for patients with PTC that distinguish between AYAs and patients aged ≥40 years.

▶ The role of age at presentation is a well-established prognostic factor in well-differentiated thyroid cancer. There is a clear disparity in the course of the disease as well as overall outcomes between adolescents and young adults compared with patients who are aged 40 years or older at presentation. The reason behind this age-related disparity in biological tumor behavior has never been elucidated and has recently become a focus of research targeting the oncogenetics of this cancer. This selected study is important because it has for the first time identified several candidate genes that are expressed differently in papillary thyroid cancers in individuals aged more than 40 years compared with adolescents and young adults. These genes may play an important role in determining the biological behavior of papillary thyroid carcinoma. Through such genomic research, new avenues may open for screening, diagnosis, and treatment of well-differentiated thyroid cancer. I recommend this article to otolaryngologists with an interest in thyroid cancer.

M. Gapany, MD

Diagnostics

Clinical Implications of Bilateral Lateral Cervical Lymph Node Metastasis in Papillary Thyroid Cancer: A Risk Factor for Lung Metastasis

Lee YS, Lim YS, Lee J-C, et al (Pusan Natl Univ School of Medicine and Med Res Inst, Republic of Korea)
Ann Surg Oncol 18:3486-3492, 2011

Background.—Distant metastasis to the lung in papillary thyroid cancer (PTC) is rarely detected, but it is known to be an important prognostic factor associated with survival. We investigated risk factors for lung metastasis in PTC.

Materials and Methods.—We performed a retrospective review of patients with PTC ($n = 977$) who were treated from January 2006 to August 2009. Enrolled patients received radioablation therapy followed by a radioiodine whole body scan. Lung metastasis was screened out with whole body scan or positron emission tomography/computed tomography (PET/CT) and confirmed with chest CT. Age, gender, extrathyroidal extension, central lymph node metastasis, lateral lymph node metastasis, and bilateral lateral cervical lymph node metastasis (BLNM) were investigated to analyze the relationship with lung metastasis.

Results.—In total, 949 patients were enrolled. The median age was 49 years (± 13 years) with 829 women. Lung metastasis was found in 20 patients (2.1%). Patients were divided into three groups by tumor size (≤ 1 cm, $1-2$ cm, >2 cm); the groups comprised 47.3%, 28.5%, and 24.1% of the patients, respectively. BLNM was identified in 4.4% ($n = 43$). In a univariate analysis, male gender, old age, large tumor, extrathyroidal extension, lymph node metastasis, lateral lymph node metastasis, and BLNM were significantly related to lung metastasis ($P < 0.05$). In a multivariate analysis, BLNM appeared to be the only significant risk factor for lung metastasis ($P = 0.026$; odds ratio $= 10.219$).

Conclusions.—BLNM may be a risk factor for lung metastasis. This indicates that careful examinations, including chest CT and positron emission tomography (PET), are recommended during the follow-up period when BLNM is suspected.

▶ This selected large retrospective study evaluated the risk factors associated with distant metastases in papillary thyroid cancer. While distant metastases are rare in well-differentiated cancer, they are associated with poor prognosis. Because of their rare occurrence, it is not customary to routinely work up newly diagnosed papillary cancers for potential distant metastases. Typically, they are discovered later in the course of the disease. The results of this study are very interesting; in a multivariate analysis, the authors found a statistically significant correlation between distant metastases and bilateral cervical lymph node metastases. While other studies are definitely needed to confirm this finding, there can be some immediate implications on how clinicians use positron emission tomography/computed tomography (PET/CT) for workup of well-differentiated thyroid cancer.

PET/CT is not routinely performed in patients with well-differentiated thyroid carcinoma. It is usually recommended in cases in which elevated or increasing thyroglobulin levels are detected despite negative radioiodine uptake. It can also be useful to better define positive radioiodine uptake in distant sites, such as lungs and bones. Based on the results of this study, it is probably reasonable to obtain PET/CT in patients who present with bilateral cervical lymph node metastases as part of their initial workup of well-differentiated thyroid cancer or shortly after the thyroidectomy and cervical lymphadenectomy at the time of the diagnostic administration of radioiodine.

M. Gapany, MD

Role of core needle biopsy and ultrasonographic finding in management of indeterminate thyroid nodules

Park KT, Ahn S-H, Mo J-H, et al (Bundang Hosp, Seoul, Korea)
Head Neck 33:160-165, 2011

Background.—Thyroid fine-needle aspiration (FNA) is used as a screening test of choice for evaluation of thyroid nodules. However, approximately 15% to 25% of the cases are classified as indeterminate, posing dilemmas in decision-making. This study was designed to compare the diagnostic performances of second FNA and core needle biopsy of indeterminate nodules by initial FNA.

Methods.—From February 2005 through June 2009, 258 patients who completed scheduled follow-ups were enrolled and the follow-up results were analyzed.

Results.—Nondiagnostic results were obtained in 41.8% of the second FNA group and in 1.7% of the core needle biopsy group ($p < .001$; chi-square). The nodules that show borderline features in preoperative ultrasonography had a malignancy rate of 18.3% and could be identified successfully with core needle biopsy.

Conclusion.—Core needle biopsy is a better method for evaluating indeterminate nodules by initial FNA than second FNA, especially in patients with ultrasonographic findings of a borderline nodule.

▶ I selected this article because it reminds us that core needle biopsy can still have a role in diagnostic workup of thyroid nodules. Frankly, I was not even aware that core needle biopsy was still used for this purpose. As far as I was concerned, fine-needle aspiration (FNA) had shown a very high degree of agreement with core needle biopsy in previous studies, and therefore had completely replaced it in clinical practice. The authors of this study show, however, that in cases where initial FNA was indeterminate, core needle biopsy (under ultrasound guidance for small nodules) was significantly more informative than repeated FNA, and could be a good complementary tool for assessing indeterminate nodules before surgical excision was recommended. The problem with core needle biopsy is that it is much more invasive than FNA and is associated with higher incidence of complications. Furthermore, very few clinicians still have the experience and the skill to successfully incorporate this diagnostic modality into their practice.

M. Gapany, MD

Outcomes

Does Mediastinal Extension of the Goiter Increase Morbidity of Total Thyroidectomy? A Multicenter Study of 19,662 Patients

Testini M, Gurrado A, Avenia N, et al (Univ Med School of Bari, Italy; Univ Med School of Perugia, Italy; et al)
Ann Surg Oncol 18:2251-2259, 2011

Purpose.—To compare the outcome in patients with cervical goiters and cervicomediastinal goiters (CMGs) undergoing total thyroidectomy using the cervical or extracervical approach.

Methods.—This was a retrospective study conducted at six academic departments of general surgery and one endocrine-surgical unit in Italy. The study population consisted of 19,662 patients undergoing total thyroidectomy between 1999 and 2008, of whom 18,607 had cervical goiter (group A) and 1055 had CMG treated using a cervical approach (group B, $n = 986$) or manubriotomy (group C, $n = 69$). The main parameters of interest were symptoms, gender, age, operative time, duration of drain, length of hospital stay, malignancy and outcome.

Results.—A split-sternal approach was required in 6.5% of cases of CMG. Malignancy was significantly more frequent in group B (22.4%) and group C (36.2%) versus group A (10.4%; both $P < .001$), and in group C versus group B ($P = .009$). Overall morbidity was significantly higher in groups B + C (35%), B (34.4%) and C (53.5%) versus group A (23.7%; $P < .001$). Statistically significant increases for group B + C versus group A were observed for transient hypocalcemia, permanent hypocalcemia, transient recurrent laryngeal nerve (RLN) palsies, permanent RLN palsies, phrenic nerve palsy, seroma/hematoma, and complications classified as other. With the exception of transient bilateral RLN palsy, all of these significant differences between group B + C versus group A were also observed for group B versus group A.

Conclusions.—Symptoms, malignancy, overall morbidity, hypoparathyroidism, RLN palsy and hematoma are increased in cases of substernal goiter.

▶ Multiple reports in the literature have shown the feasibility and relative safety of the transcervical approach to resecting substernal goiters. Despite their large size and at times significant involvement of mediastinal structures, these goiters in the vast majority of cases can be removed without sternotomy or thoracotomy. However, the increased incidence of postoperative complications and increased morbidity of substernal thyroidectomy is known to be associated with thyroidectomy for substernal goiter and has been previosly reported in the literature. This selected large multicenter study confirms these former reports. It is known that substernal goiters can remain asymptomatic despite their large size and seemingly significant compression of the trachea, esophagus, and other mediastinal structures. It is therefore important for surgeons who perform this operation to be aware of the data presented in this article and use them when weighing the risk-to-benefit ratio of substernal thyroidectomy and when counseling patients who are candidates for this operation.

M. Gapany, MD

Disease-Related Death in Patients Who Were Considered Free of Macroscopic Disease After Initial Treatment of Well-Differentiated Thyroid Carcinoma
Nixon IJ, Ganly I, Palmer FL, et al (Memorial Sloan Kettering Cancer Ctr, NY)
Thyroid 21:501-504, 2011

Background.—Death from well-differentiated thyroid cancer (WDTC) is rare, and over the past century there has been a trend away from local recurrence as the primary cause of death. The objective of our study was to report the cause of death from thyroid cancer in patients with WDTC treated with curative intent with surgery ± adjuvant radioactive iodine.

Methods.—An institutional database of 1811 patients with WDTC treated surgically for WDTC between 1986 and 2005 was analyzed and identified 165 (9.4%) who had died. Case records were studied to determine the cause of death in each patient.

Results.—Of the 165 deaths, 17 (10%) patients were confirmed to have died of thyroid cancer and 6 (4%) died of an unknown cause but had thyroid cancer present at the time of last follow-up. The remaining 142 (86%) died from other causes and were considered free of thyroid cancer at their last follow-up. We therefore identified only 23 cause-specific deaths from the entire cohort (1.3%). Of the 17 patients known to have died of thyroid cancer, all had distant recurrence. Ninety-four percent had pulmonary metastases. Of these, 47% also had bony metastasis at the time of death. Two patients had recurrent disease in the neck at the time of death, but both also had distant disease. Of the six patients (4%) who died of unknown causes but had thyroid cancer at last follow-up, four (67%) had distant disease alone, one (17%) had local and regional recurrence, and one had local and distant recurrence at last follow-up.

Conclusion.—After successful resection of WDTC, we report a low disease-specific death rate (1.3%). In contrast to earlier reports, death caused by central compartment disease in this recent series is very rare, with metastatic disease accounting for almost all fatalities.

▶ This is an important study from a highly reputable institution providing us with much-needed data on disease-related mortality from well-differentiated thyroid cancer. It is important to note that only patients with complete macroscopic eradication of the disease were included in this study. Several important facts emerge from this study. First, there is a remarkably low incidence of disease-related death of only 1.3%. Second, there is an extremely low rate of neck recurrence as a cause of disease-related death. Third, only 17% of patients at the time of death had disease in the central neck compartment. Fourth, in the majority of patients distant metastases and not local-regional recurrence were considered the cause of death. Lastly, all patients who died of well-differentiated thyroid cancer were either in the intermediate- or high-risk groups. These data lend support to the following emerging concepts. First, there is no reason to overtreat patients who fall into the favorable prognostic category, because they do not die of thyroid cancer. Second, there is no reason to overoperate on the central compartment, because it rarely contributes to death from thyroid cancer. Lastly, aggressive therapy of metastatic pulmonary disease with newly emerging chemotherapy agents, such as tyrosine kinase inhibitors, might positively affect already low mortality from well-differentiated thyroid cancer.

M. Gapany, MD

Central Compartment Reoperation for Recurrent/Persistent Differentiated Thyroid Cancer: Patterns of Recurrence, Morbidity, and Prediction of Postoperative Hypocalcemia

Roh J-L, Kim J-M, Park CI (Univ of Ulsan College of Medicine, Seoul, Republic of Korea; Chungnam Natl Univ College of Medicine, Daejeon, Republic of Korea)
Ann Surg Oncol 18:1312-1318, 2011

Background.—Incidence rates of hypoparathyroidism and vocal cord paralysis are high following central compartment reoperation, but few prospective studies have assessed morbidities and factors predictive of hypocalcemia after reoperation. We investigated recurrence patterns, morbidity, and factors predictive of postoperative hypocalcemia in patients undergoing central compartment reoperation for recurrent/persistent differentiated thyroid cancer (DTC).

Methods.—We prospectively evaluated 45 consecutive patients with recurrent/persistent DTC. Thyroid remnants or recurrent cancers were removed in 16 patients, the unilateral or bilateral central compartment was cleared in all patients, and the lateral compartment on the diseased side was comprehensively removed from 24 patients. Recurrence patterns were assessed histopathologically, morbidities were monitored, and serum concentrations of calcium and intact parathyroid hormone (iPTH) were measured in all patients.

Results.—Eleven patients (24.4%) had tumor invasion into the recurrent laryngeal nerve and/or the tracheoesophagus. Central nodal involvement occurred frequently (86.7%), and the ipsilateral jugular nodes of the lateral compartment were frequently involved. Temporary and permanent vocal cord paralysis developed in 10 (22.2%) and 8 (17.8%) patients, respectively, due primarily to intentional nerve resection following tumor invasion. Of 41 patients without preoperative hypoparathyroidism, 21 (46.3%) had temporary and 2 (4.9%) had permanent hypocalcemia.

Multivariate analysis showed that bilateral central compartment dissection and low iPTH levels (<12.0 pg/ml) were independent predictors of postoperative hypocalcemia.

Conclusions.—Most patients with recurrent/persistent DTC harbor lesions in the central compartment. Central compartment reoperation may lead to high rates of morbidity, including hypoparathyroidism, which can be predicted by surgical extent and low serum iPTH levels.

▶ Reoperation in the thyroid bed or the central compartment of the neck presents a serious challenge even for the most experienced thyroid surgeon. This selected article focuses on the morbidity associated with reoperation for recurrent/ persistent well-differentiated thyroid cancer in the central neck. There is some controversy whether reoperation in the central neck compartment is in fact associated with higher incidence of hypoparathyroidism and recurrent laryngeal nerve injury. The authors, who claim that reoperation is safe, usually tend not to routinely perform central neck dissections in the absence of radiographic or clinical evidence of central compartment lymphadenopathy. On the other hand, investigators who find increased incidence of complications at reoperation urge to perform routine central compartment lymphadenectomy to avoid reoperation. The authors prospectively enrolled 45 patients with central compartment recurrence into their study. They reported meticulous surgical technique (although intraoperative laryngeal nerve monitoring was not performed and intraoperative parathyroid hormone levels were not measured) and an effort to avoid morbidity. Nevertheless, the incidence of permanent recurrent laryngeal nerve paralysis was 17.8%, and the incidence of permanent hypocalcemia was 4.9%.

This article makes a good case for avoiding reoperation of the central neck compartment.

M. Gapany, MD

Initial therapy with either thyroid lobectomy or total thyroidectomy without radioactive iodine remnant ablation is associated with very low rates of structural disease recurrence in properly selected patients with differentiated thyroid cancer

Vaisman F, Shaha A, Fish S, et al (Memorial Sloan-Kettering Cancer Ctr, NY)
Clin Endocrinol 75:112-119, 2011

Objective.—To describe the risk of structural disease recurrence in a cohort of patients with differentiated thyroid cancer selected for treatment with either thyroid lobectomy or total thyroidectomy without radioactive iodine remnant ablation (RRA).

Design.—Retrospective review.

Patients.—A total of 289 patients were selected for either thyroid lobectomy (*n* = 72) or total thyroidectomy (*n* = 217) without RRA and followed with modern disease detection tools in a tertiary referral centre. Most patients had papillary thyroid cancer (89%) without clinically evident lymph node metastases (91%). However, 55% (156/289) of patients had primary tumours that were >1 cm and 10% (28/289) had minor extrathyroidal extension.

Measurements.—The primary endpoint was detection of recurrent/persistent structural disease.

Results.—After a 5-year median follow-up, structural disease recurrence was detected in 2·3% (5/217) of patients treated with total thyroidectomy without RRA, and in 4·2% (3/72) of patients treated with thyroid lobectomy. Size of the primary tumour, the presence of cervical lymph node metastases and American Thyroid Association risk category were all statistically significant predictors of recurrence. Changes in serum thyroglobulin were not helpful in identifying the presence of persistent/recurrent structural disease. Importantly, 88% (7/8) of the patients that had recurrent disease were rendered clinically disease free with additional therapies.

Conclusions.—Initial risk stratification is able to identify a cohort of patients with differentiated thyroid cancer with a very low risk of structural disease recurrence following treatment with either thyroid lobectomy or total thyroidectomy without RRA. Our data strongly support a selective approach to the initial management of thyroid cancer.

▶ I have selected this retrospective study because of its very important message, the importance of risk stratification when selecting patients for less aggressive therapy. It is my opinion that patients with differentiated thyroid cancer who fall into the favorable prognostic category are often overtreated. Very solid epidemiologic studies show that patients with complete microscopic eradication of the disease have a remarkably low incidence (1.3%) of disease-related death. Furthermore, all patients who died of thyroid cancer were in either intermediate or high-risk groups. Lastly, in most patients who died of thyroid cancer, the cause of death was distant metastases and not local-regional recurrence. Hence, there is no reason to be overly aggressive in treating patients who fall into the good prognostic category because they do not die of well-differentiated cancer. In those patients, complete microscopic eradication of the disease through appropriate thyroidectomy (partial or total) without prophylactic central or lateral compartment neck dissection and without radioactive iodine therapy is adequate to secure good long-term outcome.

M. Gapany, MD

Efficacy of Ultrasound-Guided Percutaneous Ethanol Injection Treatment in Patients with a Limited Number of Metastatic Cervical Lymph Nodes from Papillary Thyroid Carcinoma

Heilo A, Sigstad E, Fagerlid KH, et al (Oslo Univ Hosp HF, Norway)

J Clin Endocrinol Metab 96:2750-2755, 2011

Context.—Repeated neck explorations can be a difficult task in patients with recurrent metastatic cervical lymph nodes from papillary thyroid carcinoma (PTC).

Objective.—The aim of this retrospective study has been to assess the efficacy of ultrasound (US)-guided percutaneous ethanol injection (PEI) as treatment of metastatic cervical lymph nodes from PTC.

Materials and Methods.—Sixty-nine patients who previously had undergone thyroidectomy for PTC were selected for inclusion. However, three patients were later excluded due to lack of follow-up. Lymph node status was determined by US-guided fine-needle aspiration biopsy and/or by raised levels of thyroglobulin in washouts from the cytological needle. Guided by US, 0.1—1.0 ml of 99.5% ethanol was injected into the metastatic lymph nodes.

Results.—Three patients (eight metastatic lymph nodes in total) were reassigned to surgery due to progression (multiple new metastases), leaving 63 patients and 109 neck lymph nodes to be included. Mean observation time was 38.4 months (range, 3—72). A total of 101 of the 109 (93%) metastatic lymph nodes responded to PEI treatment, 92 (84%) completely and nine incompletely. Two did not respond, and four progressed. Two lymph nodes previously considered successfully treated showed evidence of malignancy during follow-up. No significant side effects were reported.

Conclusion.—US-guided PEI treatment of metastatic lymph nodes seems to be an excellent alternative to surgery in patients with a limited number of neck metastases from PTC. This procedure should replace "berry picking" surgery.

▶ This is a very welcome article on a relatively rarely used method of ethanol ablation of metastatic cervical lymph nodes from well-differentiated thyroid carcinoma. While the method was introduced nearly a decade ago, the efficacy of nodal ablation with ethanol injections has not been well studied. This study has shown that 93% of injected lymph nodes have responded to therapy, while 84% responded completely. This is a very impressive result for this minimally invasive method. Reoperations of previously dissected necks, especially in the central compartment, can be very challenging and are associated with a high risk of complications. On the other hand, ultrasound-guided ethanol injection is void of any serious side effects and is quick and very cost effective. It is definitely an excellent alternative to repeated surgical excisions of recurrent neck metastases. As pointed out in the article, however, it is best performed in a setting of a team that includes an experienced radiologist and, in some institutions, an interventional radiologist.

M. Gapany, MD

Surgical Technique

Loupe Magnification Reduces Postoperative Hypocalcemia after Total Thyroidectomy

Pata G, Casella C, Mittempergher F, et al (Univ of Brescia, Italy)
Am Surg 76:1345-1350, 2010

We aimed to evaluate the impact of loupe magnification (LM) on incidental parathyroid gland removal (from pathology reports), hypocalcemia, and recurrent laryngeal nerve (RLN) injury after total thyroidectomy and answer the question of whether this tool should be always recommended for patient's safety. Between January 2005 and December 2008, 126 patients underwent total thyroidectomy with routine use of $2.5\times$ galilean loupes; their charts were compared with data on 118 patients operated on between January 1997 and December 2000 without LM (two different equally skilled surgical teams operating in the two periods). LM decreased the rate of inadvertent parathyroid glands removal (3.8 vs 7.8% of total parathyroid glands; $P = 0.01$), as well as of biochemical (20.6 vs 33.9%; $P = 0.028$) and clinical (12.7 vs 33%; $P = 0.0003$) hypocalcemia after thyroidectomy. All cases (16 of 16) of symptomatic hypocalcaemia in the LM group proved to be associated with parathyroidectomy vs 76.9 per cent (30 of 39) without LM ($P = 0.046$). A trend toward decreased RLN injury rate, although statistically insignificant, was reported, being unilateral transient, unilateral permanent, and bilateral transient palsy rates 6.8, 2.5, and 1.7 per cent, respectively, without LM vs 4.8, 2.4, and 0.8 per cent, respectively, with LM ($P = 0.69$; $P = 1$, and $P = 0.61$, respectively). Our results do support the routine use of LM during total thyroidectomy.

▶ As early as the third year of my otolaryngology residency, I trained myself to use magnifying loupes for thyroid and parotid gland surgery. On occasion, when I have inadvertently forgotten to bring my loupes to the operating room, I have struggled with the case, noting how significantly less precise my dissection had become without magnification. Although some of my colleagues were perfectly happy operating without loupes (one of them noting that he will quit operating when he needs them), I always felt uneasy operating without them. Obviously, I was excited when I came across this study, which lent support to my claim that magnification does improve the accuracy of surgical dissection, especially when it comes to preserving blood supply to the parathyroid glands. I am not aware of any previous studies that assess the efficacy of loupes for thyroid surgery, and I am certainly glad that somebody has finally decided to study this issue, albeit in a retrospective fashion. I recommend this article to all thyroid surgeons who refuse to use magnification in their daily work.

M. Gapany, MD

Randomized clinical trial on harmonic Focus shears versus clamp-and-tie technique for total thyroidectomy
Mourad M, Rulli F, Robert A, et al (Université Catholique de Louvain, Brussels, Belgium)
Am J Surg 202:168-174, 2011

Background.—The Harmonic Focus is the last ultrasonic device designed for thyroid surgery. The aim is to assess its efficacy and safety compared with traditional dissection in a prospective randomized trial of total thyroidectomy procedures.

Methods.—Total thyroidectomy was performed in 34 patients using the Harmonic Focus, and in 34 patients using the clamp-and-tie technique.

Results.—In the Harmonic Focus group, relative reductions of 29% and 46% were observed in surgical time and blood loss, respectively. The number of intraoperative instrument exchanges also decreased by 70%, and use of specific materials required to achieve hemostasis decreased significantly. Safety was found to be similar in both patient groups.

Conclusions.—Our study showed beneficial effects of Harmonic Focus use in thyroid surgery. Further studies therefore are needed to evaluate cost in the light of savings made in surgical time, materials needed for hemostasis, and human resources.

▶ As surgeons, we all have our own preferences when it comes to operative technique. Those preferences often track back to our training days; they often depend on who our mentors were or on the traditions of the institution where we trained. Through years of experience, we perfect our operative technique— make it work very well for us, achieve good surgical outcomes, and keep our complications low. So when a new technique, driven by new technology, comes around, we are reluctant to embrace it right away, dreading a new learning curve, unwilling to change "winning horses." Furthermore, data showing the advantage of a new tool or technique over the old method are most usually not available, and the technology's main advocate most of the time is the manufacturer itself. Naturally, the new technology or technique is more readily embraced by younger surgeons, who do not have as much time and effort invested in old and proven methods. Once in a while, however, a good study appears comparing the old versus the new and proving unequivocally the advantage of one over the other. This selected study happens to be one such study.

M. Gapany, MD

Meta-analysis of Minimally Invasive Video-Assisted Thyroidectomy

Radford PD, Ferguson MS, Magill JC, et al (St. Bartholomew's Hosp, London, UK; West Middlesex Univ Hosp, Isleworth, Middlesex, UK; et al)
Laryngoscope 121:1675-1681, 2011

Objectives.—The aim of this study is to compare minimally invasive video-assisted thyroidectomy (MIVAT) to conventional thyroidectomy.

Study Design.—A systematic review of the literature and meta-analysis.

Methods.—All published prospective controlled trials that compared MIVAT to conventional thyroidectomy were identified. The trials data were extracted and statistical analyzed using Statsdirect 2.5.7.

Results.—Five trials were identified. The total number of patients was 318. The primary outcome measures were pain, postoperative hypocalcaemia, and postoperative recurrent laryngeal nerve palsy. There was no difference in rates of postoperative hypocalcaemia or postoperative recurrent laryngeal nerve palsy between the techniques. Reported pain scores at 24 hours were significantly lower in MIVAT compared to conventional surgery. Pooled effect size was −4.496 (95% confidence interval [CI] = −7.146 to −2.045, P = .0004). The secondary outcome measures were operative time, blood loss, and cosmesis. There was significant improvement in patient reported scores for cosmesis with MIVAT. The pooled effect size was 3.669 (95% CI 0.636−60.702, P = .0178). MIVAT was associated with a significant increase in operative time. Pooled effect size was 1.681 (95% CI 0.600−2.762, P = .0023). There was no difference in blood loss between the groups.

Conclusions.—This study demonstrates that MIVAT is as safe as the existing gold standard operation. Furthermore, it has better cosmetic and pain outcomes for patients when compared to conventional surgery. MIVAT is a promising new technique, with obvious benefits over the established surgery, for small-volume thyroid disease that mainly affects a young female patient population.

▶ The current trend in otolaryngology emphasizes the minimally invasive approach as opposed to traditional operative techniques. In thyroid surgery, the main focus of minimally invasive operations (at least initially) was the cosmetic outcome, that is, the length of incision and the amount of postoperative scarring. With the introduction of video-assisted thyroidectomy (VAT), the surgeons using this technique observed not only improved cosmetic outcomes but, more importantly, reduced morbidity of the operation. Several recent studies have reported shortened hospital stays, decreased postoperative pain and decreased postoperative voice and swallowing impairment, presumably from less extensive surgical dissection and injury to surrounding tissue. Very importantly, complication rate in VAT has been reported to be comparable with that of conventional surgery.

This selected study is a meta-analysis of all published prospective trials comparing VAT with conventional operation. It establishes VAT not only as a safe operation but a superior one, with reduced morbidity and better cosmetic outcome when performed by experienced surgeons in a properly selected patient population. For novices, it is important to be aware that it takes at least 30 operations to get comfortable with this technique. It is therefore recommended for high-volume surgeons only.

M. Gapany, MD

Article Index

Chapter 1: Allergy and Immunology

Chapter 2: Head and Neck Surgery and Tumors

Chapter 3: Laryngology

Chapter 4: Otology

Chapter 5: Pediatric Otolaryngology

Chapter 6: Rhinology and Skull Base Surgery

Chapter 7: Thyroid and Parathyroid

Author Index

A

Abdelnoor M, 196
Acar B, 114
Adappa ND, 232
Agarwal PP, 160
Agrawal A, 19
Ahmed A, 47
Ahmed KA, 167
Ahn S-H, 253
Ali MJ, 11
Alper R, 52
Altman KW, 76
Amanatidou V, 172
Amer HE, 95
Amin MR, 80
Anastasian ZH, 128
Araki K, 17
Arasteh E, 127
Arnold A, 107
Arra I, 214
Arteau-Gauthier I, 178
Artz JCJM, 130
Attili AK, 160
Attner P, 31
Avenia N, 254

B

Bachmann-Harildstad G, 196
Badia L, 209
Batra S, 134
Bäumler M, 181
Ben-Israel N, 179
Benninger MS, 97
Bernstein LJ, 12
Beynon AJ, 130
Bhalla AS, 211
Bharti AK, 112
Bhattacharyya N, 28, 200
Bicanic G, 106
Bigorre M, 181
Bijl HP, 33
Bizaki AJ, 68
Bloom D, 183
Blumin JH, 42, 44
Bock JM, 42
Bolger WE, 227
Boomsma MJ, 33
Bozkurt MK, 138
Breur JMPJ, 169
Brook I, 201
Brown J, 12
Bucca CB, 73
Buchmann LO, 248

Bugiani M, 73
Buryk M, 183

C

Calatroni A, 1
Carson K, 134
Casella C, 259
Cattaert T, 188
Caversaccio M, 107
Chan JYK, 237
Chandra RK, 220
Chaturvedi AK, 26
Chauvin P, 123
Cheney ML, 152
Chennupati SK, 180
Chisholm EJ, 7
Chiu F-S, 241
Clary MS, 65
Cohen MS, 90
Connor M, 216
Culla B, 73
Curry WT, 190

D

da Silva LFF, 63
Daniero JJ, 65
de Graaf M, 169
de Mestral C, 88
D'Elia JB, 85
Deschler DG, 29
Deveci I, 154
Dheyauldeen S, 196
Dhiwakar M, 34
Dillman JR, 160
Dreher ME, 167
Du J, 31
Duggal N, 215
Dwivedi RC, 7

E

Early SB, 189
Eggers SDZ, 143
Einhorn E, 43
Eisele DW, 94
El-Fattah AMA, 95
El-Noueam KI, 159
El-Sayed IH, 94
Eladl HM, 234
Elmiyeh B, 7
Elmorsy SM, 234

Engels EA, 26
Erickson-Levendoski E, 52

F

Fagerlid KH, 258
Fasunla AJ, 8
Faure J-M, 181
Ferguson MS, 261
Ferlito A, 21, 25, 219
Fish S, 257
Fong N, 88
Fontaine JH, 62
Foreman A, 199
Fountas K, 172
Fournier C, 38
Francis DO, 15
Freund W, 185
Friedland PL, 116
Froehlich P, 157
Fu X, 52
Fukuda M, 131

G

Gaafar AH, 159
Gan HK, 12
Ganly I, 255
Gergen PJ, 1
Gevaert P, 188
Ghosh A, 43
Gkoritsa E, 139
Godbout A, 178
Goh E-K, 162
Goldstein NA, 177
Gopen Q, 141
Gousheh J, 127
Greene BH, 8
Griffin GR, 64
Grindle CR, 180
Grover C, 67
Guerra E, 9
Gupta G, 211
Gupta M, 115
Gurrado A, 254
Guthrie S, 161

H

Habesoglu M, 154
Habesoglu TE, 154
Haigentz M Jr, 20

271